Advances in Transfusion Safety – Volume IV

Developments in Biologicals

Vol. 127

This series «Developments in Biologicals» begins with Vol. 102 and is the continuation of IABS symposia series «Progress in Immunobiological Standardization» Vols 1-5, «Immunobiological Standardization» Vols 1-22 and «Developments in Biological Standardization» Vols 23-101.

Organized and published by the International Association for Biologicals (IABS)

KARGER

Basel · Freiburg · Paris · London · New York · Bangalore · Bangkok · Singapore · Tokyo · Sydney

Advances in Transfusion Safety – Volume IV

Sydney, Australia
11-13th October 2005

Volume editors

Elizabeth M. Dax
National Serology Reference Laboratory, Australia
Fitzroy, VIC, Australia

Albert Farrugia
Therapeutic Goods Administration
Woden, ACT, Australia

Girish N. Vyas
UCSF School of Medicine
San Francisco, CA, USA

Proceedings of an international conference organized by
the International Association for Biologicals (IABS),
the National Serology Reference Laboratory, Australia
and the Therapeutics Goods Administration

41 figures and 43 tables, 2007

KARGER

Basel · Freiburg · Paris · London · New York ·
Bangalore · Bangkok · Singapore · Tokyo · Sydney

Developments in Biologicals

Library of Congress Cataloging-in-Publication Data

IABS International Conference on Advances in Transfusion Safety (2005 : Sydney, Australia)
Advances in transfusion safety : Sydney, Australia, 11-13th October 2005 : proceedings of an international conference organized by the International Association for Biologicals (IABS), the National Serology Reference Laboratory, Australia, and the Therapeutics Goods Administration / volume editors, Elizabeth M. Dax, Albert Farrugia, Girish N. Vyas.
p. ; cm. -- (Developments in biologicals ; v. 127)
"Volume 4."
Includes bibliographical references and index.
ISBN 978-3-8055-8239-1 (soft cover : alk. paper)
1. Blood--Transfusion--Safety measures--Congresses. 2. Blood--Collection and preservation--Safety measures--Congresses. 3. Blood banks--Standards--Congresses. I. Dax, Elizabeth M. II. Farrugia, Albert. III. Vyas, Girish N. IV. International Association for Biologicals. V. National Serology Reference Laboratory (Australia) VI. Therapeutic Goods Administration (Australia) VII. Title. VIII. Series.
[DNLM: 1. Blood Banks--standards--Congresses. 2. Blood Transfusion--standards--Congresses. 3. Blood Donors--Congresses. 4. Disease Transmission--prevention & control--Congresses. 5. Safety--standards--Congresses. W1 DE997VKF v.127 2007 / WH 460 I11a 2007]
RM171.3.A3889 2007
362.17'84--dc22

2007005271

Bibliographic Indices. This publication is listed in bibliographic services, including Current Contents® and Index Medicus.

Drug dosage. The authors and the publisher have exerted every effort to ensure that drug selection and dosage set forth in this text are in accord with current recommendations and practice at the time of publication. However, in view of ongoing research, changes in government regulations, and the constant flow of information relating to drug therapy and drug reactions, the reader is urged to check the package insert for each drug for any change in indications and dosage and for added warnings and precautions. This is particularly important when the recommended agent is a new and/or infrequently employed drug.

Worldwide distribution by S. Karger AG, Basel (Switzerland).
Printed in Switzerland by Médecine et Hygiène, Genève.
ISBN-10: 3-8055-8239-0
ISBN-13: 978-3-8055-8239-1

Scientific Committee

Albert Farrugia, Chairman (TGA, Australia)
Elizabeth M. Dax, Co-Chair (NRL, Australia)
Girish N. Vyas (UCSF, USA)
Ken Davis (ANZSBT)
Jean-Pierre Allain
Michael P. Busch
Roger Y. Dodd
Jay Epstein
Peter Flanagan
Andrew Heaton
Daryl Maher
Gerald Schochetman
Rainer Seitz
Paul Strengers
Diana Teo

Organising Committee

Elizabeth M. Dax
Albert Farrugia
OzAccom

Organisation of the Meeting

Session I	Optimal Use as a Route to Blood Safety Chairs: *R. Seitz and D. Teo*
Session II	Emerging Infectious Agents Chairs: *R. Dodd and G. Schochetman*
Session III	Fitting New Techniques into the Safety Paradigm Chairs: *J.P. Allain and A. Heaton*
Session IV	Regulation as a Driver for Blood Safety Chairs: *J. Epstein and D. Maher*
Session V	Transfusion and Blood Safety in the Asia-Pacific Chairs: *Lin Che-Kit and P. Flanagan*
Session VI	Harmonising Practice and Product – The Role for Blood Safety Chairs: *M. Busch and P. Strengers*
Session VII	Emerging Risks and their Communication Chair: *A. Farrugia*

The scientific integrity of the articles contained in this volume is the sole responsibility of the authors.

Acknowledgements

The IABS International Conference on **Advances in Transfusion Safety – Volume IV** is grateful to the following organisations for their essential and enabling financial support.

Abbott Diagnostics (Gold Sponsor)

Roche Diagnostics

Chiron Blood Testing

Bio-Rad

CSL Bioplasma

Novo Nordisk

BioMérieux Industry

Baxter

AcroMetrix

Pall Medical

Advances in Transfusion Safety – Volume IV – Prologue

To many people it may seem amazing that blood transfusion is not a perfectly safe procedure. It is not well-known that blood-borne infections are still being transmitted by transfusion in some places. There are other infections, including emerging infections and besides those that for which we most commonly test, that may be transfusion transmitted. Quality management systems may not be in place in all transfusion facilities. The collection of blood may still not be from voluntary, non-remunerated donors. Publicity around blood services may be less than ideal and public communications are less than perfect. Blood, a precious commodity, may not be used as wisely as it might be. In many places, there are no regulatory processes. Quality assurance measures may be sub-optimal. Yet, all these measures if carried out through the transfusion process can present an adequate blood supply that is safe for almost all recipients. The latest information, techniques and outcome measures are presented here in this very volume. These papers are the distillation of presentations made at the IVth International Association of Biologicals (IABs) Symposium on Advances in Transfusion Safety held in Sydney, Australia in October 2005. There were nearly 200 experts in the field who contributed their thoughts and advice, questions and comments to bring these Proceedings together.

The use of blood and blood products saves millions of lives, yearly. The World Health Organisation (WHO) estimates that in 2005, 81 million blood units, across the world were collected. Of those, only 38% are collected in developing countries where 82% of the population is distributed. It was estimated that 6 million tests that should have been performed were not. It was also estimated that developing countries have access to only 20% of the world's safe blood. The need for blood is said to be 10-30 units per 1000 population. In the whole African region only 5 units per 1000 population were collected. In Southeast Asia only ~9.3 million units of blood are collected although the estimated requirement is for over 15 million units. Further, almost three quarters of that blood is utilised as whole blood.

The Proceedings are presented as they were to the participants of the IVth IABs Symposium. There were six sessions. There were also papers presented or written that encouraged the advancement of Transfusion Safety and presented frameworks by which advancement could be carried out. These papers are presented to offer a bridge to suggest ways in which all participants can carry out necessary steps to improve transfusion safety in developed and developing areas. The overall goal of quality management systems is for blood services to improve *continually*; therefore there is no end to advancing transfusion safety. In other words, there is always scope for better and safer blood services.

The literature and other information shows that in well-developed blood transfusion services or systems, the greatest threat to safety occurs once the blood or blood products leave the place of collection. Thus, blood transfusion is not without risk. Blood transfusion services now have methods to quantify such risks, providing evidence for intervention strategies. Regulation in the use of blood and blood products as precious therapeutic commodities, also enhances safety outcomes. At the same time optimal use of transfusionable products needs to be understood. What guidelines can be established to ensure most appropriate use?

Exploration is being undertaken as to where and how records of events and outcomes of blood transfusion processes should be maintained and used. These, in turn, are being utilized to create evidence bases for effective use of blood and blood products. Some of the outcomes from these analyses are "challenging convention clinical wisdom" [McClelland]. These considerations assume even greater significance in calculating the cost-effectiveness of various interventions.

The issue of supply of blood and blood products is key. The public now has a role in guiding the safety of transfusion. The public has assumed a role in demanding the levels of safety that they expect their donations and taxes to deliver. Blood services are in a position to be challenged legally if expectations are not met. This places requirements that often result in limits to supply. "The default decision paradigm of using blood" can no longer be the guide for whether to transfuse or not [Isbister]. Again, evidence bases for the ways that blood and product resources may be conserved are necessary in taking transfusion safety forward. Evidence for the potential benefit of transfusion in individual recipients, before it is carried out should become the norm. Isbister questions *where* the responsibilities lie for assuring the wise use of blood. The optimal use of transfusion as a medical procedure is being investigated further. Once evidence-bases are achieved upon which decisions can be made, questions arise on who should be making decisions around blood's use.

Fascinating questions arise concerning advances in transfusion safety, when emerging infections (that may be transmitted) are considered. Some, such as parasitic infections that can be transfused, are confined – geographically. The considerations of steps to be taken in non-endemic areas are weighty. Some present serious threats beyond their present distribution [Wendel]. Ignoring these threats could be disastrous as illustrated by the rampant West Nile Virus epidemic that spread so rapidly across the U.S. in 1999-2000. At the same time, many valuable lessons about emerging infections were developed through the American responses to the viral epidemics [Stramer].

Demand for safety in blood transfusion by patients, the public, the legal fraternity, governments and clinicians has led to a burgeoning of technologies – laboratory-based and other. Molecular-based screening for donations has reduced the rates of transmission to very low levels (single chances of viral transmission per millions of donations) - after donor screening and antibody screening in the case of transfusion transmitted viral infections. The possibilities of using micro-arrays in future is tantalizing when so many pathogens are now known to be transmitted by transfusion [Fournier – Wirth]. The technological difficulties are gradually being mastered. Further, it is becoming possible to detect multiple pathogens simultaneously by a number of technologies. Cardotti and Allain described multiplex – molecular assays that are successfully in use in resource – limited settings. New technologies are opening up which provide advances more widely and to areas where such advances could not be considered in the past. Detecting multiple pathogens in one test may improve the cost-effectiveness of screening.

An important aspect of assessing transfusion safety is the ability to estimate risk. In countries where screening for transmission of virus infections has proceeded over numbers of years the risk of infection is minute. Because the risks are so small it has become necessary to use information to model risks. Busch described a new strategy for risk estimation. The model is accepted now as accurate by blood transfusionists and regulators. Such models can also be used in cost effectiveness analyses and to inform policy debates over the merits of changing strategies. Lambert had described the use of antigen-antibody combination assays to reduce the window period in HCV testing. These combination assays for HCV may be very important for use in developing countries before a nucleic acid testing strategy is implemented. On the other hand the HCV antibody-antigen assays (combo) may confer similar ability to detect HCV as the RNA assays. With further evaluations it may be that combo assays are a reasonable alternative to nucleic assay screening generally.

Gregori and Rohwer have described an animal model for investigating infectivity of transmissible spongiform encephalopathies. In a complex series of experiments, results indicated that hamster blood could be used as a reasonable substitute for human blood in investigating component distribution of TSE infectivity in blood.

The fourth session concentrated on government regulation as a driver for blood safety. In under-resourced countries regulation is often a component of the blood safety system that is lacking. On the other hand, in countries where regulation is more sophisticated there are considerable advancements towards transfusion safety through regulation. One poignant example was described by Farrugia. The iron status of blood donors has been investigated using serum ferritin as a measure of depletion. A high incidence of iron deficiency has been reported in some groups of donors. For better safety the differentiation between the depletion of storage and functional iron needs to be supported by clinical studies. It will be the responsibility of regulators to help define these issues.

Flanagan described product traceability and look-back as a mechanism in assuring the integrity of the transfusion process. The necessity for changing requirements of traceability lies in changing nature of production and improved understanding of the range of adverse effects associated with the transfusion of blood and its products. The Council of Europe Guide *for the preparation, use and quality assurance of blood components* includes look-back and traceability as a component of hemovigilance. Other standards such as those of AABB are more prescriptive than the European Guide. Further development of the systems will ensure advances in overall safety of clinical transfusion systems. The European blood directives were described by Seitz. In Europe it is the new EC legislation that ensures the high level of quality and safety of blood and blood components. The initial directive has been supplemented with directives assuring safety in collection and testing of plasma for fractionation. Because the directives relate to twenty-five member states the directive assists in assuring a similar level of transfusion safety over the European population. This will also have the advantage of considerable input from different points-of-view to refine the directive and ensure its effectiveness in regulating transfusion safety.

In Singapore there is a single agency assuring supply and safety. The Singapore experience was described by Teo and Seah. Owing to mergers of departments the National Blood Service in Singapore is now within the same agency as the National Regulatory Body. With the joint agencies there are several possible advantages including clearly defined admissions and accountabilities, clear and transparent deliverables, checks and balances within each regulatory process, external evaluation for each agency is possible and their relationships with other organizations are enhanced. These two areas are combined with five other agencies so that the interactions are developing in effectiveness.

Because the IABs Symposium was held within the Asia Pacific region a session on transfusion and blood safety in the Asian Pacific regions was held. A new blood law implemented in Japan was described by Tadokoro. The purpose of the Law was to secure a stable supply of blood based on domestic voluntary donations and to promote its appropriate use. The Law was implemented in 2003. The Law has resulted in widespread measures to increase transfusion safety but it is recognized that further safety measures would cost significant amounts of money and the quality affected would need public understanding and support. The paper, while describing the advances, acknowledges that implementation required cooperation among the stakeholders. Malaysia is a country where the government has made blood safety a priority of the Ministry of Health [reported by Ayob]. Although the country's socio-economic status is lower than many, strategies to assure the safety of blood have been developed. A policy of self-sufficiency for blood products has been adopted since the early 1980s; helping to increase blood collection supplies. The supply of Factor 8 (F VIII) consumption was used as an example of the development of blood safety. The importance of having national strategies with regulatory systems was emphasized.

China is a vast country and Zhu described the increasing safety in plasma derivative production that has been accomplished in mainland China. The tragedy of the contamination among plasma donors in Henan Province in the early 1990s presented many challenges to the industry. As a counter, regulation of the entire blood transfusion industry has been strengthened and laws and standards have been developed along with stricter licensing regulations. The way that adverse events can shape advances was stressed. The importance in coordinating such advances on a national basis was reiterated. If transfusion advances are to be mapped, the mechanisms in individual services and across countries may be through quality assurance. Particularly quality assurance measures for following the laboratory testing for transfusion safety is of great importance in following the advances. Dax and Walker described an international quality assurance system which is aligned with the regulatory services in Australia. They showed that quality assurance is the overall mechanism that provides methods to offer the checks and balances assuring the quality of tests and testing. As the complexity of blood transfusion services increases and the number of transfusion transmissible infections grows, methods to assure quality must develop. Comparisons of test systems internationally indeed, across the world are constituting significant advances in this area. Quality Assurance offers methods to assess the effectiveness of regulatory steps as well as the testing systems themselves. Systems where information may be collected electronically over huge areas and numbers of countries will allow rapid responses when aberrations in testing systems occur.

Finally in this series of presentations, the improved security of clinical blood transfusion in four provinces of China between 1997 and 2005 were described by Whyte. The activities of the blood component of the World Health IX Programme in China was described. The Programme operated in four provinces and the presentation was made in the context of the overall improvements that have occurred in China. The programmes in each province have concentrated on recruiting voluntary, unremunerated blood donors, establishing quality programmes and improving the usage of blood. The symposium delegates were reminded that this was an excellent example of commitment of staff to achieving the very best in blood transfusion services. Thus, one important advancement that can be made for transfusion safety is to encourage the dedication of blood transfusion staff to achieving safety.

The Sixth session was entitled, *Harmonizing Practice and Product the Role for Blood Safety.* It was pointed out that modeling of disease outcomes is helpful at the level of individual patients to providing advice about the likely outcome of their intervention, as well as at the population level to model the effects of infection or outcomes in a population and on hospitalization rates and for development of cost-benefit analyses. The example of screening for HCV infection was developed by Whyte. He described the outcomes of a look-back that was conducted in Victoria, Australia. Both the short-term and long-term outcomes were described. A model of survival in recipients of transfusion with red cells was constructed and survival rates were predicted from using this model. The study illustrated the importance of careful records and preserving information from transfusion services.

Strengers discussed improving transfusion practices for donors as a safer donation process and affording maximum use of any donation. He emphasized that transfusion practice needs to be regarded as a complete chain from implementing the donation to the use of the donation. Hemovigilance is a tool for this and it was emphasized that hemovigilance has led to improvements in transfusion practice. It provides the mechanism to prevent errors, improve use and offers a mechanism for continuous feedback of results and outcomes. Assuring the integrity of the transfusion process through product traceability and look-back was also described by Flanagan. He emphasized that each individual blood donation represented a unique batch in manufacturing terms. This concept has underpinned many of the systems developed to assure quality in blood product manufacture. Because of the changing nature of production and use of blood as its products, the traceability requirements have increased enormously. Thus the need for effective systems for traceability is a significant underpinning for effective materiovigilance and hemovigilance. Flanagan concluded that further development of these systems will assist in assuring the overall safety of blood components and of clinical transfusion systems.

Finally, there were a series of papers which addressed more generally how blood transfusion services might advance safety. Dodd described emerging infections and blood safety on a global level. While major transfusion transmissible diseases are largely under control and certainly under control in developed countries, the emergence of other infections has threatened the safety of all blood transfusion services. The management of HIV and its relationship to transfusion safety shaped the way that blood transfusionists regarded the threat of transfusion transmitted infections. Although most emerging infections have not been as devastating or as threatening to safety, the responses often have been modeled of the severity of the threat that HIV imposed. The recent appearance of West Nile Virus in the USA has made it evident that effective programmes to manage the threat of emerging infections are necessary and that transfusionists need to have the programmes ready. Dodd listed in detail the possible threats. Although there is a very high standard of blood safety in countries with a high human development index (HDI; i.e. developed countries), the lower the HDI is, the less possible it is to assure the same degree of safety against emerging infections. Increasingly mobile societies generate more opportunities for diseases to be moved across boarders. This emphasizes the need for both global and local surveillance. However, it is most important that systems are generated to address the threat of emerging infection.

The risk of poor communication to non-experts, was emphasized as an important issue in management of transfusion related risks. The public demands continuous searching for maximum safety of blood products and this should remain a goal for all professionals involved in blood transfusion medicine, according to Hossenlopp. Although blood transfusion therapy is safer than it has ever been, public perceptions often suggest that the public has an opposite point of view. Therefore it is necessary for transfusion professionals to inspire confidence in their products. By understanding risk and its management, transfusionists may develop better perceptions of their products if they do this in parallel with developing better communication skills. Hossenlopp proposes that communication-skill training should be incorporated into medical school curriculae and as well as continuing education programmes.

The Symposium was opened with a lecture on blood safety in the new millennium. Starr discussed scientific purity and political reality and posed the question whether they could be synthesized for public good. Starr also identified the need for more education about blood and, particularly, updated education. Starr pointed out that many advances have been made concerning blood safety but that people generally do not understand what blood centres do and how **they** need to participate in the blood transfusion process. An important way to engender this understanding is to understand they way the media operates. People's perception of not only blood transfusion but health professionals and scientists, also needs to be understood. Particularly, the media needs to be understood in its propensity to portray on-going events as a series of crises. This presents a confusing conglomeration of information for people who are not familiar with any process that is being described in the media. The message was that "Transfusionists must develop proactive engagement with the media". Starr described an effective communication strategy and how important it was that each announcement about risk be accompanied with specific actions that people can take. The transfusion landscape now involves voluntary, unremunerated donors. Thus, the raw product of transfusion is entirely dependent on the public's goodwill. Therefore the way to preserve that goodwill is for transfusionists to engage with the public both directly and also through the media to develop each possible donor as an ally.

Elizabeth M. Dax
Albert Farrugia
Girish Vyas

Contents

Dax EM, Farrugia A, Vyas G (eds): Advances in Transfusion Safety – Volume IV.
Dev Biol (Basel). Basel, Karger, 2007, vol 127, p 1.

SESSION I

Optimal Use as a Route to Blood Safety

Chairs: *R. Seitz and D. Teo*

Dax EM, Farrugia A, Vyas G (eds): Advances in Transfusion Safety – Volume IV.
Dev Biol (Basel). Basel, Karger, 2007, vol 127, pp 3-8.

Why Do We Believe in Red Cell Transfusion?

B. McClelland

Scottish National Blood Transfusion Service, Blood Transfusion Service, Royal Infirmary, Edinburgh, U.K.

Key words: Red cell transfusion, risks, studies

Introduction

Belief in the clinical value of transfusion reflects its long history. In Edinburgh, for example, the donor service was started in the 1920's by an individual who was moved by the experience of a friend's wife dying of obstetric haemorrhage. In those days, transfusion was seen to be – and probably was – a life saving intervention when a patient suffered severe blood loss. This was, however, before we had all the modern armoury of resuscitation, anaesthesia, surgery and intensive care.

Over the second half of the 20th century, transfusion in many countries grew to be a major business, its use extended to new indications, and it became an established element of a modern health system. Publicity to motivate donors stressed the life saving properties of transfusion. This presumably sustained belief in the clinical importance of transfusion and may also have diverted attention from the risks, some of which, like hepatitis, have been well known for 50 years or more. It is only quite recently that we have begun to seriously apply the disciplines of evidence based medicine to ask, "When and for whom does red cell transfusion really contribute to a better outcome?"

What is a good haemoglobin concentration in health and in illness, and why?

Current guidelines typically propose that red cell transfusion should be given when reduced haemoglobin is judged to be contributing to inadequate oxygenation. Some intensivists describe this as "diminished physiological reserve" – perhaps technical language for a clinical opinion that the patient needs a transfusion. In practice, transfusion decisions related to blood loss tend to be based on either haemoglobin concentration, estimated blood loss or both, whereas in patients with chronic anaemia, the decision is likely to be based on haemoglobin concentration and symptoms such as fatigue. Beutler and Waalen [1] have recently published an analysis of haemoglobin data from two large American databases that update the widely quoted WHO figures. However, these normal ranges do not necessarily help to define the ideal "target" haemoglobin to be achieved by red cell transfusion in different clinical situations. It is also worth considering that transfusion guidelines generally refer to haemoglobin concentration. Textbooks tell us, and recent studies in cardiac surgery patients confirm, that patients who bleed and receive both fluids and red cell replacement may experience a fall in haemoglobin concentration but have a minimal fall in red cell mass [2]. It seems logical that the red cell mass would better reflect the oxygen delivering capacity of the circulating blood; in some situations, the concentration of haemoglobin may not be a reliable predictor.

Which Patients Receive Red Cell Transfusions?

In 27 of the 45 countries in the Council of Europe, the reported use of red cells in 2003 ranged from 0.8 to 70 units per 100 population per year – although the definition of "use" may be somewhat flexible [3]. Even among longstanding and well-to-do EU member states, red cell use ranged from 37 to 70 units per 100 population per year. It is not clear what underlies these large differences. A useful starting point would be to be to classify the patients who receive transfusions in some way that would help to identify and study clinically relevant groups. This could form the basis of "case definitions" of patients at risk of transfusion that could be used to compare patterns of blood use. Such data would also help to define situations in which clinical trials may be required. A recent example of such a study is that of Wells et al [4], during which reasons for transfusion were recorded when blood was requested from the hospital blood bank. This type of study does not adequately reflect the complicated history of many transfused patients.

To better understand the use of blood components in Scotland (population 5 million, with a single national blood transfusion service) we have recently established a data warehouse in which the records of acute hospital episodes are linked by patient identifiers to hospital blood bank computer records for blood component units "assumed transfused" to each individual. The warehouse for 2002-2003 contains all acute hospital episodes (whether transfused or not) and currently covers the blood issued for about 75 % of adults in the whole country. It contains records for 140,000 units of red cells transfused to 31,000 recipients, equivalent to a red cell use of about 37 units per thousand population per year.

We are using these data to classify patient records according to "likely reason for transfusion". The initial approach has been to employ a combination of date rules and the coded information about every patient episode, including diagnoses (ICDM 10) and procedures undergone (OPCS). The broad categories created are: Group A: Event-based transfusion episode, e.g. a major elective surgery likely to involve blood loss and transfusion such as total hip replacement; Group B: Clinical conditions (diagnoses), primarily involving the haemopoietic system e.g. leukaemia or myelodysplasia, that are likely to impair red cell production and therefore to be a factor underlying the need for any red cell transfusion given during the year. These two groups account for about 40 % of all red cell units transfused.

However, more than half of the red cell units are transfused to a population that is not easily recognisable in most transfusion guidelines. These are elderly patients with complex histories who may have many hospital episodes, many different diagnoses and interventions and many transfusion episodes in the year. Diagnosis and procedure codes strongly associated with transfusion include: alcoholic liver disease, cancer, anaemia, upper GI bleeding, upper GI endoscopy and renal failure. These patients cannot sensibly be simply categorised according to "medical or surgical" by a single diagnosis or by a single procedure. Depending on the purpose of the analysis, more relevant categories may be along the lines of "critically ill" [5] or "elderly treated for multiple pathologies," provided that robust case definitions could be agreed upon. An alternative approach is to categorise transfusion episodes according to the physiopathological condition to be corrected.

When and for whom does red cell transfusion really contribute to a better outcome? There are an increasing number of clinical studies that give some answers. These studies vary greatly in design and quality. One variable aspect is the choice of endpoint, which range from major outcome measures such as mortality or organ failure, postoperative complications such as infection or bleeding to physiological endpoints. Few studies address quality of life issues in relation to transfusion regimes.

Some large observational studies, a systematic review of randomised controlled clinical trials, and some recent RCCTs will be mentioned briefly.

Observational Studies

Recent studies

Of the five large retrospective cohort studies, the two most recent ones will be mentioned here.

Wu et al [6] examined computerised hospital records to determine the risk associated with anaemia in elderly patients admitted with myocardial infarction and to determine the effectiveness of red cell transfusion in these patients. They found that mortality was higher in anaemic patients and that transfusion was associated with a reduced mortality in patients whose haematocrit (Hct) was below 33 % but not if Hct was higher than 33 %. Their data, however, shows that in patients with Hct above 33 % transfusion was associated with a significantly higher mortality. More recently, Rao and colleagues [7] have reported an analysis of the data from 3 large RCCTS of treatment of acute coronary insufficiency, involving a total of 24,000 patients, of whom about 10 % received red cell transfusion. Mortality was higher in the transfusion recipients: this was accounted for by those with Hct above 30 %.

The conclusion that can be drawn from both of these studies is that red cell transfusion is harmful for patients with an Hct above 33 %. There are numerous factors that could account for the differences between the 2 studies in the effects of transfusion when Hct is below 30 %. While these findings are provocative, it must be borne in mind that these studies have limitations. Both are retrospective and use a limited data set. There is minimal adjustment for confounding factors, the timing of transfusion is not known, nor is the Hct threshold for transfusion or the exact relationship between the haematocrit value and the transfusion.

Studies of outcomes of red cell products with different specifications

Leucodepletion versus non leucodepletion

A recent meta analysis of trials comparing conventional and leucoreduced red cell products [8] indicates that the use of leucoreduction is associated with lower mortality and reduced post operative infection.

Short versus long storage time

A number of retrospective studies report that transfusion of red cells stored for longer periods of time is associated with higher mortality compared with the use of fresh cells [9,10]. A pilot study has demonstrated the feasibility of a trial to compare major outcomes in recipients of fresh and stored red cells [11]; the investigators plan a large trial.

Randomised controlled clinical trials of red cell transfusion

A systematic review of trials of transfusion thresholds [12] is dominated by the results of one large, randomised trial of transfusion in critically ill adult patients [5]. This compared major outcomes (mortality in ICU and 30 days after discharge) in ICU patients who were randomised to receive red cell transfusion so as to maintain Hb levels at either 100-120 g/l or 90-100g/l. The main finding was that, overall, patients did as well (or possibly better) with the more restrictive transfusion regime. There was, however, a suggestion that patients with ischaemic heart disease may have fared better with the more liberal transfusion regime. A similar trial has been performed in neonates judged to be in need of red cell transfusion, and in these patients also it seems that a liberal transfusion regime is no more effective than a conservative one [13].

These conclusions challenge conventional clinical wisdom about the indications for red cell transfusion, but they are quite consistent with studies showing that resting healthy volunteers tolerate blood loss (with isovolaemic fluid replacement) down to Hb levels around 50 g/l with no evidence of inadequate oxygenation. Extending this type of observation to critically ill patients, a recent explanatory trial found that transfusion of two units of red cells, whether fresh or stored, had no detectable effect on any measurable parameter of regional or global oxygenation in ICU patients whose Hb was below 80 g/l [3]. In a totally different context, there is evidence that a highly restrictive approach to red cell transfusion may be appropriate for children with severe acute chronic anaemia. Lackritz et al [14] were able to study children admitted to a district hospital in Kenya. They found that transfusion only improved survival if the admission haemoglobin level was below 35 g/l (or below 45g/l with specified clinical signs of hypoxaemia) and where transfusion could be given within 24 hours of admission.

We Are Expensively Preoccupied with Risks that Are Fashionable

The UK haemovigilance study, SHOT, collated reports of serious transfusion hazards for 1996-2003, during which 23m units of blood components were supplied. The incidence of serious adverse reactions (per 100,000 units of blood supplied) was: death 0.2; major morbidity 1.1, of which 0.6 were cases of transfusion related acute lung injury and 0.2 were infection (mostly bacterial). The chance in the UK that a unit of blood might transmit one of the viruses for which blood is tested from 1996-2003 is significantly lower and estimated at: HIV 0.014, HCV 0.024 and HBV 0.176 per 100,000 units.

Safety comes at a high cost: in 1995 it cost £ 250 million (at 2004 sterling values) to produce blood components and associated services. A similar quantity now costs the NHS £ 500 million. Put another way, in 1998 a unit of red cells cost £ 47, a platelet dose £90 and a unit of FFP £ 13. These have risen to £ 120, £ 198 and £ 31, mainly due to newer anti-microbial tests and processes, some of which only marginally increase safety. The hepatitis C virus RNA test, introduced in 1999, has detected one additional positive per 1.4 million donations tested at a cost of £8.3m per detection [15].

Precautionary measures against vCJD include removing leucocytes from all blood components at an annual cost of £ 70m. New processes to be available soon may reduce vCJD infectivity by perhaps 10,000 fold, but could add £ 100 million per year to the blood services bill.

Conclusion

We have a very limited body of evidence about the effectiveness of red cell and plasma [16] transfusion. This is in part because the studies needed are difficult and expensive to perform. It is difficult to understand the lengths to which we are prepared to go to improve the safety of these treatments when, up to now, we have not made commensurate efforts to rigorously evaluate the benefits that they offer.

References

1 Beutler E, Waalen J : The definition of anemia. What is the lower limit of normal of the blood haemoglobin ? Blood 2006 ; 107 : 1747-1750.

2 Slight RD, Norzeihan JB, Onyekwelu CN, Pankaj SM, McClelland DBL : Peri-operative red cell, plasma and blood volume change in patients undergoing cardiac surgery. Transfusion 2006 ; 46 (3) : 392-397.

3 van der Poel CL, Janssen M : The collection, testing and use of blood and blood components in Europe in 2003 : European Health Committee CDSP, 2004.

4 Wells AW, Mounter PJ, Chapman CE, Stainsby D, Wallis JP : Where does blood go ? Prospective observational study of red cell transfusion in north England. BMJ 2002 ; 325 : 803.

5 Hebert PC, Wells GF, Blajchman MA, et al : A multicenter, randomized, controlled clinical trial of transfusion requirements in critical care. Transfusion requirements in critical care investigators, Canadian Critical Care Trials Group. N Engl J Med 1999 ; 40 : 409-417.

6 Wu WC, Rathore SS, Wang Y, Radford MJ, Krumholz HM : Blood transfusion in elderly patients with acute myocardial infarction. New England Journal of Medicine 1999 ; 39 : 701-710.

7 Rao SV, Jollis JG, Harrington RA, Granger CB, Newby LK, Armstrong PW, Moliterno DJ, Lindblad L, Pieper K, Topol EJ, Stamler JS, Califf RM : Relationship of blood transfusion and clinical outcomes in patients with acute coronary syndromes. JAMA 2004 ; 292 : 1555-1562.

8 Fergusson D et al : A meta-analysis of clinical trials evaluating leukoreduced red blood cell transfusions in surgical patients. Can J Anesth 2004 ; 51 (5) : 417-424.

9 Purdy FR, Tweeddale MG, Merrick PM : Association of mortality with age of blood transfused in septic ICU patients. Canadian Journal of Anaesthesia 1997 ; 44 : 1256-1261.

10 Vamvakas EC, Carven JH : Transfusion and postoperative pneumonia in coronary artery bypass graft surgery : effect of the length of storage of transfused red cells. Transfusion 1999 ; 39 : 701-710.

11 Hebert PC, Chin-Yee I, Fergusson D, Blajchman M, Martineau R, Clinch J, Olberg B : A pilot trial evaluating the clinical effects of prolonged storage of red cells. Anesth Analg 2005 ; 100 (5) : 1433-1438.

12 Carson JL, Hill S, Carless P, Hebert P, Henry D : Transfusion triggers : a systematic review of the literature. Transfusion Medicine Reviews 2002 ; 16 (3) : 187-199.

13 Heddle N, et al for PINT Investigators : Conservative transfusion regimens are not associated with higher mortality or morbidity in ELBW Infants – The premature in need of transfusion (PINT) randomized controlled trial. 2004. Available from http://www.pasmeeting.org/2004SanFran/Abstracts/LateBreakers/Abstracts.htm#LB15.

14 Lackritz EM, Campbell CC, Ruebush TK 2nd, Hightower AW, Wakube W, Steketee RW, Were JB : Effect of blood transfusion on survival among children in a Kenyan hospital. Lancet 1992 ; 340 : 524.

15 McClelland B, Contreras M : Appropriateness and safety of blood transfusion. BMJ 2005 ; 330 (7483) : 104-105.

16 Stanworth SJ, Brunskill SJ, Hyde CJ, McClelland DB, Murphy MF : Is fresh frozen plasma clinically effective ? A systematic review of randomized controlled trials. Br J Haematol 2004 ; 126 : 139-152.

Dr. B. McClelland, Scottish National Blood Transfusion Service, Blood Transfusion Service, Royal Infirmary, Edinburgh EH3 9HB, U.K.
E-mail : brian.mcclelland@snbts.csa.scot.nhs.uk

Dax EM, Farrugia A, Vyas G (eds): Advances in Transfusion Safety – Volume IV.
Dev Biol (Basel). Basel, Karger, 2007, vol 127, pp 9-14.

Clinicians as Gatekeepers: What Is the Best Route to Optimal Blood Use?

J.P. Isbister

Royal North Shore Hospital of Sydney, University of Sydney, Sydney, Australia

Key words: Patient blood management, transfusion medicine, appropriateness of transfusion, transfusion economics, transfusion quality and safety.

Abstract: Maintaining the supply of allogeneic blood has always been a challenge and its optimal use difficult to ensure and monitor. Increasingly, economic pressures and public perceptions have been driving decision making in delivery of sufficient and safe blood components of high quality. On the other hand, many of the assumed benefits of allogenic blood component therapy are being questioned, and the potential hazards of transfusion have been underestimated. Indeed, recent evidence suggests that in many clinical settings there are significant under-recognised hazards of transfusion in which benefit is difficult to confirm. This paper questions the current paradigm, in which there is excessive focus on the supply side of the blood transfusion chain rather than the clinical problem facing patients and clinicians. Blood transfusion should no longer be the default therapeutic decision when evidence for efficacy is lacking and there is clinical uncertainty. The appropriateness of transfusion practices will only improve, not by expecting clinicians to be gatekeepers of the blood supply, but with better patient blood management based on a sound understanding of pathophysiology and better evidence for transfusion efficacy. Evidence-based transfusion medicine should view a patient's own blood as a valuable and unique natural resource that should be conserved and managed appropriately. Altruistically donated allogeneic blood transfusion should only be used as therapy when there is evidence for potential benefit, there are no alternatives, a quality product is available and the risks are appropriately considered and balanced against the benefits.

INTRODUCTION

Homologous blood transfusion has been one of the most significant medical advances of the 20th century, enabling a higher survival rate among patients suffering from blood loss due to injury or marrow failure resulting from disease or myelosuppressive therapy, major surgical advances and improvement of the length and quality of haemophiliacs' lives. So what's the problem? There is a growing ground swell of opinion that transfusion medicine has excessively focused on the blood component supply side of the system rather than on the patient/demand perspective. Blood supply agencies understandably want to "conserve" a precious and altruistically donated resource that should be "managed" appropriately. On the opposing side, clinicians want to conserve and manage a patient's blood appropriately. As the raison d'être for blood transfusion is a patient with a problem, the latter should be the "true" meaning of blood conservation and management. The clinical focus should be on "what is best for the patient?" not, "what is best for the blood supply?" This is not meant to deny the importance of the multiple issues and challenges facing the provision of an adequate and safe blood supply, but the primary focus must be on the needs of patients, with the supply chain responding appropriately to clinical needs.

The Problems and Contradictions

If homologous blood transfusion can be avoided, the potential hazards need not be considered. For reasons that are not obvious, the transfusion of homologous blood has been regarded as a "default" decision when there is uncertainty about the possible benefits of homologous blood transfusion. In most clinical circumstances the benefits from transfusion have been assumed and it is only in recent years with the appearance of transfusion transmitted HIV that the appropriateness of many transfusions is being questioned. It is a sobering thought to consider that in circumstances where there is uncertainty or no evidence to support improved clinical outcomes from transfusion a patient may be unnecessarily exposed to potentially major morbidity or even mortality. The decision-making process for blood component therapy can be difficult and much debate continues in relation to the indications for the use of various homologous blood components [1]. However, there are good common sense and scientific reasons to adopt a non-transfusion default position when there is no evidence for potential benefit. Primum non nocere.

There is minimal evidence indicating that the transfusion of red cells and platelets have led to improved outcomes in many clinical settings. Indeed, evidence suggests that in many of the clinical situations in which red cell concentrates are used (i.e. in surgery, ICU, critical bleeding, oncology) transfusions may be unnecessary or inappropriate and, further, may be responsible for more problems than benefits [2]. It is this evidence that is leading to a broad re-analysis of transfusion practices and a primary focus on the clinical problem and transfusion alternatives. Recent observational studies indicate that the transfusion of homologous red cells is an independent variable for increased morbidity and mortality (e.g. acute lung injury, infection, multi-organ dysfunction syndrome, increased length of hospital stay) [3-5]. Although causality is difficult to establish in observational studies, a strong case can be made implicating transfusion on the basis of immunomodulation and the clinical effects of the storage lesion [6]. Both these effects are related to leucocyte contamination of stored blood and can be minimised by pre-storage leucoreduction.

There are currently many inexplicable paradoxes and contradictions in the practice of transfusion medicine that would unlikely be tolerated or persist in other medical disciplines. The precautionary principle has been applied to the safety of the blood supply to the point that welfare of patients may be threatened due to insufficiency of the blood supply. On the other hand, the opposite of the precautionary principle (the assimilatory principle) is applied to clinical practice of transfusion. Questionable and potentially dangerous clinical transfusion practices persist despite having been demonstrated to cause harm. Not only are the greatest risks to transfusion safety for patients those of error, bacterial contamination and transfusion related lung injury (TRALI), but in many circumstances these complications may occur in a context in which there is little or no evidence for potential benefit from the transfusion.

Enormous financial resources are expended on dubious incremental improvements to the viral safety of the blood supply. Such expenditure could never be justified on a cost effectiveness analysis for any other health intervention. The concern and "outrage" from the community and "tainted blood" support groups regarding transfusion transmitted HIV and hepatitis is understandable. The initial scientific responses to these transfusion transmissible viruses were rapid, rational and cost-effective. Lessons have been learnt and strategies developed to respond to emerging infectious agents threatening blood safety, but we must move on.

Dr. Denton Cooley's courageous and pioneering "bloodless" cardiac surgery on Jehovah's Witnesses as early as the 1960's, when twelve-unit blood transfusions were the norm, should have sent a message to all who prescribe transfusions that we may be overestimating the benefits and underestimating the potential hazards of transfusion [7].

Clinicians think blood is ordinary and take blood transfusion for granted, while benefit is assumed and risks are perceived as minimal. Doctors want to give patients the most effective therapy at minimal risk. In this respect, transfusion, for inexplicable reasons, is viewed differently. This must be an issue of education and communication. Allogeneic blood transfusion can no longer be viewed as always being the "gift of life".

The supply-oriented blood bankers and transfusion medicine specialists have the knowledge and the evidence about what is really happening in transfusion safety. They need to expand their horizons beyond their own professional organisations and blood supply focus out into the broader medical and nursing community, focusing more on patient blood management.

We have a knowledgeable and committed professional group in hospital transfusion medicine laboratory scientists, whose frustration at watching from the clinical sidelines has reached a level that tempts them to run onto the "field of play". When there is a paradigm shift back to focusing on the patient and patient blood management, they will be ready to "run with the ball" in a way that could amaze us all. Analogous to the changes in pharmacy in recent decades, laboratory scientists are waiting and ready to "hug the patients". Pharmacists increasingly see their role as interacting with patients and having close liaisons with the clinical staff.

Nurses are the health professionals who actually administer the majority of blood transfusions. Their role has been one of the most underrated and underappreciated in the transfusion process. With the move towards more transfusion surveillance officers, analogous to infection control officers, they are also waiting for the transfusion paradigm to shift to one of patient blood management. The terminology tends to be negative: transfusion surveillance officers should be patient blood management coordinators. Some countries are ahead of others in this respect.

Patients think blood transfusion is special and beneficial, but have difficulty accepting small risks they cannot control. Patients and relatives demand zero risk, but want 100 % autonomy. In the patient blood management paradigm there will be honesty to patients about the benefits and risks of transfusion with the option for greater choice. In parallel with this will be informed acceptance by patients and relatives that modern medicine is practiced in a context of uncertainty in which doctors aim at maximising benefits of transfusion therapy and minimising the risks.

From a blood donor's perspective donation is such a demanding exercise that it is no wonder there are problems recruiting committed members of the community who are willing to make this precious resource available to those in need. Donors give their blood in trust that it will be used appropriately, efficiently and safely to help those in need.

The community expects a safe transfusion to be available whenever they may need it, but they have the false belief, as do many clinicians, that safety relates solely to the blood product and not to the recipient and the transfusion process.

Politicians react to community pressure, irrespective of irrational community beliefs. For politicians, perception = reality = votes = survival.

Bureaucrats respond to fiscal restraints, performance contracts and politician's demands. If and when the paradigm changes the bureaucrats should fall into line.

Technological developments in recent years are leading to major advances in several areas relevant to transfusion medicine. Near-patient testing increasingly allows real-time patient blood management. Autologous apheresis technologies, recombinant blood components and pharmacological agents for enhancing haemostasis have added to the patient blood conservation armamentarium. However, industry is frustrated when they see these advances inappropriately or underutilised.

Clinical practice guidelines too often address the indications and use of blood components for a specific form of therapy. Guidelines are more practical and successful if they focus on the patient's problem rather than the therapy (Fig. 1). The better the clinical question is defined and understood, the more likely an appropriate answer and its safe application will be found.

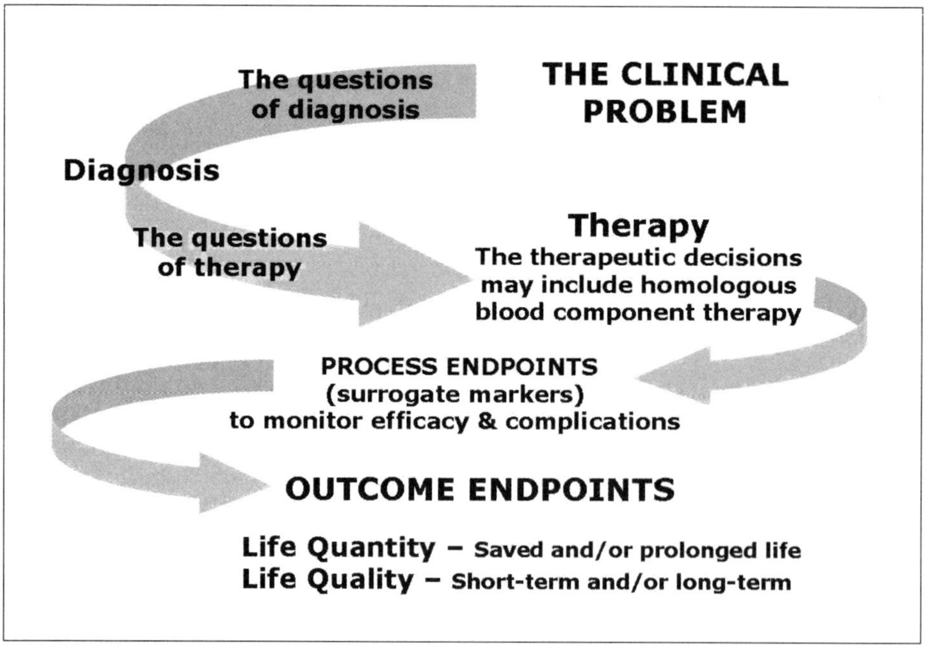

Fig. 1: Clinical practice guidelines should focus on the clinical problem and not primarily on therapeutic modalities.

Should Clinicians be Gatekeepers?

Where responsibility for appropriate use of health resources rests is a complex and at times a controversial and adversarial issue. Clinicians' primary responsibility is to their patients, ensuring they receive safe and effective evidence-based medicine. On the other hand, there are limited health resources that should be distributed in an equitable fashion. This latter responsibility rests more with the health bureaucracy. However, the lack of accurate activity-based costing restricts the development of meaningful cost effectiveness data of the various therapeutic options. As a result, there is a malalignment of the economic and clinical practice models, resulting in health care workers functioning in their own microenvironments to the detriment of the "big picture". This situation is particularly the case in transfusion medicine, as there has never been successful comprehensive activity-based costing of the whole transfusion process. The focus has generally been on the costs of the supply of blood components and the initial compatibility testing, but not on the processes of the administration and monitoring, not to mention costs associated with adverse events. Without these data, cost-effectiveness studies are not possible. Conservative estimates suggested that less than 20 % of transfusion costs relate to the cost of the blood component.

When good economic data and evidence for risk/benefit analyses are insufficient or lacking there is a tendency to adopt a gatekeeper approach to controlling usage and expenditure. Such an approach can only be regarded as a negative stop-gap measure usually of a temporary nature and associated with much angst and generation of poor relationships between professionals. Bureaucrats commonly think there is a way out by passing responsibility to clinicians at the workface. If such an approach is to be successful, appropriate economic tools, administrative resources and meaningful responsibility must be part of the process. Accountability without authority and resources is a recipe for continuing problems.

The concept of clinicians as gatekeepers for the blood supply is an oxymoron. The best route to optimal blood use of allogeneic blood is via patient blood management. For this to be successful, the clinician needs to practice scientifically-based medicine where a clinical problem is appropriately analysed, diagnosis is established and a risk/benefit assessment of therapy is made on the basis of sound evidence.

Optimal medical therapy presupposes an understanding of the pathophysiology, definition and classification of disease, accurate diagnosis, indicators for severity and natural history of untreated disease. These are all basic principles of medical practice that need to be better applied to patient blood management and transfusion medicine in conjunction with meaningful costing data. There is an urgent need for a paradigm shift away from obsession with the supply and safety of homologous blood to patient blood management [8]. Until this occurs we will continue to look for gatekeepers who either keep gates shut when they should be open or open them when they should be closed.

References

1 Isbister JP: Decision making in perioperative transfusion. Transfus Apheresis Sci 2002; 27 (1): 19-28.

2 Hebert PC, et al: A multicenter, randomized, controlled clinical trial of transfusion requirements in critical care. Transfusion Requirements in Critical Care Investigators, Canadian Critical Care Trials Group. N Engl J Med 1999; 340 (6): 409-417.

3 Madjdpour C, Spahn DR: Allogeneic red blood cell transfusions: efficacy, risks, alternatives and indications. Br J Anaesth 2005; 95 (1): 33-42.

4 Englesbe MJ, et al: Transfusions in surgical patients. J Am Coll Surg 2005; 200 (2): 249-254.

5 Spiess BD: Choose one: damned if you do/damned if you don't! Crit Care Med 2005; 33 (8): 1871-1874.

6 Blumberg N: Deleterious clinical effects of transfusion immunomodulation: proven beyond a reasonable doubt. Transfusion 2005; 45 (Suppl 2): 33S-40S.

7 Ott DA, Cooley DA: Cardiovascular surgery in Jehovah's Witnesses. Report of 542 operations without blood transfusion. Jama 1977; 238 (12): 1256-1258.

8 Isbister JP: The paradigm shift in blood transfusion. Med J Aust 1988; 148 (6): 306-308.

Dr. J.P. Isbister, Royal North Shore Hospital of Sydney, University of Sydney, Sydney, Australia.
E-mail: jisbiste@med.usyd.edu.au

Dax EM, Farrugia A, Vyas G (eds): Advances in Transfusion Safety – Volume IV.
Dev Biol (Basel). Basel, Karger, 2007, vol 127, p 15.

SESSION II

Emerging Infectious Agents

Chairs: *R. Dodd and G. Schochetman*

Dax EM, Farrugia A, Vyas G (eds): Advances in Transfusion Safety – Volume IV.
Dev Biol (Basel). Basel, Karger, 2007, vol 127, pp 17-41.

Parasitic Infections in the Blood Supply: Assessing and Countering the Threat

S. Wendel[1], *D.A. Leiby*[2]

[1] Blood Bank, Hospital Sirio Libanês, São Paulo, Brazil

[2] American Red Cross Holland Laboratory, Rockville, MD, USA

Key words: Parasites, blood transfusion, infectious diseases, malaria, Chagas disease

INTRODUCTION

In the light of current blood safety, in a time when many viral threats have been controlled, one cannot disregard the potential damage that parasites impose on the blood supply. The concept of a "Safety Tripod" (selection of appropriate and "low-risk" donors, usage of screening tests for the relevant infection marker, and elimination of pathogens residuals to the previous principles) [1] must also always be present in blood safety policy. Though most developed countries adopt this concept, higher benefits will be ascertained once properly established in the developing countries, where parasitic infections are more prevalent and incident. Given that there are still problems related to geographical distribution, pattern of emigration, high number of asymptomatic donors, lack of medical knowledge to correctly diagnose most of the cases, and pending technical refinements for laboratory screening, each country must be aware of their particular epidemiologic pattern and adopt a combination of procedures for prevention. This review intends to highlight the main parasites that can be transmitted by transfusions, with particular focus on their potential global threats.

MALARIA

Malaria is a life-threatening parasitic disease transmitted by mosquitoes [2]. Human malaria is transmitted by 4 different species: *Plasmodium falciparum, Plasmodium vivax, Plasmodium ovale* and *Plasmodium malariae*, all of which require two different hosts to complete their life cycle – an *Anopheles* mosquito (sexual stage), and humans (asexual stage). The main differences observed in each of the four species are summarized in Table I.

Table I: Major differences observed in all four *Plasmodia* species [2-5].

	***Plamodium* species**			
	P. falciparum	***P. vivax***	***P. ovale***	***P. malariae***
Merozoites	40,000	10,000	15,000	2,000
Schizonts	16	16	8	8
Erythrocytic cicle (hr)	48	48	48	72
Incubation (days)	7-12	12-17	16-18	18-40
Parasitaemia/mm^3	20,000-50,000	50,000	30,000	20,000
Relapses	Short	Variable	Variable	Long
Duration of infection (untreated, years)	1-2	1,5-5	1,5-5	3-50
Hypnozoites	No	Yes	Yes	No
Geographical predominance	Africa, Oceania, Asia, America	India, America, China	Sub-Saharan West Africa	Sub-Saharan West Africa

Induced malaria can also be transmitted by blood transfusion [6], organ transplants [7-9], sharing of intravenous drugs or needles, accidental laboratory exposure, congenitally, or, more rarely, in persons living close to or working at airports [10].

Since the first case of transfusional transmission of malaria (TxM) was reported in 1911 [11], more than 3,000 cases have been described [12], possibly representing only half of the true number of cases [13]. Though eradicated in almost all European countries [14], USA [15], Australia [1], and Japan [16], malaria was still present in 106 countries of the world in 2002, as shown in Figure 1. In this same year, WHO reported more than 120 million people infected in 72 countries, though it has been estimated that there are 350 to 515 million new cases annually, with 270 to 400 million of these due to *P. falciparum* (70 % in Africa and 20 % in South-East Asia), and nearly 1 million deaths, with 90 % in Africa south of Sahara, mostly in children. Recently, a study has claimed that the real number is almost two-fold the one predicted by WHO [17], with 515 million people affected only by *P. falciparum*. In addition, nearly 40 % of the world population, or 2 billion people (2005) still remain exposed to varying degrees of risk of malaria infection [17-19]. Comprehensive reports from annually reported cases in Europe can be found in the European Network on Imported Infectious Disease Surveillance.

Transmission by blood components is either a consequence of the sanitary conditions of a country or region, imported cases into developed, non-endemic places by immigrants or travelers from endemic areas within endemic countries or non-endemic countries (considered geographically distinct [20]) where vectorial malaria has been completely controlled [21-24], with a trend of continuous increase of imported malaria in the last two decades, mainly *P. falciparum* cases [21].

The annual incidence of TxM ranges from 0.25-0.67 cases/million units in the USA [25] and Canada [26], respectively, to more than 50 cases/million units in endemic regions [24].

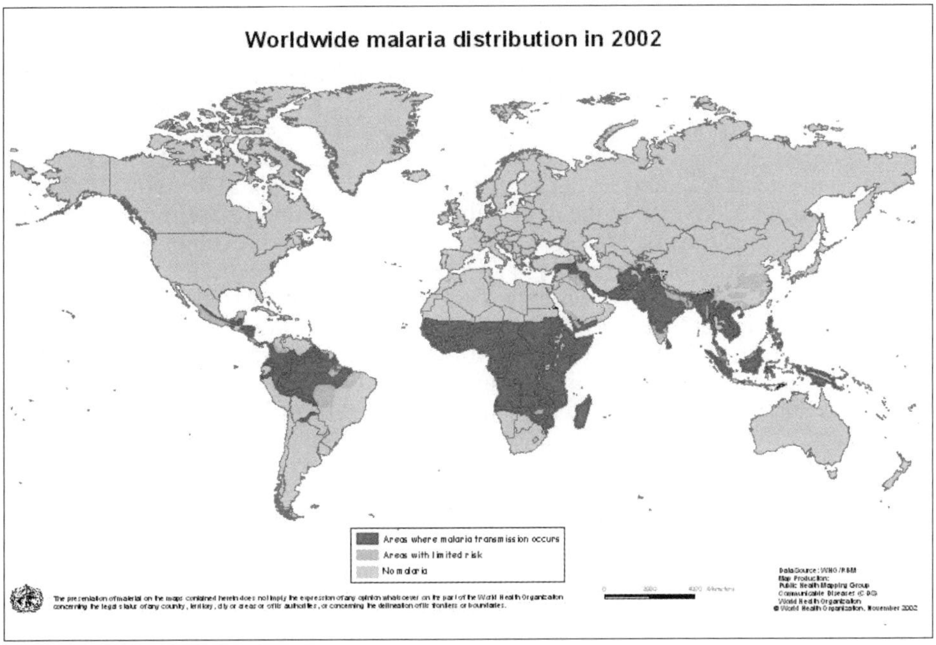

Fig. 1: Malaria distribution in the world, as defined by WHO (http://www.who.int/GlobalAtlas).

Infected blood donors may harbour parasites for years, especially those partially immunized from exposure to endemic regions where immunity renders a somewhat absence of symptoms, or after chemoprophylaxis. As listed in Table 1, different periods of infection are seen for each species. Despite the exceptionally prolonged periods for *P. falciparum*, *P. ovale* and *P. vivax*, it seems unlikely that a donor will remain infective after 5 years of infection, which is the basic element for questioning blood donors.

TxM is transmitted by asexual forms present in red blood cells, usually from asymptomatic donors who carry a low parasitaemic level, and rarely in the period between the subclinical parasitaemia and the onset of symptoms (usually associated with previous chemoprophylaxis). Gametocytes are not infective, and free merozoites are present in the bloodstream for a very short period and do not maintain viability in stored units. Chances of infection by circulating sporozoites right after the insect biting has not been associated with transfusion cases [29]. Transmission from symptomatic donors is very unlikely and, when present, usually occurs in endemic regions.

The minimum level of parasites that will lead to infection is not known. For *P. vivax*, a total of 10 parasites/µl was successful in inducing experimental transmission [24]. In addition, an infection rate of 1-2 parasites/µl will render nearly half a million parasites in a single whole blood unit, a number far from the minimum necessary to induce an active infection in the recipient [13]. Even if the real value is unknown, one can assume that one infected unit to a naïve receptor equals 100 % of infectivity [26].

Transmission occurs mainly by the use of red cell products (whole blood or packed red cells), although all other blood components (liquid or frozen, untreated fresh plasma, platelets and granulocytes concentrates) cannot be regarded as devoid of viable infective parasites [30]. No infection has been associated with blood derivatives, even if donated from potentially infected donors.

In the past 50 years, the pattern of the distribution of the causative species in several non-endemic countries has shifted from *P. malariae* and *P. vivax* [24,25,27] to *P. falciparum*. Conversely, the distribution among different endemic regions also shows a wide variation: in Africa, *P. falciparum* is the most prevalent agent [18,19], while *P. vivax* is common in India [31] and Brazil [20,32,33].

Given that migratory movements, particularly from Africa and India into Europe and from Southeastern Asia and South America into North America [13] were responsible for TxM, specific measures are taken in order to prevent it. These include 1) an accurate history including place of birth, previous residence places during lifetime, immigration and a complete account of prior travel during the past three years, 2) The use of specific questionnaires aiming at excluding three types of infected donors: i) non-immune travelers who acquired malaria abroad or asymptomatic parasitaemia following inadequate chemoprophylaxis; ii) military personnel returning from endemic areas; iii) foreign visitors or immigrants from endemic regions that are usually immune and asymptomatic.

As a general policy [30,34] travelers or residents of non-malarious areas coming from malarious areas (irrespective of chemoprophylaxis) should be deferred for a 1-year period, if free of malaria symptoms. Immigrants from endemic areas (asymptomatic) should be deferred 3 to 5 years, and the same for those who have had a diagnosis of malaria and became asymptomatic [26]. However, this is not valid for *P. malariae*, for which longer periods of infectivity are recorded [27,35], leading to the adoption of a permanent deferral for donors reporting a history of diagnosis or treatment of malaria at any time in the past in Canada [36]. Because the world malarial zone is too vast, an alphabetical list of countries reporting malaria transmission and a malarial map (provided by Roll Back Malaria – WHO) [37] should be present in every collection facility.

Unfortunately, prevention of infectious donors by questionnaires alone introduces two additional problems [38]: 1) *Low specificity*, rejecting a high number of healthy donors, calculated as 50,000 blood units in the USA [27,39] or some 40,000 blood units in Australia [1], despite recent changes in testing and selection algorithm (Albert Farrugia, personal communication); 2) *Low sensitivity,* such as reported in the USA in the period 1963-1999 [27], where failure was found in approximately two thirds of 93 cases observed; even if current guidelines were correctly applied, still a third of cases could not be prevented, mostly by *P. malariae* [15]. Also, accuracy of the donors' histories is fallible in many cases [25,40], as most of them were infected in childhood or simply do not recall being infected.

In view of these problems, some non-endemic countries have introduced a series of specific strategies aimed at reducing risk, such as temporary exclusion when returning from specific WHO-defined endemic areas, temporary/permanent exclusion of candidate donors with a positive malaria history, and specific serological screening, applicable only to selected suspected donors (immigrants or individuals born in endemic areas, and those who had had malaria from 3 to 5 years before donation) [28,30,41]. These measures have been adopted in France [42] and the UK [43] with savings of up to 95 % of non-plasma components from donors with malaria risk. Still, up to 30,000 donors might be annually lost due to a possible exposure to malaria.

In endemic countries, exclusion of previously infected donors for 3 years may be unsuitable. Also, screening tests such as detection of malarial antibodies may be inadequate, as they detect only previous infection and not the presence of circulating parasites, emphasizing the possibility of testing for malarial antigens [52].

On the other hand, in remote endemic areas, where it is virtually impossible to rely upon uninfected donors, where neither screening tests are available nor adequate blood collection facilities are present, the following procedures are recommended: a) Exclusion of candidates who had malaria in the previous 12 months or with a febrile episode in the last 30 days. This procedure has been used in the highly endemic Brazilian Amazon area [44], though a substantial number of donors might bear antibodies [33]; b) In endemic areas, where no organized BTS are available, one alternative is to introduce the use of chloroquine in donors 48 hours before donation or a single shot immediately before, and then accept a donation. This measure usually comes together with preventive chemoprophylaxis to the recipient, particularly neonates after an exchange-transfusion [45], who must be continuously treated for a month. This measure is not advisable for pregnant or breast-feeding women and is ineffective for drug-resistant *P. falciparum* strains, responsible for the worst cases [3,24]. This should be regarded as a last option measure, and should not be taken into account when recipients are from non-endemic regions (non-immune).

The use of inactivating agents such as Inactine PEN110 might be a suitable alternative in the near future [46]. However, it seems that there is still a long way to go before reduction agents can be widely used for RBC products.

Screening tests are aimed at the detection of circulating antibodies or antigens [24,31]:

- *Detection of antibodies* is based mainly on indirect immunofluorescence assay (IFA) or ELISA using *P. falciparum*, non-human parasites, purified or recombinant antigens. These tests are useful for interpreting high titered or negative sera, denoting, respectively, the presence or absence of infection. However, low titered sera must, in most cases, be supplemented with a thorough interview with the donor [13]. Though the presence of IgG antibodies correlate with the number of past malarial attacks [33], the presence of antibodies does not imply the presence of circulating parasites, especially among donors in endemic region. Antibodies detected by IFA are present in > 95 % of infected donors, usually arising 7-14 days after the onset of infection by *P. falciparum* (with longer periods for other species). They persist for several years in those who are subject to continuous exposure (immune donors from endemic countries), particularly in *P. malariae* infection. Antibodies may persist for 6-12 months after adequate treatment. IFA is highly recommended for screening donors in non-endemic countries [42], but it is unsuitable in highly endemic regions, where a high prevalence of antibody positive donors are to be found. The adoption of antigen detection in these situations is more suitable. Sensitivity in the window phase ranges from 50 to 80 % [47,48]. However, it is unlikely that donors with acute infection donate their blood, especially in non-endemic countries. In addition, if a proper and valid questionnaire is applied, most of those negative, acute phase donors will be temporarily rejected. A different approach using three recombinant antigens for *P. falciparum* and one for *P. vivax* is adopted in the UK [43]. False positive reactions are related to commercial kits using A_1 red blood cell cultures (due to binding of natural antiglobulins mainly from group O individuals) [42], or cross-reactivity to HIV antibodies, particularly in high endemic areas [49]. More recently, a new technology using flow-cytometry-based-multiplexed immunoassays was proposed [50], especially for developing countries, but validations in endemic countries are pending.

- *Detection of antigens* – The thick smear test has a limit sensitivity of 50 parasites/μl, or 0.001 % infected RBC, only achieved by highly qualified technicians. In practice, detection occurs only with 0.01 % infected RBC [51], more than the minimum necessary for transmission. However, prevention by thick smear in only 10 % of TxM and positivity in 31 % (8/26) of donors implicated in TxM was reported [25].

Parasite detection within erythrocytes is reported with the use of acridine orange by IFA [52]. Sensitivity reaches 5-50 parasites/μl, but lower levels of parasitaemia may reach up to 2.5 x 10^6 parasites in one unit of blood [24].

The description of *PfHRP-2*, a water soluble, histidine-rich antigen present in immature *P. falciparum* gametocytes [53,54] and the production of monoclonal antibodies (MAb) against it are the basis of two distinct methods for circulating antigen detection methods, the first an ELISA [55-57], and the second two similar tests utilizing a rapid lateral flow immunochromatographic test (dipstick or rapid diagnostic test – RDT). One utilizes a combination of MAb against HRP-2 and plasmodial aldolase [58], and the other is based on the detection of parasite-specific lactate dehydrogenase [59] (through a combination of one specific MAb for *P. falciparum* and two other panspecific MAb against all plasmodia LDH, allowing detection of both *P. falciparum* and *P. vivax*). Good sensitivity is achieved only when parasite concentration is > 100 parasites/μl, with specificity ranging from 40-93 % [51]. Because WHO recommends a sensitivity of up to 100 parasites/ml (0.002 % parasitaemia) [60], a high positive likelihood ratio (LR – or a high post-test probability) and low negative LR (to rule out malaria infection in negative results), this might be a suitable alternative for regions where skilled microscopy technicians are not available or where thick or thin film examination cannot be considered as first-line methods (i.e., non-endemic countries) [61]. Even though these results are problematic for *P. ovale* and *P. malariae*, which are both less frequent in the context of transfusional cases, the results are not devoid of clinical importance. More comprehensive data on rapid diagnostic tests for malaria can be found elsewhere [51,62-65]. False positive results are observed in the presence of rheumathoid factor and low-level parasitaemia (ranging from 50 to 5000/μl) [66]. A combination of testing potentially infected donors for the simultaneous presence of malarial antibodies and antigens was reported in France [67], with increased sensitivity and shortened seroconversion period (from 11.4 ± 1.6 to 5.3 ± 1.1 days) as compared with using the IFA screening method only.

A screening procedure using PCR was published that showed a sensitivity for *P. falciparum* of 1-4 parasites/50 ml, and for *P. vivax* of 40-130 parasites/50 μl (100 times more than the one achieved by blood films in Vietnamese blood donors [68]). However, its high cost, particularly in regions with limited resources, still renders this method unsuitable for routine use. In addition, non reactive PCR results are reported in donors implicated in induced malaria in developed countries [15,35,40]. More recently, a real-time PCR able to discriminate all 4 species and with a sensitivity of 30 parasites/ml was proposed [69] for use in low parasitaemia-infected travelers, for blood transfusion or transplant recipients, and possibly for blood donors, especially in endemic areas. A small study in Spain adopted PCR as a strategy for testing blood donors with a potential risk for malaria [70]. Only 4 % of cases were discarded, with some 42 % of donors returning to make another donation. No transmission was reported in recipients.

An important problem is still the definition of a gold standard for screening of blood donors. Though in many countries IFA is considered as such, 100 % sensitivity or specificity cannot be expected by this method. False positive and negative results always have to be considered, and a suitable material for preparation of this test is not readily available to many laboratories. Furthermore, they are derived only from *P. falciparum* strains, even though this is the most common species. The fact that one has to rely on cross-reactions to detect the other strains renders this method far from ideal. In addition, a recent study with recombinant EIA antigens demonstrated a superiority of results on proven cases [43]. In summary, it is clear that there is no single and standard approach to prevent malaria transmission by blood products in non-endemic and endemic countries; it is up to each country to define the most appropriate strategy to be applied [71].

American Trypanosomiasis (Chagas Disease)

American Trypanosomiasis, or Chagas disease, occurs only in the American continent. It is caused by the protozoan *Trypanosoma cruzi*. Transmission by blood transfusion was first suggested by Mazza in Argentina in 1936 [72], later supported in Brazil, Uruguay and Argentina. The first two cases of the transmission of Chagas disease were published in 1952 [73]. During that same period, the value of chemoprophylaxis with crystal violet (gentian violet) was studied [74]. Though regarded as a strictly Latin American problem, Chagas disease transmission through blood components became recognized in North America in the late 80's [75-80].

There are some 100 million people at risk of exposure in endemic areas and from 18 to 20 million possibly infected in 18 Latin American countries (it has not been described in Cuba or the Dominican Republic) [81-85]. It is estimated that 2 to 3 million people manifest chronic features (cardiac or gastrointestinal) of infection, with nearly 45,000 deaths annually [6]. That makes Chagas disease the main cause of early retirement and the leading cause of number of years lost from incapacity. Actually, when Chagas disease is measured by disability-adjusted life years (DALYs), it shows the highest DALY in all of Latin America. The remaining infectious diseases with public importance (malaria, schistosomiasis, leishmaniasis, leprosy, filariasis and onchocercosis) represent, all together, less than 25 % of the economic burden [87,88]. On a global scale, Chagas disease represents the third most important tropical disease measured by DALYs, after malaria and schistosomiasis [89].

The Southern Cone [90] and the Andean [91] Countries Initiatives have as main objective elimination of the domiciliary infestation by *Triatoma infestans* (main reduviid bug) and complete control over transfusional transmision within a time span of 10 years [92]. Rigid governmental control and serological screening is required as mandatory. This action was also enhanced by the 51st World Health Assembly, which deemed the control of Chagas disease as one of its main priorities [93].

Trypanosoma cruzi is a long and slender protozoan (order *Kinetoplastida*, family *Trypanosomatidae*), with a single nucleus, a flagellum, and a kinetoplast. A DNA particle present in the mitochondria is organized into a network of interlocked minicircles, with 20,000 to 25,000 copies per kinetoplast. There are 3 stages in its evolutive life cycle: 1) *amastigotes* are found as clusters in infected cells of vertebrates or in the invertebrate triatomine stomach; 2) *epimastigotes* are present in the foregut of the insect vector; 3) *trypomastigotes* are found in vertebrates in the bloodstream, lymph and cerebrospinal fluid. This is especially in the acute phase, while in invertebrates can be found in the duodenum and hindgut (*metacyclical trypomastigotes*). There are more than 100 different strains, each one with a particular preference for humans, domestic or sylvatic reservoirs [94]. A polymorphism is observed according to morphological criteria and also due to different isoenzymes patterns (zymodemes) [95,96], kDNA cleavage by RFLP (schyzodemes) [97], or molecular sequencing of several parasite genes [98]. Recently, the genome sequence has been characterized [99].

Invertebrates responsible for transmission of *T. cruzi* are haematophagus bugs (family *Reduvidae* and sub family *Triatominae*). They are a significant vector only in the New World (from latitude 42N – North California, Utah, Maryland – to 46S – Patagonia).

Chagas disease is also transmitted by blood transfusions [94], congenital transmission, vertically through breast-feeding, accidental laboratory contamination, organ transplants [100,101], or by accidental ingestion of infected food [102].

Because the American continent comprises more than 20 different countries, a wide array of prevalence in infected donors is observed in different regions. This ranges from as low as 0.01 % in the USA to 60 % in certain Bolivian cities [81,83,94,103-108]. There has been a progressive decrease in the prevalence of *T. cruzi* among Latin American blood donors.

With the exception of blood derivatives, all blood components are infective. *T. cruzi* remains viable at 4°C for at least 18 days [109] or up to 250 days when kept at room temperature [110]. Frozen strains are infective for longer periods [110,111]. The viability of the parasite is somewhat lower in frozen components (up to 24 hours), though several haemophiliacs treated only with cryoprecipitate have been infected [112-114].

In many places, blood transfusion is recognized as the second most common way of transmission of Chagas disease; on the other hand, it can be recognized as the main route in industrialized countries (e.g. Canada, USA and Spain) [75-78,115]. The true number of reported cases is grossly underestimated, since no more than 300 cases have been published in the literature [82,94,116,117].

Although the reported cases in countries of the Northern hemisphere is quite low, there is intense Latin American emigration in these countries, with some 12.400,000 to the USA, 500,000 to Europe, 500,000 to Japan and 100,000 to Australia. It is expected that 50,000 to 370,000 immigrants in North America are infected with *T. cruzi* [118], and nearly 75,000 of them may have some cardiac manifestation [119].

The possibility of infection by blood components depends on several factors: amount of transfused blood, the parasite strain, presence of parasitaemia at the time of donation, recipient immune status and screening tests) [94,105,120]. Data derived in the 1960´s and 1970´s demonstrated that the real infectivity rate from one infected whole blood unit is around 12-25 % [113,122,123]. A higher value (46.7 %) was observed in Bolivia [124]. It may be that low parasitaemia (less than 1 parasite/20 ml whole blood) and the concomitant presence of antibodies in donor´s bloodstream are partially responsible for incomplete infectivity. In addition, there are no data to demonstrate different patterns of infectivity in different components. Although sensitivity of tests is still far from that observed for viral screening tests (97-99 %) [125], universal screening has dramatically changed the transfusional risks associated in Latin America in the past few years. In countries where screening strategies have been fully implemented, the residual risk if infection is calculated to be around 1 : 200,000 units [120,126], with clustered spatial geographic distribution.

A recent Brazilian survey [127] derived from a cluster sampling method to produce a national panel (n = 13,383 samples) represented over 15 million whole blood donations. Original screening tests were compared with two screening methods (indirect hemagglutination and ELISA) in a reference laboratory. All positive results by at least one screening test and 1.5 % of negative sera were used to produce a reference panel (n = 273) that was tested against 4 reference (confirmatory) tests (TESA blot, Indirect immunofluorescence, RIPA, and a trypomastigote chemoluminescent test). After correction of verification bias, the estimated prevalence of *T. cruzi* infected donors ranged from 0.1-0.2 %, with a crescent age-related positivity. Interpolation by ordinary anisotropic point kriging analysis resulted in risk areas in the country both for false positive and negative data in 4 different regions (where vectorial activity is still found) and the presence of a possible new risk area in the Amazon region, with national estimates of 0.9 to 7.4 false negative results per 100,000 whole blood donations. This translates to 0.44 to 2.75 infectious blood components per 100,000 being presented to recipients. This survey concluded that the residual risk of transmition of *T. cruzi* by blood transfusion in Brazil is presently some 10 to 15-fold greater than for HIV, HBV or HCV, with spatial concentrations.

The incubation period of acute Chagas disease following an infected blood unit varies from 20 to 40 days (ranging from 8 to 120 days). Fever is the most common sympton and sometimes the only manifestation of disease. Lymphadenopathy and hepatosplenomegaly may also be present and the association of these latter symptoms must always be suspected as Chagas disease in recipients transfused from untested donors.

Cardiac arrhythmia (disturbances of atrioventricular conduction, ECG alterations or reduction of ejection fraction), pericardial effusion and/or cardiac arrest can be observed. Sometimes this is fatal, but mostly in immunocompromised recipients.

The central nervous system can also be affected: somnolence, fatigue and tremors are the most common symptoms. Myoclonus, seizures, meningitis or meningoencephalitis, though very rare, occur mainly in immunocompromised patients.

The gastrointestinal system is usually spared in acute Chagas disease. Approximately 20 % of infected recipients are completely asymptomatic, raising no suspicion of diagnosis. In fact, in non-endemic areas from industrialized countries, this rate might be somewhat higher than in endemic countries.

A spontaneous recovery will ensue 6-8 weeks (but may extend up to 4 months) after the acute phase. Thereafter, the disease follows its natural course through a phase of undetermined length (persisting for years or decades), occurring in the majority of cases. In the chronic phase, cardiac, gastrointestinal or neurological symptoms are observed after several years. Usually these are not linked to an acute phase. A more comprehensive data set about the chronic manifestations of Chagas disease can be found elsewhere [82,84,94,116].

One of the key issues concerning the clinical findings among blood donors infected with *T. cruzi* is that the vast majority are asymptomatic. These can be subdivided into three main groups: 1) *Serological Chagas disease*, where only antibodies are found, without any evidence of symptoms, comprising 60 % to 80 % of all infected donors; 2) *Latent chronic phase*, with visceral abnormalities, as evidenced by different diagnostic tests (X-ray, CT Scan, ECG), but still asymptomatic; 3) *Symptomatic donors*, representing the minority of cases.

Prevention of transmission of Chagas disease can be accomplished by three different strategies [128]: 1) *Anamnesis and questionnaires to the donors* – there is a trend to find more infected donors among those with a higher age, first time donors or those who have spent a certain length of time of living in endemic areas [126,129,130]. In endemic and non-endemic regions, donors who lived in infested dwellings or acknowledge being bitten by the bug must be deterred from donation; 2) *Serological tests* – several methods are available for screening in Latin America, but unfortunately, none has yet been licensed in the USA (although a major movement has been recently observed to accomplish this); 3) *Chemoprophylaxis* – crystal violet was used in the past at a concentration of 1:4,000 or 200 µg/ml (0.6 m*M*) [74,131-133] and is proven to be effective against all parasite stages and several different strains [131,135]. The Brazilian experience confirmed the efficacy of crystal violet treatment [134]. However, this compound is not devoid of effects on red blood cells and platelets. Thus, as a principle for universal pathogen reduction, other methods have been extensively evaluated in the past few years, and among the several new agents tested are amotosalen-HCL [136] and INACTINE Pen-110 [46], both of which have have been proven to be satisfactory. However, these products are still not globally used.

Detection of parasites via direct examination in the peripheral bloodstream, or indirect methods (culture systems such as xenodiagnosis or hemocultures), though still regarded as the gold standard for diagnosis, cannot be considered as practical on a daily or routine basis. In addition, a negative result still does not exclude infection, given that the sensitivity of these methods rarely reaches 85 % [137,138]. Both methods require up to 120 days for full and conclusive results.

Due to the relative low sensitivity and technical problems observed by xenodiagnosis and hemoculture on chronically infected patients, PCR was considered as an alternative. However, the main difficulty in chronic patients derives from the low and intermittent parasitaemia observed in a significant percentage. In order to obviate that, investigators have focused on DNA sequences largely represented on the *T. cruzi* genome present on the parasite mitochondria kDNA [139-143], on ribosomal RNA (rRNA) [144], or on the Paraflagellar Rod genes (PFR) [145]. However, the need of chaotropic agents (guanidine HCl) for better DNA extraction [139], as well as the assay's variable sensitivity (45 to 100 %) [146-156] precluded its adoption as a gold standard to date. Also, false positive results may be more common than expected [140,143,146,157].

Thus, as a practical procedure, one has to rely on detection of parasite antibodies. Assays are easy to perform and are at relative low cost and high sensitivity (though with variable specificity). There are several methods commercially available in Latin America [15,159], mostly based on ELISA [160-166], Indirect Hemagglutination [167-169] or Indirect Immunofluorescence Assay (IFA) [170,171], using whole parasites or crude lysates as the antigen source. There is intense research on the development of synthetic peptides or recombinant antigens. *Trypanosoma cruzi* antibody titers or concentrations are quite variable in infected people and usually bear no relationship with clinical symptoms. They also vary in the same individual during their lifetime.

The current serological methods also are prone to cross reaction with sera containing antibodies against other infectious agents such as yeasts, *Leishmania spp.*, *T. rangeli* (a non pathogenic agent found in Venezuela, Colombia, Peru, Ecuador, Panama and Costa Rica), *T. gambiensis* (the agent of the sleeping sickness or African Trypanosomiasis), *H. muscarum, L. seymoury, C. fasciculata* and other tripanosomatids. In addition, non-specific IgM directed against phosphocoline [172], an antigenic fraction widely present in several mycobacteria and parasites, is also responsible for cross reactivity. It also has to be considered that doubtful sera are seen in approximately 3-5 % of all blood donors, characterized by a reactive result in only one assay (usually with clear negative or very low titer in a second test).

These events usually pose a major problem for the Blood Bank scenario, as far as counseling of donors are concerned. For this reason, supplemental assays are also highly necessary in order to confirm the screening tests. Though several methods have been advocated for their potential role as confirmatory tests [173-181], common cross-reactivity has also been demonstrated. Perhaps only two methods deserve some attention at this point: 1) *Western blot* using highly purified trypomastigote excreted-secreted antigens (TESA) [182-184]; 2) *Radioimmuneprecipitation Assay (RIPA)* when lysed cultured epimastigotes containing a radioisotope (^{125}I or ^{35}S) are tested against serum, displaying two major glycoprotein bands (gp 72 and gp 90) [185,186]. However, both methods showed some flaws in a Brazilian survey [126,188], where a national panel (n = 273) originated from over 150 collection facilities representing more than 1.5 million donations (initially screened by a combination of hemagglutination – IH – and ELISA tests from several different brands) displayed a wide range of reactivity in screening methods, ranging from 28 to 60 samples. When these reactive sera were tested by TESA and RIPA confirmatory methods, positive results varied from 24 to 33 samples, with kappa index ranging from 0.711 to 0.920. Given that reactions were variable amongst confirmatory methods, their reciprocal behaviour by ROC curves also gave a wide discrepancy in results, as studied by the area under the curve – AUC (0.8361-0.9587), sensitivity (0.6667-0.9286) and specificity (0.9580-0.9918). Both putative gold standard methods recognized reactive samples that were missed by the other, leading to the possibility that they still should be considered only as "*imperfect gold standard*" [189].

In summary, though vectorial Chagas disease is under intense control in Latin America, recent emigration movements to many countries in the world pose a new threat to the safety of the blood supply. It requires stringent and adequate control measures to prevent transfusion transmission in many countries until considered free from any risk.

Babesiosis

Babesia spp. are intra-erythrocytic protozoan parasites resembling *Plasmodium*, and are the etiologic agents of babesiosis. It was first described in Yugoslavia in 1957 [190]. Since then, hundreds of cases of have been reported in humans, primarily in the USA and Europe [191-193]; cases have also been observed in other countries. The main agents of disease in the United States and Europe are *B. microti* and *B. divergens*, respectively [193-198]. In addition, there are several *Babesia*-like agents described in the United States (WA-1, CA-1, MO-1) and Europe (EU-1) [199]. Like Lyme disease, it is transmitted by the tick vector *Ixodes scapularis* (USA) or *I. trianguliceps* and *I. ricinus* (Europe).

Babesia microti is a pear-shaped, oval or round parasite 1-5 mm in length. They only reproduce in red cells, and can therefore be easily misdiagnosed as *Plasmodium falciparum*. The life cycle of the tick vector, *Ixodes* spp., is quite complex and involves larval and nymphal stages, both feeding mainly upon the white-footed mouse (primary natural reservoir). The adult phase feeds upon the white-tailed deer, which does not become infected but serves only as a blood meal source and transport host.

Human infections occur following the bite of a *Babesia*-infected nymphal tick, and the risk of transmitting infection is related, in part, to the infection level of not only the tick but also the mouse on which it fed. Clinical symptoms begin 1-4 weeks after exposure and severity of disease is influenced by the host's immune status and the infecting babesial species. The infection induces fever, chills, headache, hemolytic anemia and hemoglobinuria, and in many cases resembles malarial infection [192]. Some infections are fatal. However, most infections (60-65 %) are asymptomatic or subclinical and self-limiting.

The prevalence of *B. microti* antibodies among blood donors ranges from 0.3-4.3 % in the USA [200,201], half of which have demonstrable parasitaemia. In Germany, two studies reported a prevalence of *B. divergens and B. microti* antibodies ranging from 0.8-8.0 % [202,203].

Diagnosis is based on: a) identification of intra-erythrocyte parasites in the bloodstream by examination of thick or thin smears, but is usually only effective with high parasitaemias and hemolytic episodes; b) infecting hamsters or mice with *B. microti* or rodents and gerbils with *B. divergens*; or c) identification of *B. microti* antibodies using IFA (the gold standard method) [204], though this approach is not a feasible option for screening a large number of blood units, leaving a promising space for ELISA tests in the future [205]. Molecular methods using highly conserved sequences of small-subunit rRNA (ss-rRNA) gene have been employed as the target of sensitive and specific PCR assays [206], but currently, nucleic acid-based technologies for *Babesia* spp. have not been developed for blood bank use.

Infected donors may remain asymptomatic for as long as 1 year. There are over 50 transmission cases reported for blood recipients from all ages [207], mainly in the USA [208,209] but also in Japan and Canada [210]. However, like all transfusion-transmitted parasites this is likely an underestimate. Most cases involving *B. microti* are the result of transfusion of red cell units and platelets contaminated with viable red cells. The parasite can persist in red cell products at 4° C for up to 35 days or under freezing conditions (glycerolized red cells) for several years [209,211]. Implicated donors were asymptomatic in most cases, with no recollection of tick bites. Incubation periods in blood recipients are generally 1 to 9 weeks post transfusion, with variable severity.

The risk of transmission by red cells seems to be 1 in 600 to 1 in 1,800 based on local seroprevalence (0.3-1.4 %), parasitemia (56 %), and transmission rate (26 %) estimates [212]. On the other hand, questionnaires aimed at identifying specific risk factors among blood donors lack sensitivity, and are therefore of limited value. Avoiding collection of blood units in endemic areas during high peak seasons, though theoretically sound, produces localized blood shortages and does not prevent collection of chronically infected donors in non-endemic areas. Donors who report a history of previous infection must be permanently deferred.

Toxoplasmosis

Toxoplasmosis is a zoonosis caused by *Toxoplasma gondii*, an obligate intracellular protozoan parasite. Felines are the definitive hosts, and birds and other mammals (including humans) are the intermediate hosts. Their life cycle involves three separate stages: bradyzoites, tachyzoites and oocysts. It is estimated that about one third of the human population worldwide is infected with *T. gondii* [213], with an annual incidence of new cases ranging from 1-5 %.

Infection in humans may occur by one of the following ways: a) Ingestion of cysts contained within raw or undercooked meat of infected livestock (e.g. pork, lamb or beef); b) Accidental ingestion of oocysts after contact with water or food sources infected with faeces from household cats, usually present in litter or in the soil; c) Congenitally, from infected mothers to their babies [214]; d) Direct contamination of open wounds, organ transplantation [215], and blood transfusion [216-218].

There are several factors that support the possibility of acquisition of toxoplasmosis by transfusion of blood components. Fourteen months to four years after the onset of infection, the organism may be recovered from asymptomatic donors or from infected persons [216,218,219], and the agent is able to survive at 4° C for up to 50 days in citrated blood [220]. Perhaps transmission cases are not recognized, but given the high rate of exposure among the general population, many blood recipients may be immune to re-infection unless they are naïve or immunocompromised.

The majority of infected recipients are asymptomatic. Occasionally lymphadenopathy, malaise, fever, headache, cutaneous rashes and sore throat may be found, the illness resembling a mononucleosis-like syndrome. Usually this is not recognized as toxoplasmosis by the attending physician. Severe cases have only been found in immunosuppressed recipients who have usually received large amounts of leukocytes from chronic myelogenous leukemia donors [216,219], though in one case an infection was described in a platelet recipient [221]. Some patients may develop severe symptoms such as meningoencephalitis, myocarditis, hepatitis, retinochoroiditis or posterior uveitis, with permanent damage or even death.

The seroprevalence of donors shows a wide distribution ranging from 8-60 %, according to geographic regions [213,222,223]. This increases with age, most likely because of increased exposure over time.

Although the direct identification of parasites has been described (histological analysis of blood smears and tissue biopsies, in vitro culture of the parasite from blood or body fluids, inoculation of mice with blood or biopsy materials or by PCR) [213,224] as highly specific, these techniques have limited sensitivity because the parasite is generally present in blood and tissues at low concentrations. Perhaps PCR is the only practical detection method in the blood bank environment, particularly for acute or "window period" infections since several target sequences are routinely used in *T. gondii* nested PCR assays [225-227]. From a practical point of view, serological tests (*T. gondii* antibodies) are still more appropriate for routine use. There are several methods for *T. gondii* antibody detection, including IFA, ELISA and Western blots [228-230]. The IgG avidity test, which measures the functional affinity of IgG antibodies, can be used to differentiate between recent and past infections [231,232]. Antibody affinity increases with time; thus, IgG affinity measurements for past *T. gondii* infections would be high, whereas recent infections would demonstrate IgG antibodies with low affinity. Taken together, the persistence of antibodies in a large portion of the general population, combined with the difficultly in differentiating between recent and past infections, make a blood screening intervention for *T. gondii* unlikely at this time.

Owing to the relatively low risk for recipients, except for those who are immunosupressed and receiving large amounts of leukocytes, or perhaps unexposed pregnant women (though no congenital cases have been described where blood components are the cause), it seems unlikely that routine blood screening procedures need to be implemented for *T. gondii*. When there is a chance of transfusing blood components to high-risk recipients, especially those receiving leukocytes, one can establish a panel of anti-*Toxoplasma* negative blood donors [233]. With the advent of leukoreduction, and since the parasite is an obligate intracellular organism, *T. gondii* infected cells may be removed by the filtration process. In the event of a transfusion to bone marrow transplant recipients involving granulocytes derived from donors stimulated with cytokines, the above measures and preventive chemoprophylaxis could be effective.

Leishmaniasis

The *Leishmania* are obligate, intracellular, protozoan pathogens of human blood cells of the monocyte lineage. The parasite is endemic primarily to tropical and subtropical regions worldwide, where it causes leishmaniasis. Leishmaniasis is spectral in nature, ranging from self-curing cutaneous lesions to more serious visceral forms of disease associated with cells and organs of the reticuloendothelial system. Globally, 350 million people are estimated to be at risk for infection with *Leishmania*, and 2 million new infections are reported each year [234].

Visceral leishmaniasis (Kala-azar) is caused by *Leishmania donovani* or *L. infantum* infections in the Old World and *L. chagasi* in the New World through the bite of sand-flies. The result is a chronic infection with fever, anemia, lymphadenopathy and hepatosplenomegaly that affects approximately 12 million people in tropical and sub-tropical areas. The parasite is found in the reticuloendothelial cells and in leukocytes and can be transmitted to blood recipients from asymptomatic donors.

Despite the intracellular niche of *Leishmania* and the parasite's ability to survive in stored blood products (25 days at 4° C), there are few transfusion cases reported in the literature. Most involve newborns and immunosupressed patients [235,236]. In most instances, reported cases were associated with visceral forms of *Leishmania*, which is not surprising considering the chronic nature of these infections and the identification of infected cells in the peripheral blood. Though very rare, donors with a history of visceral leishmaniasis must not be accepted as donors.

Because Kala-azar has been diagnosed in American soldiers serving in international military units and a viscerotropic form of *L. tropica* was found among the military personnel who served during the Gulf War in the 1990´s [237], concerns have been expressed about the potential of transmitting *Leishmania* by transfusion. Indeed, recent reports that nearly 850 parasitologically confirmed cases of leishmaniasis have been reported in personnel serving in and around Iraq, coupled with reports of leishmaniasis in military personnel serving in Afghanistan, have led to the implementation of a 1 year deferral for all military or civilian personnel who return to the United States from Iraq and adjacent locations [238]. While the likelihood of *Leishmania* transmission appears low, previous reports of viscerotropic forms of cutaneous leishmaniasis have led the military and U.S. blood banks to be cautious.

Serologic assays (IFA, ELISA) as testing options for visceral forms of *Leishmania* in the blood bank environment are limited not by technology, but by demand in the face of the associated low risk. Alternatively, given that the *Leishmania* are localized to monocytes, the potential application of leukoreduction filters to minimize transfusion-transmission warrants further study.

Because leishmaniasis is a vector borne disease, the primary risk factor for acquiring infection is exposure to a *Leishmania*-infected sand-fly. In general, this will restrict exposures to those areas in which *Leishmania* is endemic. For non-endemic areas such as the United States and much of Europe, the primary risk factor (much like malaria) will be travel to areas where *Leishmania* is endemic.

References

1 Farrugia A: The mantra of blood safety: time for a new tune? Vox Sang 2004; 86: 1-7.

2 Warrell DA, Gilles HA, Gilles HM: Bruce-Chwatt's essential malariology, 4 th Edition. London, UK, Edward Arnold, 2002.

3 Tabor E: Infectious complications of blood transfusion. New York, USA, Academic Press, 1982.

4 WHO: The biology of malaria parasites – Technical Report Series 743, World Health Organization, Geneva, Switzerland, 1987.

5 López-Antuñano FJ, Schmunis G (eds): Diagnosis of malaria. Scientific Publication No 512. Washington DC, USA, Pan American Health Organization, 1990.

6 Wendel S: The protozoal parasites, malaria and chagas´ disease, in Linden JV, Bianco C (eds): Blood Safety and Surveillance. Marcel Dekker, Inc. New York, 2003, pp 355-398.

7 Salutari P, Sica S, Chiusolo P, Micciulli G, Plaisant P, Nacci A., Antinori A, Leone G: Plasmodium vivax malaria after autologous bone marrow transplantation: an unusual complication Bone M Transpl 1996; 18: 805-806.

8 Talabiska DG, Komar MJ, Wytock DH, Rubin RA: Post-transfusion acquired malaria complicating orthotopic liver transplantation. Am J Gastroenterol 1996; 91: 376-379.

9 Tran VB, Tran VB, Lin KH: Malaria infection after allogeneic bone marrow transplantation in a child with talassemia. Bone M Transpl 1997; 19: 1259-1260.

10 Thellier M, Lusina D, Guiguen C, Delamaire M: Is airport malaria a transfusion-transmitted malaria risk? Transfusion 2001; 41: 301-302.

11 Woolsey G: Transfusion for pernicious anaemia: two cases. Ann Surg 1911; 53: 132-135.

12 Turc JM: Malaria and blood transfusion, in Westphal RG, Carlson KB, Turc JM (eds): Emerging global patterns in transfusion-transmitted infections. Arlington, VA, USA, AABB, 1990, pp 31-43.

13 International Forum: which are the appropriate modifications of existing regulations designed to prevent the transmission of malaria by blood transfusion, in view of the increasing frequency of travel to endemic areas? Vox Sang 1987; 52: 138-148.

14 Rouger P: Du paludisme au paludisme post-transfusionnel. Transf Clin Biol 1999; 6: 72-74.

15 Shah S, Filler S, Causer LM, Rowe AK, Bloland PB, Barber AM, Roberts JM, Desai M, Parise ME, Steketee RW: Malaria surveillance, United States, 2002. MMWR 2004; 53 (SS01): 21-34. Also available as www.cdc.gov/mmwr/PDF/ss/ss5301.pdf.

16 Kano S, Kimura M: Trends in malaria cases in Japan. Acta Tropica 2004; 89: 271-278.

17 Snow RW, Guerra CA, Noor AM, Myint HY, Hay SI: The global distribution of clinical episodes of Plasmodium falciparum malaria. Nature 2005; 434: 214-217.

18 WHO – World malaria situation in 1990. Weekly Ep. Record 1992; 67: 161-168 (Part I).

19 WHO – World malaria situation in 1990. Weekly Ep. Record 1992; 67: 169-176 (Part II).

20 Alves MJCP, Rangel O, Souza SSAP: Malária na região de Campinas, São Paulo, Brasil, 1980 a 1994. Rev Soc Bras Med Trop 2000; 33: 53-60.

21 Bradley DJ, Warhurst DC, Blaze M, Smith V, Williams J: Malaria imported into the United Kingdom in 1996. Eurosurveillance 1998; 3:40-42

22 Frey-Wettstein M, Maier A, Markwalder K, Münch U: A case of transfusion transmitted malaria in Switzerland. Swiss Med Wkly 2001; 131: 320.

23 Bellmann R, Sturm W, Pechlaner C, Weiss G, Bellman-Weiler R, Wiedermann J, Patsch JR: Imported malaria: Six cases of severe Plasmodium falciparum infection in Innsbruck, Austria, within a period of five weeks (February/March 1999). Wien Klin Wochenschr 2000; 112: 453-458.

24 Bruce-Chwatt LJ: Transfusion malaria revisited. Trop Dis Bull 1982; 79: 827-840.

25 Nahlen BL, Lobel HO, Cannon SE, Campbell CC: Reassessment of blood donor selection criteria for the United States travellers to malarious areas. Transfusion 1991; 31: 798-804.

26 Shehata N, Kohli M, Detsky A: The cost-effectiveness of screening blood donors for malaria by PCR. Transfusion 2004; 44: 217-228.

27 Mungai M, Tegtmeier G, Chamberland M, Parise M: Transfusion-Transmitted malaria in the United States from 1963 through 1999. N Engl J Med 2001; 344: 1973-1978.

28 Kitchen A, Mijovic A, Hewitt P: Transfusion-transmitted malaria: current donor selection guidelines are not sufficient. Vox Sang 2005; 88: 200-201.

29 Fairley NH: Trans R Soc Trop Med Hyg 1947; 40: 621-676.

30 Council of Europe: Guide to the preparation, use and quality assurance of blood components – 2005 (11th edition), available at www.coe.int.

31 Wells L, Ala FA: Malaria and blood transfusion. Lancet 1985; i: 1317-1318.

32 Andrade JCR, Wanderley DMV: Malária induzida no Estado de São Paulo, Brasil. Rev Soc Bras Med Trop 1991; 24: 157-161.

33 Ferreira MV, Camargo LMA, Carvalho ME, Ninomia RT, Garcia LAV, Santos FR: Prevalence and levels of IgG and IgM antibodies against Plasmodium falciparum and P. vivax in blood donors from Rondonia, Brazilian Amazon. Mem Inst Oswaldo Cruz 1993; 88: 263-269.

34 Standards for Blood Banks and transfusion services. Bethesda MD, USA, AABB, 23rd ed, 2005.

35 Purdy E, Perry E, Gorlin J, Jensen K: Transfusion-transmitted malaria: unpreventable by current donor exclusion guidelines? Transfusion 2004; 44: 464.

36 Slinger R, Giulivi A, Bodie-Collins M, Hindieh F, St. John R, Sher G, Goldman M, Ricketts M, Kain KC: Transfusion-transmitted malaria in Canada. Can Med Assoc J 2001; 164: 377-379.

37 Roll Back Malaria. World Health Organization (WHO), http://mosquito.who.int/malariacontrol.

38 Sazama K: Prevention of transfusional-transmitted malaria: is it time to revisit the standards (Editorial). Transfusion 1991; 31: 786-788.

39 Custer B, Johnson ES, Sullivan SD, Hazlet TH, Ramsey SD, Hirschler N, Murphy EL, Busch MP: Quantifying losses to donated blood supply due to deferral and miscollection. Transfusion 2004; 44: 1417-1426.

40 Arafat R, Long S, Perry M, Marsh S, Wilson M, Avashia S, Filler S: Probable Transfusion-Transmitted malaria. Houston, Texas, MMWR 2003; 52: 1076-1076.

41 Chiodini PL, Hartley S, Hewitt PE, Barbara JAJ, Lalloo K, Bligh J, Voller A: Evaluation of a malaria antibody ELISA and its value in reducing potential wastage of red cell donations from blood donors exposed to malaria, with a note on a case of transfusion-transmitted malaria. Vox Sang 1997; 73: 143-148.

42 Soler CP, Gerome P, Soullié B, Tissedre F, Bejan H, Yvetot J, Joussemet M: Comparaison de techniques de depistage des anticorps anti-paludiques utilisées en transfusion. Med Trop 2003; 63: 587-589.

43 Kitchen AD, Lowe PHJ, Lalloo K, Chiodini PL: Evaluation of a malarial antibody assay for use in the screening of blood and tissue products for clinical use. Vox Sang 2004; 87: 150-155.

44 Brazilian Ministry of Health, Resolution 153, 2004.

45 Ibhanesebor SE, Otobo ES, Ladipo OA: Prevalence of malaria parasitemia in transfused donor blood in Benin City, Nigeria. Ann Trop Ped 1996; 16: 93-95.

46 Zavizion B, Pereira M, Jorge MM, Serebryanik D, Mather TN, Chapman J, Miller NJ, Alford B, Bzik DJ, Purmal A: Inactivation of protozoan parasites in red blood cells using INACTINE PEN110 chemistry. Transfusion 2004; 44: 731-738.

47 Draper CC, Sirr SS: Serological investigation in retrospective diagnosis of malaria. Br J Med 1980; 2: 1575-1576.

48 Assal A, Kauffmann-Lacroix C, Rodier MH, Dardé ML, Houssay D, Jacquemin JL: Comparison de deux techniques de détection des anticorps anti-Plasmodium falciparum: Falciparum-spot IF® (Boimérieux) et Malaria IgG Celisa® (BMD). Résultats préliminaires. Transf Clin Biol 1999; 6: 119-123.

49 Fonseca MO, Pang L, Ávila SLM, Arruk VG, Ferreira AW, Sáez-Alquezar A, Boulos M: Cross-reactivity of anti-Plasmodium falciparum antibodies and HIV tests. Trans Roy Soc Trop Med Hyg 2000; 94: 171-172.

50 Jani IV, Janossy G, Brown DWG, Mandy F: Multiplexed immunoassays by flow cytometry for diagnosis and surveillance of infectious diseases in resource-poor settings. Lancet Infect Dis 2002; 2: 243-250.

51 Moody A: Rapid Diagnostic Tests for malaria parasites Clin Microbiol Rev 2002; 15: 66-78.

52 Choudhury N, Jolly JG, Mahajan RC, Dubey ML, Kalra A, Ganguly NK: Selection of blood donors in malaria endemic countries. Lancet 1988; ii: 972-973.

53 Rock EP, Marsh K, Saul SJ, Wellems TE, Taylor DW, Maloy WL, Howard RJ: Comparative analysis of the Plasmodium falciparum histidine-rich proteins HRP1, HRP2, and HRP3 in malaria diagnosis of diverse origin. Parasitology 1987; 95: 209-227.

54 Parra ME, Evans CB, Taylor DW: Identification of Plasmodium falciparum Histidine-Rich Protein 2 in the Plasma of Humans with Malaria. J Clin Microbiol 1991; 29: 1629-1634.

55 Taylor DW, Voller A: The development of a simple antigen detection ELISA for Plasmodium falciparum malaria. Trans R Soc Trop Med Hyg 1993; 87: 29-31.

56 Namsiriponpun V, Wilde, H, Pamsandang P, Tiersansern P: Field study of an antigen-detection ELISA specific for Plasmodium falciparum malaria. Trans R Soc Trop Med Hyg 1993; 87: 32-34.

57 Davidson N, Woodfield G, Henry S: Malarial antibodies in Auckland blood donors. N Z Med Journal 1999; 112: 181-183.

58 Meier B, Dobeli H, Certa U: Stage-specific expression of aldolase isoenzymes in the rodent malaria parasite Plasmodium bergei. Mol Biochem Parasitol 1992; 52: 15-27

59 Piper RC, Vanderjagt DL, Holbrook JJ, Makler M: Malaria lactate dehydrogenase: target for diagnosis and drug development. Ann Trop Med Parasitol 1996; 90: 433.

60 World Health Organization (WHO): Malaria Rapid Diagnosis. Making it work. Meeting Report 20-23.01.2003 (RS/2003/GE/05 (PHL)), available at http://mosquito.who.int.

61 De Monbrison F, Gérome P, Chaulet JF, Wallon M, Picot S, Peyron F: Comparative diagnostic performance of two commercial rapid tests for malaria in a non-endemic area. Eur J Clin Microbiol Infect Dis 2004; 23: 784-786.

62 Playford EG, Walker J: Evaluation of the ICT malaria P.f./P.v. and the OptiMal rapid diagnostic tests for malaria in febrile returned travelers. J Clin Microbiol 2002; 40: 4166-4171.

63 Bell D: Malaria Rapid Diagnostic tests: one size may not fit all (letter). Clin Microbiol Rev 2002; 15: 771-772.

64 Craig MH, Bredekamp BL, Vaughan Williams CH, Rossouw EJ, Kelly VJ, Kleinschmidt I, Martineau A, Henry GFJ: Field and laboratory comparative evaluation of ten rapid malaria diagnostic tests. Trans R Soc Trop Med Hyg 2002; 96: 258-265.

65 Seed CR, Kitchen A, Davis TME: The current status and potential role of laboratory testing to prevent transfusion-transmitted malaria. Transf Med Rev 2005; 19: 229-240.

66 Orton SL, Virvos VJ, Williams AE: Validation of selected donor-screening questions: structure, content, and comprehension. Transfusion 2000; 40: 1407-1413.

67 Silvie O, Thellier M, Rosenheim M, Datry A, Lavigne P, Danis M, Mazier D: Potential value of Plasmodium falciparum-associated antigen and antibody detection for screening of blood donors to prevent transfusion-transmitted malaria. Transfusion 2002; 42: 357-362.

68 Vu TT, Phan NT, Le TT, Luong VH, O'Brien E, Morris GE: Screening donor blood for malaria by polymerase chain reaction. Trans R Soc Trop Med Hyg 1995; 89: 44-47.

69 De Monbrison F, Angei C, Staal A, Kaiser K, Picot S: Simultaneous identification of the four human Plasmodium species and quantification of Plasmodium DNA load in human by real-time polymerase chain reaction. Trans Royal Soc Trop Med Hyg 2003; 97: 387-390.

70 Barea L, Gonzalez R, Bueno JL, Castro E: Strategy for the acceptance of blood donors coming from malaria areas. Transfusion 2001; 41 (Suppl): 75S.

71 International Forum: Are current measures to prevent transfusion-associated protozoal infections sufficient? Vox Sang 2004; 87: 125-138.

72 Mazza S, Montana A, Benitez C, Juzin E: Transmisión de "Schizotrypanum cruzi" al niño por leche de la madre con enfermedad de Chagas. Publ MEPRA 1936; 28: 41-46.

73 Freitas JLP, Amato V, Sonntag R, Biancalana A, Nussenszweig V, Barreto JG: Primeiras verificacões de transmissão acidental da molestia de Chagas ao homem por transfusão de sangue. Rev Paul Med 1952; 40: 36-40.

74 Nussenzweig V, Sonntag R, Biancalana A, Freitas JLP, Amato Neto V, et al: Ação de corantes tri-fenilmetanicos sobre o Trypanosoma cruzi in vitro. Emprego da Violeta de Genciana na profilaxia da transmissão da Moléstia de Chagas por transfusão de sangue. O

75 Geiseler PJ, Ito JI, Tegtemeier BR, Kerndt PR, Krance R: Fulminant Chagas' disease in bone marrow transplantation. 27th Intersc Conf on Antimicro Agents and Chemoter. Washington, Am Soc for Microbiol (Abstract), 1987, 418.

76 Grant I, Gold JWH, Wittnee M, et al: Transfusion associated acute Chagas' disease acquired in the United States. Ann Intern Med 1989; 111: 849-851.

77 Nickerson P, Orr P, Schoeder MC, Sekla L, Johnson J: Transfusion associated Trypanosoma cruzi infection in a non endemic area. Ann Inter Med 1989; 111: 851-853.

78 Cimo PL, Luper WE, Scouros MA: Transfusion-associated Chagas' disease in Texas: Report of a case. Tex Med 1993; 89: 48-50.

79 Leiby DA, Yund J, Read EJ, Lenes BA, Dodd RY: Risk factors for Trypanosoma cruzi infection in seropositive blood donors. Transfusion 1996; 36 (Suppl 9S): S228.

80 Galel S, Wolles S, Stumpf R: Evaluation of a selective donor testing strategy. Transfusion 1997; 37 (Suppl 9S): S296.

81 Leiby DA, Jensen NC, Fucci MC, Stumpf RJ: Prevalence of Trypanosoma cruzi antibodies in a blood donor population at low risk. Transfusion 1997; 37 (Suppl 9S): S297.

82 Schmunis GA: American Trypanosomiasis as a Public Health Problem, in PAHO: Chagas' disease and the Nervous System. Washington DC, USA, Scientific Publication, 1994, vol 547, pp 3-29.

83 Umezawa ES, Stolf AMS, Corbett CEP, Shikanai-Yasuda MA: Chagas'disease. Lancet 2001; 357: 797-799.

84 Prata A: Clinical and epidemiological aspects of Chagas disease. Lancet Infect Dis 2001; 1: 92-100.

85 World Health Organization (WHO): Chagas disease. TDR strategic direction, February, 2002, http://www.who.int/tdr/diseases/chagas/direction.htm.

86 Hayes RJ, Schofield CJ: Estimación de las tasas de incidencia de infecciones y parasitosis crónicas a partir de la prevalencia: La enfermedad de Chagas en America Latina. Bol Of Sanit Panam 1990; 108: 308-316.

87 World Bank: The World Bank Development Report 1993. Investing in Health. World development indicators. Washington, University Press, 1993.

88 Silveira AC: Introdução, in O controle da doença de Chagas nos países do Cone Sul da América. História de uma Iniciativa Internacional 1991/2001, OPS, 2002, pp 16-41.

89 Moncayo A: Chagas'disease. Tropical disesase Research. Progress 1991-92. Eleventh Programme Report of the UNDP/World Bank/WHO Special Programme for Research and Training in Tropical Diseases (TDR). Worl Health Organization, Geneva, 1993, pp 67-75.

90 Panamerican Health Organization: I Reunión de la Comisión Intergubernamental del Cono Sur para la Eliminación de T. infestans y la Interrupción de la Transmision de la Tripanosomiasis Americana Transfusional, OPS, 1992 OPS/HCP/HCT/PNSP/92.18.

91 Panamerican Health Organization: Va. Reunión de la Comisión Intergubernamental (CI) de la Iniciativa Andina de Control de la Transmisión Vectorial y Transfusional de Chagas – Guyaquil, Ecuador, Mayo 2003 – OPS, 2003 (available at http://www.paho.org/Spanish/AD/DPC/CD/dch-v-inicandina.htm).

92 Panamerican Health Organization: Iniciativa del Cono Sur. VI Reunión Intergubernamental para la eliminación de Triatoma infestans y la interrupción de la tripanosomiasis americana por transfusión. Documento OPS/HPC/HCT 98/102, 1997, 83 p.

93 World Health Assembly: Resolution WHA.51.14, Geneva, 1998.

94 Wendel S, Brener Z, Camargo M, Rassi A (eds): Chagas disease (American Trypanosomiasis): its impact on transfusion and clinical medicine. ISBT, Brasil '92, SBHH, 1992.

95 Miles MA: Further enzymic characters of Trypanosoma cruzi and their evaluation for strain identification. Trans Roy Sci Trop Med Hyg 1980; 74: 221-237.

96 Miles MA: The epidemiology of South American Trypanosomiasis, biochemical and immunological approaches and their relevance to control. Trans Roy Soc Trop Med Hyg 1983; 77: 5-23.

97 Morel C, Chiari E, Plessman-Camargo E, Mattei D, Romanha AJ, Simpson L: Strains and clones of Trypanosoma cruzi can be characterized by pattern of restriction endonuclease products of kinetoplast DNA minicircles. Proc Natl Acad Sci USA 1980; 77: 6810-6814.

98 Avila H, Gonçalves AM, Nehme NC, Morel CM, Simpson L: Schizodeme analysis of Trypanosoma cruzi stocks from South and Central America by analysis of PCR-amplified minicircle variable region sequences. Molec Biochem Parasitol 1990; 42: 175-188.

99 El-Sayed NM, Myler PJ, Bartholomeu DC, et al: The genome sequence of Trypanosoma cruzi, etiologic agent of Chagas disease. Science 2005; 309: 409-415.

100 Chocair PR, Sabbaga E, Amato Net V, Shiroma M, Goes GM: Transplante de rim: nova modadlidade de transmissão da doença de Chagas. Rev Med Trop S Paulo 1981; 23: 282-282.

101 Ferraz AS, Figueiredo JFC: Transmission of Chagas'disease through transplanted kidney: ocurrence of the cute form of the disease in two recipients from the same donor. Rev Inst Med Trop S Paulo 1993; 35: 461-463.

102 Valente SAS, Valente VC, Fraiha Neto H: Considerations on the Epidemiology and Transmission of Chagas Disease in the Brazilian Amazon. Mem Inst Oswaldo Cruz 1999; 94 (Suppl I): 395-398.

103 Dias JCP, Brener Z: Chagas' disease and blood transfusion. Mem Inst Oswaldo Cruz 1984; 79: 139-147.

104 Schmuñis GA: Trypanosoma cruzi, the etiologic agent of Chagas' disease: status in the blood supply in endemic and non endemic countries. Transfusion 1991; 31: 547-557.

105 Wendel S, Gonzaga AL: Chagas disease and blood transfusion: a new world problem? Vox Sang 1993; 64: 1-12.

106 Wendel S: Doença de Chagas Transfusional, in Dias JCP, Coura JR (eds): Clínica e terapêutica da Doença de Chagas. Rio de Janeiro, Brasil, Editora Fiocruz, 1997, pp 411-427.

107 Appleman MD, Shulman IA, Saxena S, Kirchhoff LV: Use of a questionnaire to identify potential blood donors at risk for infection with Trypanosoma cruzi. Transfusion 1993; 33: 61-64.

108 Barea L, Cañavate C, Flores M, Rodriguez M, Bueno JL, Gozales R, Gárate T, Castro E: Seroprevalence of anti-Trypanosoma cruzi in blood donors coming from Chagas´s diasease endemic countries. Vox Sang 2004; 87 (Suppl 3): Abstract W 01.03.

109 Sullivan TS: Viability of Trypanosoma cruzi in citrated blood stored at room temperature. J Parasitol 1944; 30: 200.

110 Weinman D, MacAlister J: Prolonged storage of human pathogenic protozoa with conservation of virulence. Am J Hyg 1947; 45: 102-121.

111 Filardi LS, Brener Z: Cryopreservation of Trypanosoma cruzi bloodstream forms. J Protozool 1975; 22: 398-401.

112 Schlemper Jr BR: Estudos experimentais de quimioprofilaxia de transmissão da doença de Chagas por transfusão sangüínea. Rev Patol Trop 1978; 7: 55-111.

113 Cerisola JA, Rabinovich A, Alvarez M, Di Corleho CA, Pruneda J: Enfermedad de Chagas y la transfusion de sangre. Bol of Sanit Panam 1972; 63: 203-221.

114 Lorca M, Lorca J, Child R, Atias A, Conales M, et al: Prevalencia de la infección por Trypanosoma cruzi en pacientes politransfundidos. Rev Med Chile 1988; 116: 112-116.

115 Villalba R, Fornés G, Alvarez MA, Román J, Rubio V, Fernandez M, Garcia JM, Viñals M, Torres A: Acute Chagas' disease in a recipient of a bone marrow transplant in Spain: case report. Clin Inf Dis 1992; 14: 594-595.

116 Kirchhoff LV: Trypanosoma cruzi: a new threat to our blood transfusion supply (Editorial). Ann Intern Med 1989; 111: 773-775.

117 Kirchhoff LV: American trypanosomiasis (Chagas disease). A tropical disease now in the United States. N Engl J Med 1993; 329: 639-644.

118 Kirchhoff LV, Neva FA: Chagas' disease in Latin American immigrants. JAMA 1985; 254: 3058-3060.

119 Milei J, Mautner B, Storino R, Sanchez JÁ, Ferrans VS: Does Chagas'disease exist as an undiagnosed form of cardiomyopathy in the United States? (Editorial) Am H Journ 1992; 123: 1732-1735.

120 Schmunis GA, Cruz JR: Safety of the blood supply in Latin America. Clin Microbiol Rev 2005; 18:12-29.

121 Wendel S: Chagas disease: an old entity in new places (Editorial). Int J Art Organs 1993; 16: 117-119.

122 Coura JR, Nogueira ES, Silva JR: Índices de transmissão da doença de Chagas por transfusão de sangue de doadores na fase crônica da doença. O Hospital 1966; 69: 115-122.

123 Rohwedder RW: Infección chagásica en doadores de sangre y las probabilidades de transmitirla por medio de la transfusion. Bol Chile Parasitol 1969; 24: 88-93.

124 Zuna H, Recacoechea M, Bermudez H, Romero A, Castedo J: Transmissión de la enfermedad de Chagas por via transfusional en Santa Cruz de la Sierra, Bolivia. Bol Inf CENENTROP 1979; 5:49-56.

125 Luquetti AO. – Diagnóstico etiológico da doença de Chagas. Rev Pat Trop 2000; 29 (supl.): 145-149.

126 Wendel S: Risco residual da transmissão da infecção por Trypanosoma cruzi por via transfusional no Brasil, PhD Thesis. Faculdade de Medicina da Universidade de São Paulo, Brazil, USP/FM/SBD-20/05, 2005.

127 Wendel S, Yasuda MAS, Silva GR: Residual risk for Trypanosoma cruzi transmission by transfusions in Brazil. Transfusion 2005; Suppl Abstract S50-030J.

128 Wendel S: Blood Banking preventive approaches for Chagas disease. Mem Inst Oswaldo Cruz 1993; 88 (suppl.): 59-60.

129 Zicker F, Martelli CMT, Andrade ALLS, Silva SA: Trends of T. cruzi infection based on data from blood bank screening. Rev Inst Med Trop S Paulo 1990; 39: 132-137.

130 Wendel S, Biagini S: Absence of serological surrogate markers for Trypanosoma cruzi infected blood donors. Vox Sang 1995; 69: 44-49.

131 Docampo Moreno SNJ, Muniz RP, Cruz FS, Mason RP: Light-enhanced free radical formation and Trypanocidal action of Gentian Violet (Crystal Violet). Science 1983; 220: 1292-1295.

132 Docampo R, Moreno SNJ: Free radicals metabolites in the mode of action of chemotherapeutic agents and phagocytic cells on Trypanosoma cruzi. Rev Inf Dis 1984; 6: 223-238.

133 Docampo R, Gadelha FR, Moreno SNJ, Benaim G, Hoffman ME, Vercasi AE: Disruption of Ca + 2 homeostasis in Trypanosoma cruzi by crystal violet. J Eur Microbiol 1993; 40: 311-316.

134 Souza HM: The present state of chemoprophylaxis in transfusional Chagas' disease (Editorial) Rev Soc Bras Med Trop 1989; 22:1-3.

135 Schlemper Jr BR: Estudos experimentais de Quimio-profilaxia de transmissão da doença de Chagas por transfusão sangüínea. Rev Pat trop 1978; 7:55-111.

136 Van Voorhis WC, Barrett LK, Eastman RT, Alfonso R, Dupuis K: Trypanosoma cruzi inactivation in human platelet concentrates and plasma by a psoralen (amotosalen HCl) and long-wavelength UV. Antimicrob Agents Chemother 2003; 47: 475-479.

137 Chiari E: Diagnostic tests for Chagas disease, in Wendel S, Brener Z, Camargo ME, Rassi A (eds): Chagas disease (American Trypanosomiasis): Its impact on transfusion and clinical medicine. São Paulo, ISBT Brazil'92, pp 153-164.

138 Wendel S, Takaoka DT, Fachini R, Oliveira LC, Lima LP, Tibbals MA, Leiby DA: Serological screening tests for Trypanosoma cruzi antibodies: the role of supplemental methods. Transfusion 1997; 37 (suppl): S298.

139 Avila HA, Sigman DS, Cohen LM, Millikan RC, Simpson L: Polymerase Chaín reaction of Tripanosoma cruzi kinetoplast minicircle DNA isolated from whole blood lysates: diagnosis of chronic Chagas disease. Mol Biochem Parasitol 1991; 48: 211-222.

140 Avila H, Pereira JB, Thiemann O, Paiva E, Degrave W, Morel CM, Simpson L: Detection of Trypanosoma cruzi in blood specimens of chronic chagasic patients by polymerase chain reaction amplification of kinetoplast minicircle DNA: comparison with serology and xenodiagnosis. J Clin Microbiol 1993; 31: 2421-2426.

141 Wincker P, Britto C, Pereira JB, Cardoso MA, Oelemann W, Morel C: Use of a simplified polymerase chain reaction procedure to detect Trypanosoma cruzi in blood samples from chronic chagasic patients in a rural endemic area. Am J Trop Med Hyg 1994; 51: 771-777.

142 Britto C, Cardoso MA, Ravel C, Santoro A, Borges Pereira J, Coura JR, Morel CM, Wincker P: Trypanosoma cruzi: parasite detection and strain discrimination in chronic chagasic patients from Northeastern Brazil using PCR amplification of kinetoplast DNA and nonradioactive hybridization. Exp Parasitol 1995; 81: 462-471.

143 Gomes ML, Galvão LMC, Macedo AM, Pena SDJ, Chiari E: Chagas'disease diagnosis: comparative analysis of parasitologic, molecular and serologic methods. Am J Trop Med Hyg 1999; 60: 205-210.

144 Souto RP, Zingales B: Sensitive detection and strain classification of Trypanosoma cruzi by amplification of a ribosomal RNA sequence. Mol Biochem Parasitol 1993; 62: 45-52.

145 Clark AK, Kovtunovych G, Kandikar S, Lal S, Stryker GA: Cloning and expression analysis of two novel paraflagellar rod domain genes found in Trypanosoma cruzi. Parasitol Res 2005; 96: 312-320.

146 Brenière SF, Bosseno MF, Revollo S, Rivera MT, Carlier Y, Tibayrenc M: Direct identification of Trypanosoma cruzi natural clones in vectors and mammalian hosts by polymerase chain reaction amplification. Am J Trop Med Hyg 1992; 46: 335-341.

147 Britto C, Cardoso MA, Ravel C, Santoro A, Borges Pereira J, Coura JR, Morel CM, Wincker P: Trypanosoma cruzi: parasite detection and strain discrimination in chronic chagasic patients from Northeastern Brazil using PCR amplification of kinetoplast DNA and nonradioactive hybridization. Exp Parasitol 1995; 81: 462-471.

148 Silber AM, Búa J, Porcel BM, Segura EL, Ruiz AM: Trypanosoma cruzi: specific detection of parasites by PCR in infected humans and vectors using a set of primers (BP1/BP2) targeted to a nuclear DNA sequence. Exp Parasitol 1997; 85: 225-232.

149 Zingales B, Souto RP, Mangia RH, Lisboa CV, Campbell DA, Coura JR, Jansen A, Fernandes O: Molecular epidemiology of American trypanosomiasis in Brazil based on dimorphisms of rRNA and mini-exon gene sequences. Intern J Parasitol 1998; 28: 105-112.

150 Antaz PRZ, Medrano-Mercado N, Torrico F, Ugarte-Fernandez R, Gómez F, Oliveira RC, Chaves ACL, Romanha AJ, Araújo-Jorge TC: Early, intermediate, and late acute stages in Chagas' disease: a study combining anti-galactose IgG, specific serodiagnosis, and polymerase chain reaction analysis. Am J Trop Med Hyg 1999; 61: 308-314.

151 Lages-Silva E, Crema E, Ramirez LE, Macedo AM, Pena SD, Chiari E: relationship between Trypanosoma cruzi and human chagasic megaesophagus: blood and tissue parasitism. Am J Trop Med Hyg 2001; 65: 435-441.

152 Marcon GEB, Andrade PD, Albuquerque DM, Wanderley JS, Almeida EA, Guariento ME, Costa SCB: Use of a nested polymerase chain reaction (N-PCR) to detect Trypanosoma cruzi in blood samples from chronic chagasic patients and patients with doubtful serologies. Diagn Microbiol Infect Dis 2002; 43: 39-43.

153 Galvão LMC, Chiari E, Macedo AM, Luquetti AO, Silva SA, Andrade ALSS: PCR assay for monitoring Trypanosoma cruzi parasitemia in childhood after specific chemotherapy. J Clin Microbiol 2003; 41: 5066-5070.

154 Virreira M, Torrico F, Truyens C, Alonso-Vega C, Solano M, Carlier Y, Svoboda M: Comparison of polymerase chain reaction methods for reliable and easy detection of congenital Trypanosoma cruzi infection. Am J Trop Med Hyg 2003; 68: 574-582.

155 Vera-Cruz JM, Magallón-Gastelum E, Grijalva G, Rincón AR, Ramos-García C, Armendáriz-Borunda J: Molecular diagnosis of Chagas disease and use of an animal model to study parasite tropism. Parasitol Res 2003; 89: 480-486.

156 Salomone OA, Basquiera AL, Sembaj A, Aguerri AM, Reyes ME, Omelianuk M, Fernández RA, Enders J, Palma A, Barral JM, Madoery RJ: Trypanosoma cruzi in persons without serologic evidence of disease, Argentina. Emerg Infect Dis 2003; 9: 1558-1562.

157 Castro AM, Luquetti AO, Rassi A, Rassi GG, Chiari E, Galvão LMC: Blood culture and polymerase chain reaction for the diagnosis of the chronic phase of human infection with Trypanosoma cruzi. Parasitol Res 2002; 88: 894-900.

158 Cura E, Wendel S (eds): Manual de Procedimientos de Control de Calidad para los Laboratorios de Serologia de los Bancos de Sangre. PAHO/HPC/HPT/94.21, Washington DC USA, 1994.

159 Ferreira AW: Serological diagnosis: Tests for Chagas disease serodiagnosis: a review, in Wendel S, Brener Z, Camargo ME, Rassi A (eds): Chagas disease (American Trypanosomiasis): Its impact on transfusion and clinical medicine. São Paulo, ISBT Brazil'92, pp 179-193.

160 Voller A, Draper C, Bidwell DE, Bartlett A: A micro-plate enzyme-linked immunosorbent assay (ELISA) for Chagas disease. Lancet 1975; 1: 426-429.

161 Wendel S, Lopes VHG, Batemarchi MV, Takaoka DT, Neitzert E: High levels of false positive reaction for Trypanosoma cruzi antibodies tests used for blood donors screening. Transfusion 1993; 33 (suppl) Abstract S155: 41S.

162 Carvalho MR, Krieger MA, Almeida E, Oelemann W, Shikanai-Yasuda MA, Ferreira AW, Pereira JB, Sáez-Alquézar A, Dorlhiac-Llacer PE, Chamone DF, Goldenberg S: Chagas' disease diagnosis: evaluation of several tests in blood bank screening. Transfusion 1993; 33: 830-834.

163 Ferreira AW, Belem ZR, Moura MEG, Camargo ME: Aspectos da padronização de testes sorológicos para a Doença de Chagas: Um teste imunoenzimático para a triagem de doadores de sangue. Rev Inst Med Trop S Paulo 1991; 33: 123-128.

164 Brashear RJ, Winkler MA, Schur JD, Lee H, Burczak JD, Hall HJ, Pan AA: Detection of antibodies to Trypanosoma cruzi among blood donors in the southwestern and western United States. I – Evaluation of the sensitivity and specificity of an enzyme immunoassay for detecting antibodies to T. cruzi. Transfusion 1995; 35: 213-218.

165 Houghton RL, Benson D, Skeiky Y, Sleath P, Lodes M, Badaró R, Krettli A, Reed SG: Multi-epitope peptide elisa for detection of serum antibodies to Trypanosoma cruzi in patients with treated and untreated Chagas'disease. Transfusion 1996; 36 (suppl): S137.

166 Hoffman A, Jaczko B, Jones J, Tursi N, Lee SR: Evaluation of a prototype screening ELISA and supplemental analysis for the serological identification of Chagas disease. Transfusion 1997; 37 (suppl): S181.

167 Luquetti AO: Use of Trypanosoma cruzi defined proteins for diagnosis. Multicentre trial, serological and technical aspects. Mem Inst Oswaldo Cruz 1990; 85: 497-505.

168 Zicker F, Smith PG, Luquetti AO, Oliveira OS: Mass screening for Trypanosoma cruzi infections using the immunofluorescence, ELISA and hemagglutination tests on serum samples and on blood eluates from filter paper. Bull WHO 1990; 68: 465-471.

169 Andrade ALSS, Martelli CMT, Luquetti AO, Oliveira OS, Silva SA, Zicker F: Serologic screening for Trypanosoma cruzi among blood donors in central Brazil. Bull Pan Am Health Organ 1992; 26: 157-164.

170 Fife Jr EH, Mushel LH: Fluorescent antibody technique for serodiagnosis of Trypanosoma cruzi infection. Proc Soc Exp Biol (NY) 1959; 101: 540-543.

171 Camargo ME, Souza SL: The use of filter paper blood smears in a practical fluorescent test for American trypanosomiasis serodiagnosis. Rev Inst Med Trop S Paulo 1966; 8: 255-258.

172 Lal RB, Ottesen EA: Phosphocoline epitopes on helminth and protozoal parasites and their presence in the circulation of infected human patients. Trans Roy Soc Trop Med Hug 1989; 83: 652-655.

173 Lanar DE, Manning JE: Major surface proteins and antigens on the different in vivo and in vitro forms of Trypanosoma cruzi. Mol Biochem Paras 1984; 11: 119-131.

174 Rosfjord EC, Mikhael KS, Rowland EC, Powell MR: Analysis of antibody cross-reactivity in experimental American trypanosomiasis. J Parasitol 1990; 76: 698-702.

175 Chiller TM, Samudio MA, Zoulek G: IgG antibody reactivity with Trypanosoma cruzi and Leishmania antigens in sera of patients with Chagas' disease and leishmaniasis. Am J Trop Med Hyg 1990; 43: 650-656.

176 Malchiodi EL, Chiaramonte MG, Taranto NJ, Zwirner NW, Margni RA: Cross reactivity studies and differential serodiagnosis of human infections caused by Trypanososma cruzi and Leishmania spp; use of immunoblotting and Elisa with purified antigen (Ag 163B6). Cin Exp Immunol 1994; 97: 417-423.

177 Reed SG, Badaró R, Lloyd RMC: Identification of specific and cross-reactive antigens of Leishmania donovani chagasi by human infection sera. J Immunol 1987; 138: 1598-1601.

178 Sabino EC, Salles N, Stoops E, Santos ML, Saez-Alquezar A: Evaluation of Chagas Innolia assay as a confirmatory test for Chagas disease. Mem Inst Oswaldo Cruz 1997; 92: Suppl 1, 266.

179 Costa GCV, Teixeira MGM, Borges-Pereira J, Castro JAF, Coura JR, Vanderborght BOM, Stroops E, Zrein M, Peralta JM, Oelemann WMR: A recombinant antigen and peptide line immunoassay (LIA) as na alternative diagnostic test for Chagas'disease. Mem Inst Oswaldo Cruz 1997; 92: (Suppl 1) 267.

180 Almeida IC, Ferguson MAJ, Schenkman S, Travassos LR: Lytic anti-alpha-galactosyl antibodies from patients with chronic Chagas disease recognise novel O-linked oligosaccharides on mucin-like GPI-anchored glycoproteins of Trypanosoma cruzi. Biochem J 1994; 304: 793-802.

181 Almeida IC, Covas DT, Soussumi LMT, Travassos LR: A highly sensitive and specific chemiluminescent enzyme-linked immunosorbent assay for diagnosis of active Trypanosoma cruzi infection. Transfusion 1997; 37: 850-857.

182 Umezawa E, Nascimento NS, Kasper NJR, Coura JR, Borges-Pereira J, Junqueira AC, Camargo ME: Immunoblot assay using excreted-secreted antigen of Trypanosoma cruzi in serodiagnosis of congenital, acute, and chronic Chagas disease. J Clin Microbiol 1996; 34: 2143-2147.

183 Silveira-Lacerda EP, Silva AG, Junior SF, Souza MA, Kesper N, Botelho-Filho A, Umezawa ES: Chagas'disease: application of TESA-blot in inconclusive sera from a Brazilian blood bank. Vox Sang 2004; 87: 204-207.

184 Kesper N, Almeida KA, Stolf MS, Umezawa ES: Immunoblot analysis of trypomastigote excreted-secreted antigens as a tool for characterization of T. cruzi strains and isolates. J Parasitol 2000; 86: 862-867.

185 Winkler MA, Brashear RJ, Hall HJ, Schur JD, Pan AA: Detection of antibodies to Trypanosoma cruzi among blood donors in the southwestern and western United States. II – Evaluation of a supplemental enzyme immunoassay and radioimmuneprecipitation assay for confirmation of seroreactivity. Transfusion 1995; 35: 219-225.

186 Kirchhoff LV, Gam AA, Gusmão RA, Goldsmith RS, Rezende JM, Rassi A: Increased specificity of serodiagnosis of Chagas'disease by detection of antibody to the 72- and 90-kilodalton glycoproteins of Trypanosoma cruzi. J Infect Dis 1987; 155: 561-564.

187 Leiby DA, Wendel S, Takaoka DT, Fachini RM, Oliveira LC, Tibbals MA: Serologic testing for Trypanosoma cruzi: comparison of radioimmunoprecipitation assay with commercially available indirect immunofluorescence assay, indirect hamagglutination assay, and enzyme-linked immunosorbent assay kits. J Clin Microbiol 2000; 38: 639-642.

188 Wendel S, Yasuda MAS, Silva GR, Leiby DA, Umezawa E, Almeida I: Confirmatory serological methods for T. cruzi antibodies screening tests: should they be considered as imperfect gold standards? Transfusion 2005; Suppl Abstract S49-030J.

189 Zhou XH, Obuchowski NA, McClish DK: Statistical Methods in Diagnostic Medicine. New York, John Wiley & Sons, 2002.

190 Skrabalo Z, Deanovic Z: Piroplasmosis in man: report of a case. Doc Med Geogr Trop 1957; 9:11-16.

191 Scholtens RG, Braff EH, Healy GR, Gleason N: A case of babesiosis in man in the United States. Am J Trop Med Hyg 1968; 17: 810-813.

192 Homer MJ, Aguilar-Delfin I, Telford SR, Krause PJ, Persing DH. Babesiosis. Clin Microbiol Rev 2000; 13: 451-469.

193 Zintl A, Mulcahy G, Skerrett HE, Taylor SM, Gray JS: Babesia divergens, a bovine blood parasite of veterinary and zoonotic importance. Clin Microbiol Rev 2003; 16; 622-636.

194 Meer-Scherrer L, Adelson M, Mordechai E, Lattaz B, Tilton R: Babesia microti infection in Europe. Curr Microbiol 2004; 48: 435-437.

195 Saito-Ito A, Tsuji M, Wei Q, He S, Matsui T, Kohsaki M, Arai S, Kamiyama T, Hioki K, Ishihara C: Transfusion-acquired, autochthonous human babesiosis in Japan: Isolation of Babesia microti-like parasite with hu-RBC-SCID mice. J Clin Microbiol 2000; 38: 4511-4516.

196 Shih CM, Liu LP, Chung WC, Ong SJ, Wang CC: Human babesiosis in Taiwan: asymptomatic infection with a Babesia microti-like organism in a Taiwanese women. J Clin Microbiol 1997; 35: 450-454.

197 Michael SA, Morsy TA, Montasser MF: A case of human babesiosis (preliminary case report in Egypt). J Egypt Soc Parasitol 1987; 17: 409-410.

198 Bush JB, Isaäcson M, Mohamed AS, Potgieter FT, de Waal DT: Human babesiosis – a preliminary report of 2 suspected cases in southern Africa. S Afr Med J 1990; 78: 699.

199 Herwaldt BL, Cacciò S, Gherlinzoni F, Aspöck H, Slemenda SB, Piccaluga P, Martinelli G, Edelhofer R, Hollenstein U, Poletti G, Pampiglione S, Löschenberger K, Tura S, Pieniazek NJ: Molecular characterization of a non-Babesia divergens organism causing zoonotic babesiosis in Europe. Emerg Infect Dis 2003; 9: 942-948.

200 Popovsky MA, Lindberg LE, Syrek AL, Page PL: Prevalence of Babesia antibody in a selected blood donor population. Transfusion 1988; 28: 59-61.

201 Linden JV, Wong SJ, Chu FK, Schmidt GB, Bianco C: Transfusion-associated transmission of babesiosis in New York State. Transfusion 2000; 40: 285-289.

202 Hunfeld KP, Allwinn R, Peters S, Kraiczy P, Brade V: Serologic evidence for tick-borne pathogens other than Borrelia burgdorferi (TOBB) in Lyme borreliosis patients from Midwestern Germany. Wien Klin Wochenschr 1998; 119: 901-908.

203 Hunfeld KP, Lambert A, Kampen H, Albert S, Epe C, Brade V, Tenter AM: Seroprevalence of Babesia infections in humans exposed to ticks in Midwestern Germany. J Clin Microbiol 2002; 40: 2431-2436.

204 Herwaldt BL, McGovern PC, Gerwel MP, Easton RM, MacGregor RR: Endemic babesiosis in another eastern state: New Jersey. Emerg Infect Dis 2003; 9: 184-188.

205 Lodes MJ, Houghton RL, Bruinsma ES, Mohamath R, Reynolds LD, Benson DR, Krause PJ, Reed SG, Persing DH: Serologic expression cloning of novel immunoreactive antigens of Babesia microti. Infect Immun 2000; 68: 2783-2790.

206 Krause PJ, Spielman A, Telford SR, Sikand VK, McKay K, Christianson D, Pollack RJ, Brassard P, Magera J, Ryan R, Persing DH: Persistent parasitemia acute babesiosis. N Engl J Med 1998; 339: 160-164.

207 Leiby DA, Gill JE: Transfusion-transmitted tick-borne infections: a cornucopia of threats. Transfusion Med Rev 2004; 18: 293-306.

208 Reddy RL, Delmasso AP: Transfusion acquired babesiosis in Minnesota. XXIst Congress, International Society of Blood Transfusion (ISBT)/AABB, Los Angeles, USA, 1990, Abstract S447, pp 112.

209 Mintz ED, Anderson JF, Cable RG, Hadler JL: Transfusion-transmitted babesiosis: a case report from a new endemic area. Transfusion 1991; 31: 365-368.

210 Jassoum SB, Fong IW, Hannach B, Kain KC: Transfusion-transmitted babesiosis in Ontario: first reported case in Canada. Can Commun Dis Rep 2000; 26: 9-13.

211 Eberhard ML, Walker EM, Steurer FJ: Survival and infectivity of Babesia in blood maintained at 25 C and 2-4 C. J Parasitol 1995; 81: 790-792.

212 Gerber MA, Shapiro ED, Krause PJ, Cable RG, Badon SJ, Ryan RW: The risk of acquiring Lyme disease or babesiosis from a blood transfusion. J Inf Dis 1994; 170: 231-234.

213 Montoya JG, Liesenfeld O: Toxoplasmosis. Lancet 2004; 363: 1965-1976.

214 Dunn D, Wallon M, Peyron F, Petersen E, Peckham C, Gilbert R: Mother-to-child transmission of toxoplasmosis: risk estimates for clinical counseling. Lancet 1999; 353: 1829-1833.

215 Rynin FW, McLeod R, Maddox JC, Hunt S, Remington JS: Probable transmission of Toxoplasma gondii by organ transplantation. Ann Intern Med 1979; 90: 47-49.

216 Siegel SE, Lunde MN, Gelderman AH, Halterman RH, Brown JA, Levine AS, Graw RG. Transmission of toxoplasmosis by leukocyte transfusion. Blood 1971; 37: 388-394.

217 Beauvais B, Garin JF, Lariviere M, Languillat G, Galal H: Toxoplasmose et transfusion. Ann Parasitol Hum Comp 1976; 51: 625-635.

218 Räisänen S: Toxoplasmosis transmitted by blood transfuions. Transfusion 1978; 18: 329-332.

219 Roth JA, Siegel SE, Levine AS, Berard CW: Fatal recurrent toxoplasmosis in a patient initially infected via a leukocyte transfusion. A J C P 1970; 56: 601-605.

220 Talice RV, Gurri J, Royal J, Perez-Moreira L: Investigaciones sobre la Toxoplasma gondii en sangre destinado a transfusion. Ann Fac Med Univers, Montevideo 1957; 42: 143-147.

221 Nelson JC, Kauffmann JH, Ciavarella D, Senisi WJ: Acquired toxoplasmic retinochoroiditis after platelet transfusions. Ann Ophtamol 1989; 21: 253-254.

222 Jones JL, Kruszon-Moran D, Wilson M, McQuillan G, Navin T, McAuley JB: Toxoplasma gondii infection in the United States: seroprevalence and risk factors. Am J Epidemiol 2001; 154: 357-365.

223 Galván-Ramírez ML, Covarrubias X, Rodríguez R, Troyo R, Alfaro N: Toxoplasma gondii antibodies in Mexican blood donors. Transfusion 2005; 45: 281-282.

224 Remington JS, Thulliez P, Montoya JG: Recent developments for diagnosis of toxoplasmosis. J Clin Microbiol 2004; 42: 941-945.

225 Burg JL, Grover CM, Pouletty P, Boothroyd JC: Direct and sensitive detection of a pathogenic protozoan, Toxoplasma gondii, by polymerase chain reaction. J Clin Microbiol 1989 27; 1787-1792.

226 Homan WL, Vercammen M, De Braekeleer J, Vershueren H: Identification of a 200- to 300-fold repetitive 529 bp DNA fragment in Toxoplasma gondii, and its use for diagnostic and quanititative PCR. Int J Parasitol 2000; 30: 69-75.

227 Costa JM, Pautas C, Ernault P, Foulet F, Cordonnier C, Bretagne S: Real-time PCR for diagnosis and follow-up of toxoplasma reactivation after allogeneic stem cell transplantation using fluorescence resonance energy transfer hybridization probes. J Clin Microbiol 2000; 38: 2929-2932.

228 Walton BC, Benchoff BM, Brooks WH: Comparison of the indirect fluorescent antibody test and methylene blue dye test for detection of antibodies to Toxoplasma gondii. Am J Trop Med Hyg 1966; 15: 149-152.

229 Balsari A, Poli G, Molina V, Dovis M, Petruzzelli E, Boniolo A, Rolleri E: ELISA for toxoplasma antibody detection: a comparison with other serodiagnostic tests. J Clin Pathol 1980; 33: 640-643.

230 Remington JS, Araujo FG, Desmonts G: Recognition of different Toxoplasma antigens by IgM and IgG antibodies in mothers and their congenitally infected newborns. J Infect Dis 152: 1020-1024.

231 Hedman K, Lappalainen M, Seppala I, Makela O: Recent primary Toxoplasma infection indicated by a low avidity of specific IgG. J Infect Dis 1989; 159: 736-739.

232 Liesendfeld O, Montoya JG, Kinney S, Press C, Remington JS: Effect of testing for IgG avidity in the diagnosis of Toxoplasma gondii infection in pregnant women: experience in a US reference laboratory. J Infect Dis 2001; 183: 1248-1253.

233 McDonald CP, Barbara JAJ, Contreras M, Brown S: Provision of a panel of Anti-Toxoplasma-Negative blood donors. Vox Sang 1989; 57: 55-58.

234 Herwaldt BL. Leishmaniasis. Lancet 1999; 354: 1191-1199.

235 Chung HL, Chow KK, Lu JP: The first two cases of transfusion Kala-azar. Chin Med J 1948; 66: 325-326.

236 Andre R, Brumpt L, Dreyfus B: Cutaneous leishmaniasis, cutaneous glandular leishmaniasis and trasfusional Kala-azar. Trop Dis Bull 1958; 55: 379.

237 Kostman R, Barr M, Bengtssom E, Garnham PCC, Hult G: Kala-azar transferred by exchange blood transfusion in two Swedish infants. Proceeding of the Seventh International Congress of Tropical Medicine and Malaria, 1963, vol 2, 384p.

238 Anonymous: Defense Department drops question on leishmaniasis for blood donor. Blood Bank Week 1993; 10 (45): 4-5. http://www.pdhealth.mil/downloads/Leishmaniasis_Information__28% 20April%2005.pdf.

Dr. S. Wendel, Blood Bank, Hospital Sirio Libanês, Rua Adma Jafet 91, São Paulo, Brazil 01308-050.
E-mail: snwendel@uninet.com.br

Dax EM, Farrugia A, Vyas G (eds): Advances in Transfusion Safety – Volume IV.
Dev Biol (Basel). Basel, Karger, 2007, vol 127, pp 43-58.

Reacting to an Emerging Safety Threat: West Nile Virus in North America

S.L. Stramer

American Red Cross Biomedical Services, Gaithersburg, MD, USA

Key words: West Nile virus, neuroinvasive disease, blood donation, nucleic acid testing.

Abstract: West Nile virus (WNV) entered North America in 1999 and in 2002 was shown to be transfusion transmitted. With competent mosquito and bird vectors throughout the United States and Canada, WNV clinical disease continues at epidemic proportions. Due to these facts, blood donor screening was implemented prior to the 2003 mosquito season and occurs using a variety of strategies. A combination of minipool (MP) nucleic acid amplification testing (NAT) during the " non-season, " coupled with the conversion to the more sensitive individual donation (ID) NAT in epidemic locations during epidemic times, has been successful in detecting approximately 1500 infected blood donors. Assuming that each donation was infectious and manufactured into 1.45 blood components, testing has therefore prevented close to 2200 recipient infections and potential clinical disease. During this same time, transfusion transmission has occurred from seven MP NAT-nonreactive/ID NAT-reactive units (6 in 2003 and 1 in 2004), or a total of 30 transfusion transmitted cases since WNV has been identified in North America. Because WNV occurs in infected blood donors at low concentrations (i.e., lower viral loads than HIV or HCV with the highest viral load of 580,000 copies/mL observed in a blood donor), a trigger strategy that is used in most of the US consisting of two NAT-reactive donations detected by MP NAT and a frequency of 1 : 1000 or greater has been developed. Since the full implementation of the MP to ID NAT trigger strategy, there have been no documented WNV transfusion transmissions. Because WNV is an acute infection that only occurs seasonally, other strategies have been proposed, such as seasonal testing, which has been implemented successfully in Canada (Quebec), coupled with a screening question used in the " non-season " of whether the donor has been in the US during the past 56 days; if so, WNV NAT is performed. WNV is an example of an emergent agent in which a rapid series of interventions has been successful in controlling transmission through blood transfusion.

Introduction

Documented human clinical disease caused by West Nile virus (WNV) in North America first appeared in 1999 in New York City, although human infection was first described in the West Nile region of Uganda in 1937 [1]. WNV is now the leading cause of arboviral (i.e., arthropod-borne virus) encephalitis in the United States [2]. WNV is a small (50-nm), spherical, single-stranded, positive-sense, RNA-containing, enveloped flavivirus with many characteristics in common with HCV, including its susceptibility to viral inactivation methods used for plasma-derived products [3].

The route of introduction of WNV into the US is unknown but likely occurred via an infected exotic bird imported to a New York zoo. The number of neuroinvasive disease cases caused by this flavivirus was relatively low and limited to the northeastern US in 1999 (59 cases in four states) and in 2000 (19 cases in 12 states plus the District of Columbia, DC). By 2001 the virus spread to the southeastern US with a total of 66 neuroinvasive disease cases reported in 27 states and DC, and by 2002 it had reached across the Ohio River valley, Midwest and through the central plains to the leading edge of the Rockies with a total of 4156 clinical cases and 2942 neuroinvasive disease cases in 44 states and DC. Although the agent was quiescent in 2000 and 2001, the 2002 WNV epidemic represented the largest arbovirus outbreak documented in North America and the largest WNV outbreak ever recorded [4]. WNV has remained present in epidemic proportions in subsequent years and spread throughout the contiguous US, with neuroinvasive disease cases totaling 2866 in 46 states plus DC in 2003, 1142 neuroinvasive disease cases in 47 states plus DC and Puerto Rico in 2004, and in 2005, 1242 neuroinvasive disease cases in 42 states, as reported to the US Centers for Disease Control and Prevention (CDC) through February 14, 2006 [5]. In 2005, WNV had expanded into 21 US counties that had not previously reported transmission to humans or animals and recurred in 1196 counties where transmission had been reported in previous years [2]. In contrast with previous years, the highest number of clinical disease cases reported to the CDC was in California (871 cases), representing 31 % of the total. The spread of WNV in the US is shown in Figure 1 (courtesy of Lyle Petersen, CDC; modified from [1]).

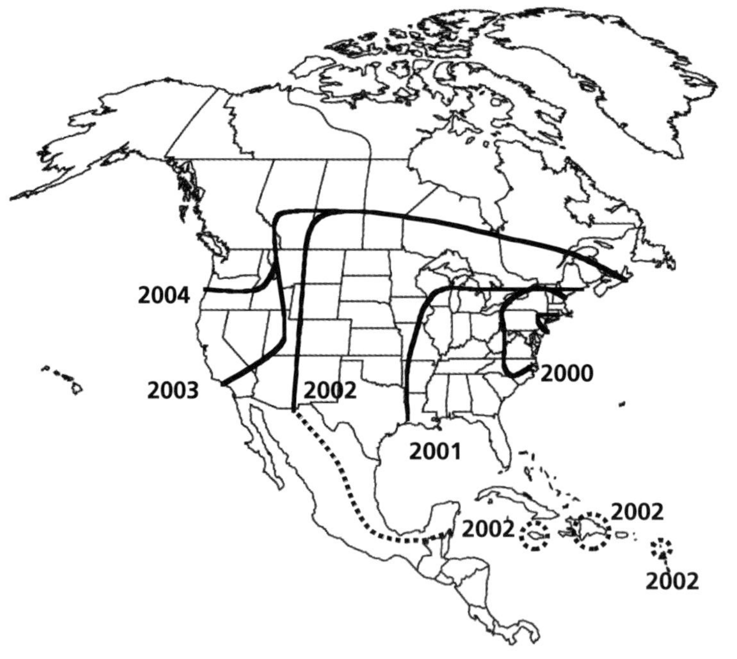

Fig. 1: Published reports on the distribution of West Nile virus. (Courtesy of Lyle Petersen, CDC).

Predictions regarding the further spread and persistence of WNV in North America are difficult, but the increase in the number of reported disease cases in 2005 compared with 2004 suggests that the endemic transmission of WNV in the US will continue for the foreseeable future [2]. A closely related flavivirus also in the Japanese encephalitis serogroup, St. Louis Encephalitis (SLE), has been responsible for epidemics of neuroinvasive disease in the US. Epidemics of SLE appeared sporadically in the US from 1932-2004 with major epidemics in the mid 1950's and 1960's, with the largest occurring in 1975. Of interest is that the distribution of neuroinvasive disease cases occurring in the 1975 SLE epidemic was very similar, even to the county level, to that observed for WNV in 2002.

Other mosquito-transmitted agents also represent emerging threats, either as newly introduced agents or re-introduced agents, including dengue and malaria, respectively. For both agents, the mosquitoes responsible for transmission occur in the US (species of *Aedes* and *Anopheles*, respectively). Unexplained cases of malaria have occurred throughout the US as documented from 1957-1994 [6]; in fact, the more recent cases of US-borne malaria have been identified in the same areas that experienced epidemic malaria earlier in US history. Regarding dengue virus, this agent has reached epidemic levels outside North America, especially in subtropical and tropical areas, but from 1963-present, the number of dengue fever and dengue hemorrhagic fever cases have been increasing (personal communication, CDC, Puerto Rico). Dengue is recognized as one of the world's major infectious disease threats, and although few transfusion-transmitted cases have been documented (with the exception of a ProMED listing on October 11, 2002, of a case in Hong Kong), there is no reason to believe that this agent should not be as effectively transmitted by blood as is WNV.

WNV in North America has been documented to occur in 58 different mosquito species and 288 avian species; however, *Culex* mosquito species are the principle vectors of WNV transmission in over 98 % of cases; of these, less than 10 species are the primary vectors. The top three transmitting species include *Culex pipiens* (the northern household mosquito), *C. quinquefasciatus* (the southern household mosquito) and *C. tarsalis*, which transmits primarily in the western US [2,7]. The virus over-winters in infected females that then transmit WNV into their eggs that initiate the next WNV season. The life cycle of WNV is dependent on both competent mosquito vectors and susceptible bird species that serve as a reservoir for the virus. Virus levels vary in infected birds but may reach high enough levels in some species to cause mortality rates in excess of 40 % [2,7]; in these cases, virus may be recovered from oral swabs and feces. The most susceptible bird species are corvids, common grackles, house finches and house sparrows; corvids (especially the American crow and blue jay) account for 72 % of dead birds reported in the US from 1999-2005. Non-human animal species (at least 18 different species) are only infected incidentally: that is, the mosquito-bird cycle is the primary amplifying cycle, but spill-over to other animals occurs when the numbers of infected mosquitoes and birds become high. The most effective preventive measure for human infection and disease is control of *Culex* mosquitoes and use of mosquito repellents (e.g., DEET); vaccines for human use are in development; there is a vaccine for horses [8].

Careful epidemiologic studies during the WNV epidemic of 2002 led to the identification of new modes of transmission, including blood transfusion and organ transplantation, breast feeding, mother to child transplacentally, and percutaneously in health care workers [1,9-11]. Transfusion transmission was investigated in 61 recipients of blood products in 2002, with 23 cases of transfusion-transmitted WNV infection confirmed [12]. The 23 confirmed cases included 13 neuroinvasive disease cases, two with West Nile fever (WNF), the remainder being asymptomatic cases identified since these individuals received co-components from the same donors as those having more severe disease. The onset of illness of 2-21 days (median of 10 days) following transfusion could be documented in 14 cases. Of those reporting more severe symptoms, seven died; however, it was unclear if the exact cause of death was related to their WNV infection or underlying disease. A total of 16 donors (donations) were identified retrospectively as having transmitted WNV to the 23 recipients; each of the 16 donors was viremic at the time of donation, and all were negative for antibody (IgM/IgG). Donors were identified as implicated if virus could be recovered from one of the components of their index donation by donor seroconversion, and if a co-component from their index, viremic donation transmitted WNV to another recipient. Seven of the 16 donors were linked to greater than one recipient with WNV infection, and one recipient received components from two different viremic donors. Donors were queried about their symptoms retrospectively, and based on the responses of nine of 14 donors who reported WNV-related symptoms before or following donation, the US Food and Drug Administration (FDA) developed guidance for industry to defer blood donors who had headache with fever in the seven days prior to donating (recognizing that 20 % or fewer WNV infections result in identifiable disease symptoms).

Approximately 80 % of all WNV infections are asymptomatic: 20 % cause WNF and less than 1 % cause neuroinvasive disease [13]. Neuroinvasive disease caused by WNV has been a notifiable disease in the US since 2002 [1]. Incidence of neuroinvasive disease and death increase with age and are highest for persons over 60 years and slightly higher for males [1,7,8,14]. Based on the number of neuroinvasive disease cases and an estimated ratio of 1 : 150 for the number of neuroinvasive disease cases to total cases, it may be estimated that greater than 1 million persons were infected with WNV during the 2002 epidemic [13]. For the 2003 epidemic year, other investigators estimated a ratio of 1 : 256 (95 % confidence interval of 112-401) for the relationship between neuroinvasive disease cases and total number of WNV infections. From these calculations, it was estimated that 735,000 (95 % confidence interval 322,000-1,147,000) WNV infections occurred in 2003 in the US. The estimates were based on a derived relationship between the number of infected blood donors in the US in 2003 that were identified by minipool nucleic acid amplification testing (MP NAT), or 944 based on participating blood center counts, a calculated 7-day MP NAT detectable period (6.9 days, 95 % confidence interval 3.0-10.7), IgM seroprevalence, and the number of neuroinvasive disease cases reported in the US [15].

WNV investigational blood donation screening began for the first time in 2003 (see below) as a model program of cooperation among public health agencies, regulators, manufacturers, and the blood-supply system [16].

Materials and Methods

Prior to the initiation of blood donation screening for WNV, the FDA provided guidance to blood centers to encourage donors to report post-donation illnesses that could be associated with infection by WNV and, at that time, for donors to be deferred for 28 days if post-donation information was received. WNV blood donor screening was initiated starting in June of 2003 under FDA approved investigational new drug (IND) protocols. Two different NAT assays based on different testing methodologies have been used: real-time quantitative reverse transcriptase polymerase chain reaction (RT-PCR) in minipools of 6 (TaqScreen using the Cobas Ampliprep and Taqman system; Roche Molecular Systems) used at 13 sites in the US and all Canadian sites, and transcription-mediated amplification (TMA; Gen-Probe/Chiron) in minipools of 16 used by the American Red Cross, Blood Systems Laboratories and 24 other sites. In addition to MP NAT, some sites screen individual donations (ID) rather than pooling; ID NAT is used during epidemic periods in epidemic locations (see below). The WNV TMA enhanced semi-automated platform (eSAS) is the same as used for HIV-1/HCV TMA; however, many sites also use an automated platform (TIGRIS) under the IND protocol. Following initial reactive test results on a single donation, either from MP NAT resolution testing or from ID NAT, donations are considered confirmed positive if the WNV NAT reactivity repeats by the same technology or an alternate WNV NAT method, or following the demonstration of WNV antibody (usually IgM) in the index or a follow-up sample [17,18]. For users of the TMA assay, the result of screening expressed as a signal-to-cut-off (S/CO) ratio is very predictive of a confirmed positive test result. Data collected by the American Red Cross and Blood Systems indicate that donations having an S/CO value of equal to or greater than 17 have an 88 % chance of confirming as positive. The first FDA licensure of a WNV NAT assay was granted to Gen-Probe's TMA assay using the eSAS platform on December 1, 2005 [19].

There are also WNV IgM/IgG assays cleared by the FDA [11]; however, many blood centers use antibody tests that are covered under specific IND protocols, including the use of the US state public health laboratories. Validation of all tests prior to use is necessary; for example, the American Red Cross uses the licensed Focus IgM/IgG test, but qualification studies comparing the Focus test to the previously used IgM assay (Abbott) indicated that comparable results required the use of a reduction in the cutoff of the Focus test [17].

NAT assays used for blood donation screening have been shown to have 50 % lower limits of detection that range from 3.4 to 29 copies per mL; when diluted to their operational MP NAT pool size, the 50 % limit of detection is reduced to 43 to 309 copies per mL [20]. Detection of viremia via MP NAT is compromised for seropositive units, which is likely due to the lower viral loads in individuals following seroconversion; of those samples studied, 13-24 % had viral loads below the 50 % detection of MP NAT screening assays [20].

WNV blood donation screening in the US occurs year-round. The WNV "season" is defined from May 1 to November 30 in the US (i.e., cases identified in blood donors during that period) [11] (Table 1 and Fig. 2). The peak season for each epidemic year has been from the end of July through the first week of September [17,18]. The season abates as female mosquitoes enter a dormant state and stop biting [1]. However, WNV activity in birds and mosquitoes has been documented year-round in states with warm winter climates. Human infection in these areas is a theoretical risk at all times of the year, and therefore screening in the US has occurred even through the winter months. In contrast, Hema-Quebec, serving the province of Quebec in Canada, tests all donations only during the summer months and from December 1 to June 1 asks each donor if they have been to the US within the prior 56 days: if so, those donations are WNV tested. WNV testing is likely to continue for the foreseeable future due to the continued presence of WNV in North America through the continued presence of competent mosquito and avian vectors. Because of low viral loads in infected humans (lower than HIV or HCV), WNV ID NAT screening would be a more sensitive testing strategy; however, ID NAT is not feasible for all WNV testing, and therefore triggers have been developed such that conversion from MP to ID NAT can occur in those areas having epidemic proportions of WNV [17,18]. Typically, the maximum capacity that each organization has for ID NAT is 10-20 % or 1000 donations tested individually per day, depending on the organization. This level of increased testing cannot be sustained for long periods of time (e.g., in excess of two to three months). Some capacity issues for the TMA users have been addressed with the introduction of an automated platform referred to as the TIGRIS, which can process 1000 samples in a 14-hour shift [21], but cost and reliability have limited the use of this instrument. The reliability issues are being addressed by the manufacturer, and FDA licensure of this automated platform is expected by the end of 2006-early 2007. Therefore, sites using TIGRIS at the present time continue under IND [22].

All organizations must be prepared to "trigger", i.e. convert from MP to ID NAT since the time and location of a WNV epidemic, and hence the need for ID NAT, are unknown. The development/validation of triggers has been a subject for debate, but most organizations have used both an absolute number of cases (usually two) and a frequency that exceeds 1: 1000. The derivation of these numbers is based on retrospective studies using donations collected in 2002 from epidemic areas and tested by both ID and MP NAT. These studies determined that for every four WNV RNA positive donations detected by MP NAT, one additional donation required ID NAT for detection. This number was used in combination with a frequency of 1: 1000 that had been predicted (and later observed through retrospective testing) for the same locations and time [23,24]. The sensitivity of this method was increased by using two WNV-reactive donations in place of four [25]. For 2003-2005, ID NAT has detected 27-32 % of all WNV RNA-positive donations, of which 5-10 % are antibody negative and therefore pose the greatest threat to blood safety (see below).

The results presented include data summaries for the 2003-2005 WNV seasons compiled through an internet-based arbovirus surveillance system, referred to as ArboNet, managed by the state health departments and the CDC [2,4]. Blood centers provide numbers of WNV-reactive donors (with or without confirmation) to their local/state public health departments, who in turn report the data to the CDC. In addition, included is the compilation of the same three years of WNV NAT screening results obtained by the major blood collection/testing programs in the US (the American Red Cross, Blood Systems Laboratories and the 13 Roche sites); data have been generously shared by these organizations for use in this review.

Table 1: WNV RNA detection in US blood donors.

	2003	2004	2005	*Total*
Total donations screened (1st-last positive)	4,529,248	4,185,419	4,355,885	*13,070,552*
Donations screened by ID NAT (during epidemic period)	34,465 (0.8 %)	233,908 (5.6 %)	229,298 (5.3 %)	*497,571 (3.8 %)*
Date range (1st-last positive)	6/25-12/1	5/3-11/29	5/26-11/30	*5/3-12/1*
# Confirmed positive	721	256	352	*1329*
Frequency per 10,000 donations	1.59	0.61	0.81	*1.02*
# Presumptive viremic donors reported to ArboNET (CDC)	818	224	399	*1441*

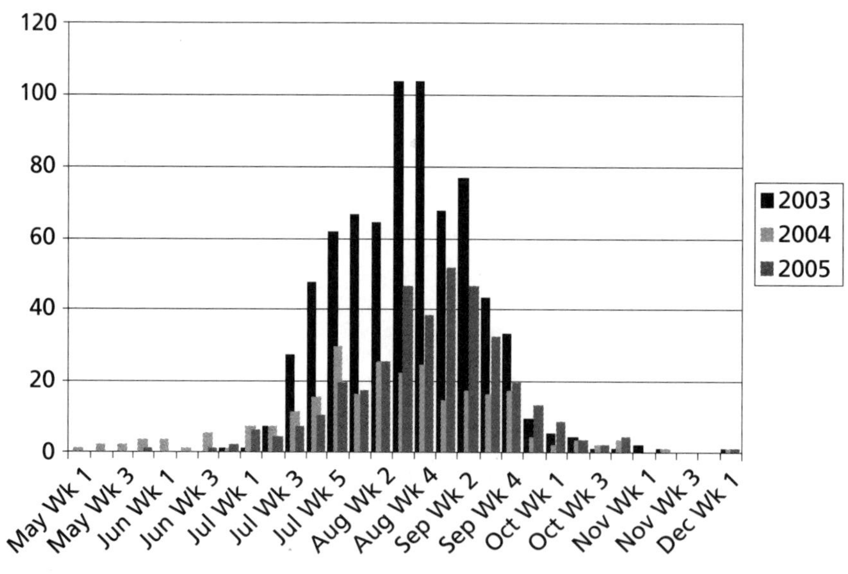

Fig. 2: Number of WNV RNA positive donors reported by Week, 2003-2005.

Results

Of 818 presumed viremic donors (PVDs), defined as WNV NAT-reactive donations that repeated using the same test or had elevated S/CO values, reported to CDC in 2003, 78 % came from six US states: Colorado, Kansas, Nebraska, North Dakota, South Dakota and Texas; in contrast, in 2004, only 224 PVDs were reported with 75 % from five states: Arizona, California, Colorado, Louisiana, and New Mexico [26]. Finally, in 2005, 399 PVDs were reported with 67 % coming from six states: Arizona, California, Kansas, Louisiana, Nebraska and Texas (Table 1, as reported to the CDC). In some cases, WNV-related disease could be documented in donors post donation. For example, less than 2 % reported neuroinvasive disease, and 30 % reported WN fever in 2004. Blood center survey data from the American Red Cross documented higher numbers of donors reporting WNV-related symptoms (61 %) in the three years of testing. However, in all cases, donors who were questioned knew that they tested WNV-NAT reactive so that recall bias may have artificially elevated these observations [14].

Transfusion transmission in 2003, in spite of WNV MP NAT screening of all blood donations, occurred in six cases; in each case one blood component was identified that contained a WNV viremic donation, and in five of six, symptoms compatible with WNV-related illness occurred [26-28]. The concentrations of WNV determined in these donations from which samples were available for viral quantitation ranged from 0.06-0.5 pfu per mL (or 24-200 copies/mL, where 1 pfu equals 400 copies). In contrast, in 2002, prior to WNV donor screening, the viral loads in the 16 donations implicated in transfusion transmission ranged from 0.8-75.1 pfu per mL (or 320-30,040 copies/mL) [12,26]. In 2004, there was a single probable case of WNV transfusion transmission documented in Arizona [29] that occurred just prior to the conversion from MP to ID NAT. In all cases, WNV screening was performed in a MP NAT format, where all the implicated donations were nonreactive; in each case where additional testing occurred retrospectively, viral levels were consistent with detection as individual donations and all were antibody negative at index. In each case, the donor seroconverted when followed. In contrast, in 2005, no transfusion transmissions were documented; however, transmission of WNV to recipients of four organs occurred from an infected donor who was WNV-antibody positive [30]. Similarly, WNV in plasma containing antibody can infect Vero cells and monocyte-derived macrophages in culture, as evidenced by cytopathic effects or WNV-specific RNA by RT-PCR following passage [31,32]. Therefore, the issue of transmission of WNV from antibody-positive blood in which case infectious virus may persist, although not documented for four WNV seasons, is still a theoretical possibility. Thus far, the data are limited: 30 recipients infected from WNV RNA-positive, antibody-negative components and no infection in four recipients transfused with WNV RNA-positive, antibody-positive components [17,18]. Recipients of organs who are highly immunosuppressed may be at the greatest risk of infection with low level virus, even in the presence of antibody, resulting in severe disease [30].

Combined blood center data summarizing WNV donor testing results for the three major collection/testing systems in the US during the 2003-2005 WNV seasons represent greater than 80 % of all blood collected in the US and are summarized on Table 1 [33]. WNV NAT screening began in 2003 prior to the epidemic for that year; in that and the subsequent two years, all US programs performed WNV MP NAT, or in epidemic periods/locations ID NAT. These data represent donations tested by either the Gen-Probe WNV Assay (TMA) in pools of 16 or in pools of 6 by the Roche TaqScreen Assay (RT-PCR). Confirmation of WNV infection in donors of index and follow up samples were performed by repeating the same NAT method, an alternate NAT method (in house or by a reference laboratory) and by antibody testing (using both IgM and IgG).

According to the data compiled, 1329 donations confirmed positive of 13.07 million donations screened during the three WNV seasons for an overall frequency of 1.02 per 10,000 donations and a range of 0.6 in 2004 to 1.6 in 2003 (Table 1 and Fig. 2). Although blood is screened by MP NAT year round, as stated, the numbers here represent the "WNV season." Of all blood donations included in the 13.07 million, ID NAT was used for approximately 4 % of the donations tested. The first detected confirmed positive donation in any season occurred May 3 and the last positive on December 1. The total of 1329 WNV confirmed-positive donors identified (for the 80 % of US data collected) is comparable to the 1441 reported by the CDC. The duration of the three WNV seasons is presented in Figure 2 by week of WNV-positive collection date highlighting the peak season from July through September. Figures 3-6 detail the three individual and combined seasons by the number of confirmed positive donors by their state if residents in the US. ID NAT was required to detect 291 of 1329 (22 %) confirmed positives; 67 (5 %) of the 291 were antibody negative and therefore most likely infectious (Table 2). At index, a total of 344 donations of the 1329 total (26 %) were antibody positive, while 74 % were antibody negative. Of the total 985 antibody-negative donors at index, 766 (58 %) were followed to seroconversion. The specific data are not shown, but using a confirmatory algorithm of index donation testing by repeat NAT (same or alternate method) and antibody resulted in 99.24 % sensitivity of index NAT confirmation, with only 10 donors requiring follow up for confirmation. Using a stricter criterion for confirmation of antibody seroconversion limits the calculation to only those 766 donors who seroconverted; this results in a sensitivity of index confirmation of 98.6 % (756/766). Of the 1329 confirmed positive donations, 756 of 1013 tested (75 %) had viral loads of greater than 100 copies per mL, of which 704 (93 %) were antibody negative (Fig. 7). The highest viral loads observed in data from the American Red Cross was 580,000 copies per mL, with higher viral loads for those donors who were antibody negative (5,800 copies/mL median) than those who were antibody positive (<100 copies/mL median) [17]. In the composite data set, antibody negative donors seroconverted at a median of 14 (IgM) to 17 (IgG) days; NAT positivity persisted in 54 % for a median of 14 and maximum of 98 days based on the algorithm presented. If additional replicates of follow-up samples from donors who tested WNV NAT nonreactive but WNV antibody positive at follow up are tested, additional viremic samples may be identified. This indicates viral loads that are lower than the 95 % detection limit of the NAT assay [11].

In contrast to rates of confirmed positivity, rates of false positivity decreased from 1.0 to 0.28 per 10,000 donations screened over the three years. False positivity may be attributed to user unfamiliarity with the new test; however, this is unlikely due to the same system being used for HIV-1/HCV as used for WNV for the majority of donations tested, as well as the use of automated systems by some facilities. False positivity may also be attributable to quality of the reagents or samples. The cause of most false positivity is related to the use of ID NAT, in which any reactive donation based on a single test is not transfused and the donor deferred. False positivity associated with ID NAT accounted for a total of 69 % of all false positives reported.

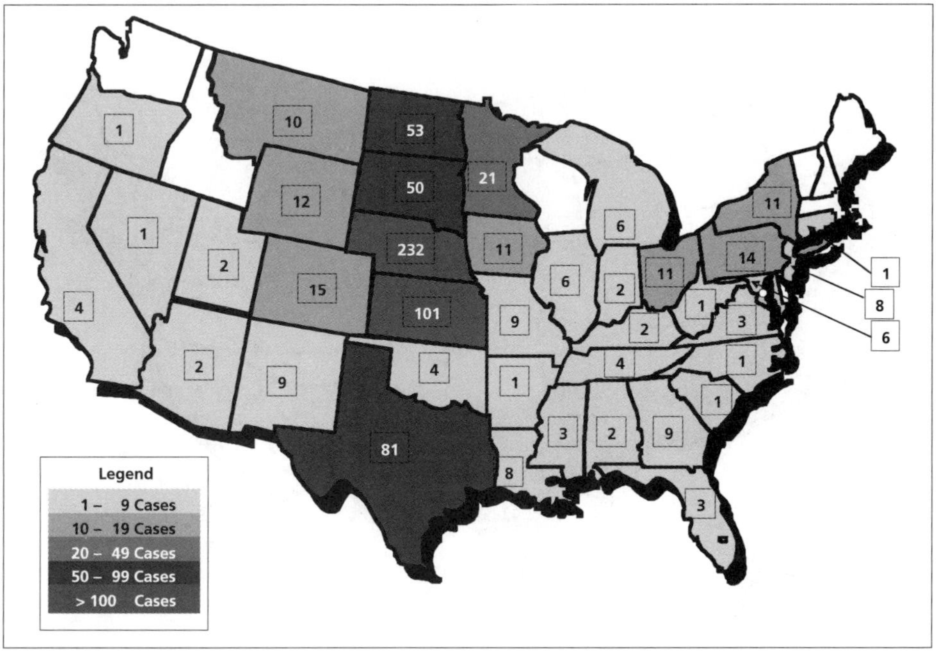

Fig. 3: Total WNV RNA confirmed positive donors. 2003 (N = 721).

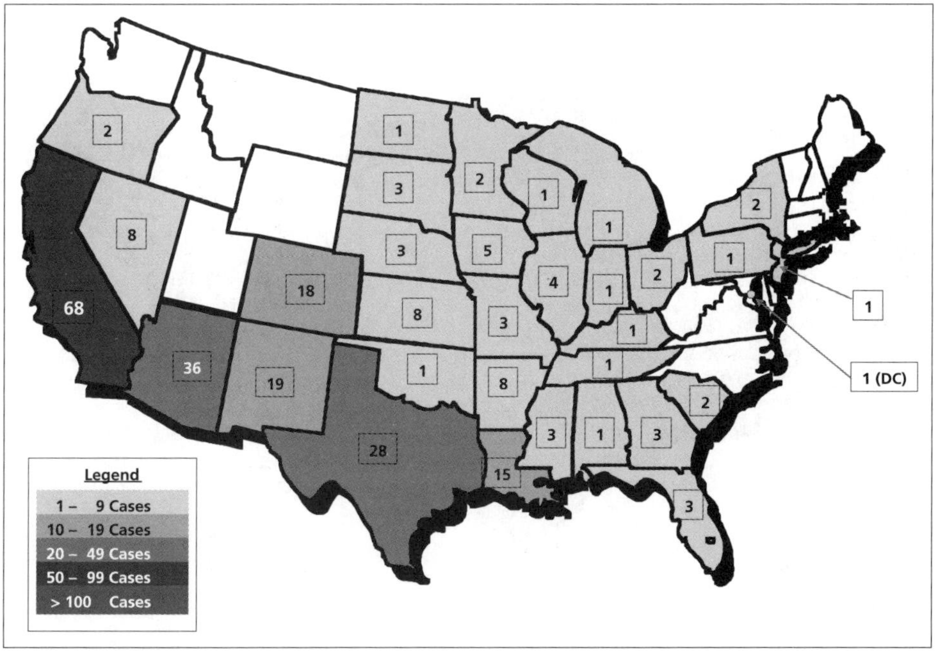

Fig. 4: Total WNV RNA confirmed positive donors. 2004 (N = 256).

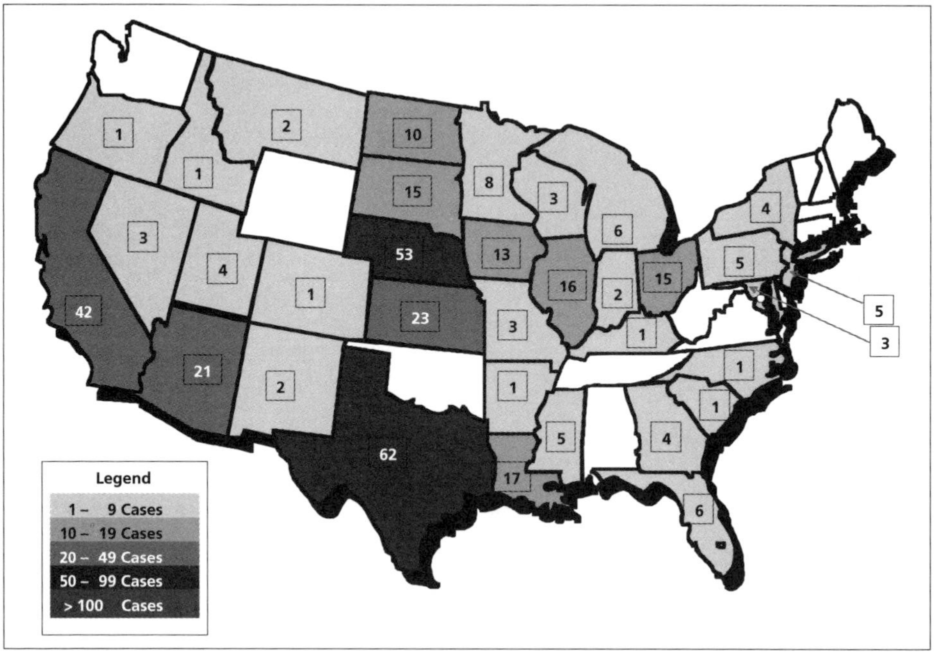

Fig. 5: Total WNV RNA confirmed positive donors. 2005 (N = 352).

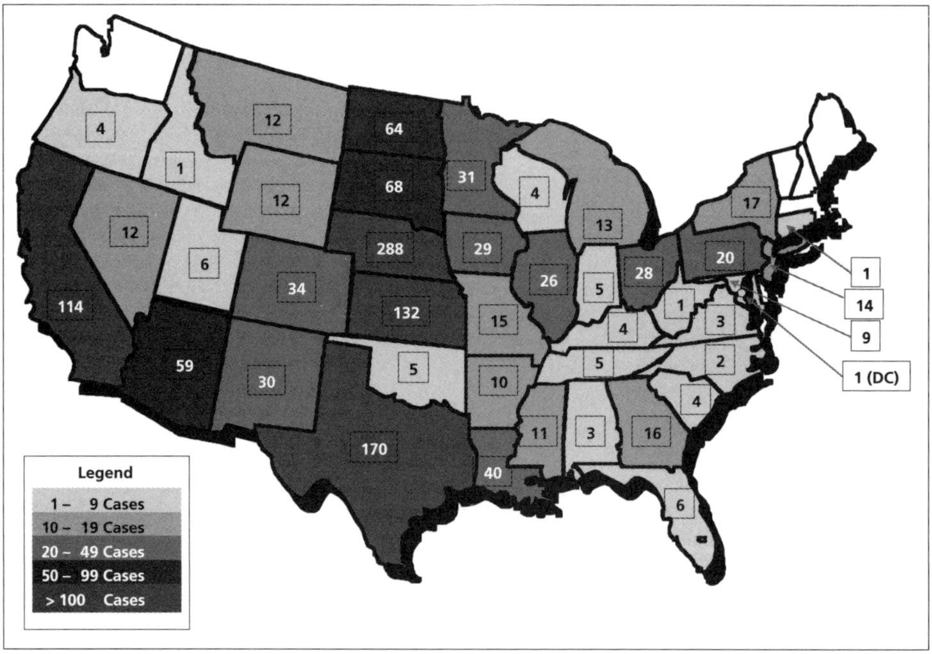

Fig. 6: Total WNV RNA confirmed positive donors. 2003, 2004 & 2005 (N = 1329).

Table 2: WNV confirmed positives sorted by detection method (MP or ID NAT required) coupled with presence/absence of antibody.

ID NAT	MP NAT	Ab	2003	2004	2005	*Total*	
+	-	-	14	32	21	*67 (5 %)*	Ab Neg: 985 (74%)
+	+	-	534	145	239	918 (69 %)	
+	+	+	55	23	42	*120 (9 %)*	Ab Pos: 344 (26 %)
+	-	+	118	56	50	*224 (17 %)*	
Total			721	256	352	*1329*	

67 + 224 = 291 (22 %) required ID NAT for detection.

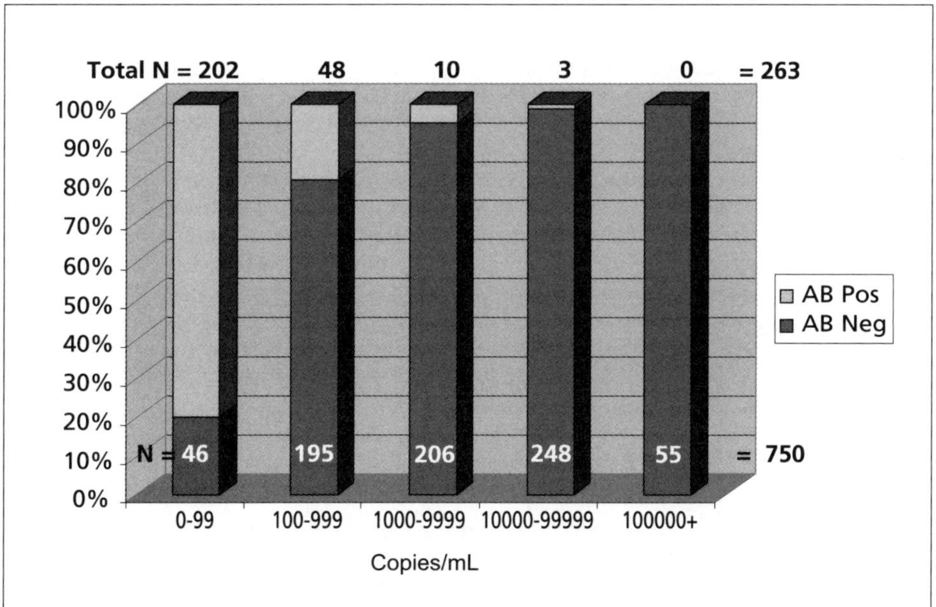

Fig. 7: Index donation viral loads of WNV confirmed positives 756/1013 (75 %) have quantifiable virus of which 704 (93 %) are antibody negative.

The WNV pre-clinical incubation period is thought to range from 2-14 days following mosquito bite, with viremia beginning at 1-3 days and lasting 1-11 days (with a mean of 6 days) [11]. Studies in blood donors who have participated in follow-up studies as part of the INDs have been designed to determine the dynamics of WNV infection and clearance. These studies have demonstrated longer periods of viremia than previously documented, especially in the presence of IgM. As mentioned above, it is unknown if blood components manufactured from viremic donations that are antibody positive are infectious. The longest period of viremia in a donor is 104 days after initial detection by NAT. Studies performed by the American Red Cross from follow up of 186 seroconverting donors in 2003 have shown that low level viremia persists for a median of 20.5 days (range of 6.5 to 56.4 days, representing 99 % of the observed population based on modeling studies [34]; Fig. 8). In the model, virus detection was extrapolated to 1 copy per mL (representing the initiation of viremia, or time 0, t_0) from donors having ramp-up viremia in the absence of antibody, or a 2.2-day interval from time 0 to ID NAT detection and a 4.8-day interval from time 0 to MP NAT detection. Data from seroconverting donors was fit to the model demonstrating that 7.9 days occur following the initiation of viremia to index donation, and 15-16 days from the initiation of viremia to IgM (6.5-day lower bound) and IgG (10.5-day lower bound). Studies performed by Blood Systems demonstrated the longest viremic observations in donors who are IgM positive (for 2003 at 49 days and 2004 at 104 days); replicate tests of five were performed, indicating that a single nonreactive WNV NAT result does not indicate complete viral clearance.

Based on the above data, the FDA published guidance recommending 120-day donor deferral for those donors testing WNV reactive with an investigational screening test (whether confirmed positive or not) as well as those donors suspected of, or being diagnosed with WNV infection [11]. Donors may be reentered after 120 days from the date of their reactive donation unless a follow-up sample is reactive, in which case the donor must then be deferred for 120 days past the date of the last reactive WNV NAT result.

IgM in WNV-infected blood donors persists for 100 days or longer in 89 % (166) of followed donors and 60 % of those followed for greater than 1 year (IgM was demonstrated at 398 days or longer) [17]; these data are consistent with other

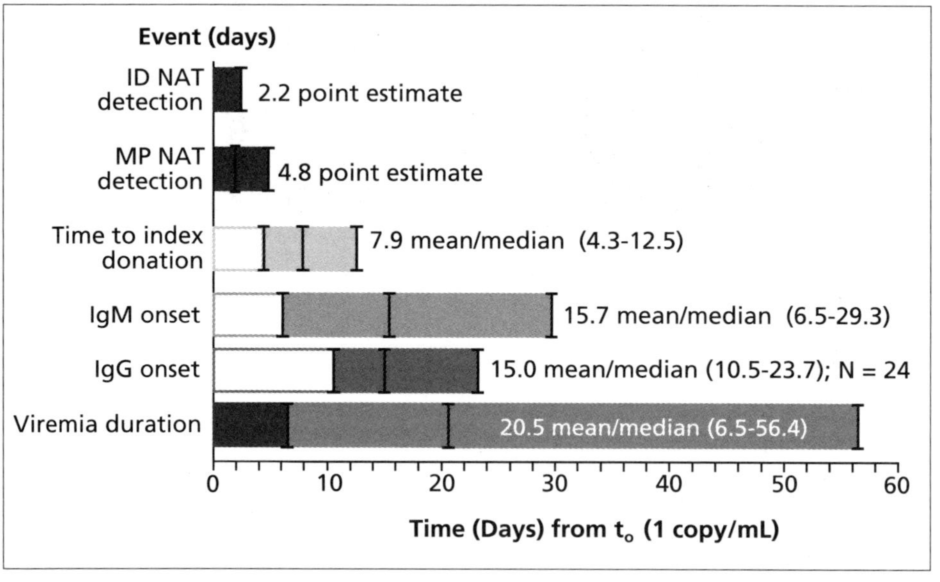

Fig. 8: Modeled WNV dynamics of infection from 1 copy/mL (estimated time 0, t_0). N = 186 donors with multiple follow-up samples.

reports [35]. In another study [36] of 89 donors followed for up to 440 days, 88 % remained IgM positive by linear regression analysis to 218 days. Therefore, it appears that IgM persists for greater than 6 months after infection and is a useful tool in confirmation of WNV-reactive donors.

Data presented at the FDA's Blood Products Advisory Committee meeting in October of 2004 indicated that self-reported fever with headache in the past week before donation did not appear to be predictive of WNV infection and did not correlate with peak periods or locations of WNV incidence as determined by WNV NAT detection in blood donors. The analysis included 550,000 donations collected between June 1 and December 31 of 2003 at five American Red Cross regions. Regions with epidemic levels of WNV-infected donors (20.5-30 per 10,000 donations) were compared to those regions having no WNV-infected donors. Although the number of deferrals due to a "yes" response to the fever with headache question prior to donation was low in all regions, the number of "yes" responses to deferrable symptoms reported before donation did not agree with the number of WNV-positive donors by time or location of the epidemic [14]. WNV NAT-reactive donors who participated in follow up studies conducted by the American Red Cross during the 2003 and 2004 WNV epidemics were also invited to participate in a study that included a demographic, symptom and date-of-symptom questionnaire (i.e., symptoms pre-donation or on the day of, or post donation [14]). Cases (389) were defined as WNV-reactive donors who confirmed positive, whereas those donors who were determined to be false positives were used as controls (387). The demographic characteristics of infected donors reflected the rural nature of the 2003 and 2004 epidemics, as observed by others [4]. Symptoms were reported by 61 % of cases versus 20 % of controls with 74 % of symptoms reported by cases within the 14 days after donation. The frequency of headache and fever reported together in the seven days before donation was not significantly different between cases and controls; only the individual frequencies of headache, eye pain and new rash during this time were significantly different, and, consequently, asking donors about pre-donation headache and fever had no detectable contribution to blood safety [37-39].

Discussion

WNV screening using a combination of MP NAT during the "non-season" coupled with the conversion to the more sensitive individual donation (ID) NAT in epidemic locations during epidemic times detected approximately 1500 infected blood donors. Assuming that each donation was infectious and manufactured into 1.45 blood components [40], testing has therefore prevented close to 2200 possible recipient infections and potential clinical disease. During this same time, transfusion transmission has occurred from seven MP NAT-nonreactive/ID NAT-reactive units (6 in 2003 and 1 in 2004), or a total of 30 transfusion-transmitted cases since WNV has been identified in North America. Because WNV occurs in infected blood donors at low concentrations (i.e., lower viral loads than HIV or HCV, with the highest viral load observed in a blood donor at 580,000 copies/mL), a trigger strategy that is used in most of the US consisting of two NAT-reactive donations detected by MP NAT and a frequency of 1 : 1000 has been developed. Since the full implementation of the MP to ID NAT trigger strategy, there have been no documented WNV transfusion transmissions. Because WNV is an acute infection that only occurs seasonally, other strategies have been proposed, such as seasonal testing, which has been implemented successfully in Canada (Quebec) coupled with a screening question used in the "non-season" of whether the donor has been in the US during the past 56 days, in which case WNV NAT is performed. WNV is an example of an emergent agent in which a rapid series of interventions has been successful in controlling transmission through blood transfusion.

Cost effectiveness for various WNV prevention strategies has been estimated. Custer and colleagues [41] determined that for the 2003 WNV season in the US, which was the largest of the three screening seasons thus far, the cost of MP NAT was $ 483,000 per quality-adjust life year (QALY) versus $ 897,000 if ID NAT was performed. The MP/ID NAT targeted (trigger) strategy cost was $ 520,000 per QALY. The cost of any of these strategies is ultimately dependent on WNV prevalence. Due to the high cost and relative poor cost effectiveness of WNV screening using the MP/ID NAT approach, other prevention strategies have been proposed that minimize or eliminate testing [42]. In addition to seasonal testing, selective testing for only immunocompromised patients or the use of questionnaires to eliminate at-risk donors was proposed. These additional strategies, however, did not fully consider regulation, cost or logistics. Although WNV screening of blood donations is not yet required in the US by the FDA, testing is controlled via the IND or licensure process. The FDA perspective is one of risk versus benefit as opposed to cost versus benefit [43]. It is clear that the US cannot use the same approach as Canada since the Canadian approach to testing in the "off season" is dependent on travel to the US. In a seasonal or geographic model where fewer reagents are used, it is not clear that a proportional reduction in cost would occur. The proposed strategies of Korves [42] of WNV symptom-related pre-donation questioning and/or transfusion of WNV-screened components to at-risk recipients ignored the other factors involved in system cost such as labor and computer systems that can manage tested versus non-tested components [44,45]. Also, as discussed, the use of a pre-donation questionnaire would not have detected the 74 % of donors who later developed symptoms [14]. Stratifying recipients based on need is also problematic, as not all recipients who developed WNV clinical disease were strictly classified as immunocompromised. Lastly, the maintenance of a dual-tiered blood inventory is a source of potential errors. Selective transfusion protocols create operational difficulties and frequently fail to meet their objectives in that patients who need a specific component may not necessarily receive it [46]. The MP/ID NAT targeted testing strategy serves as a bridge between no testing and very expensive year-round ID NAT and may serve as a model for testing new agents if the disease epidemiology is clearly related to specific geographic regions. This approach may not be the least costly, but it does achieve blood safety and public health goals [45]. The real proof of the effectiveness of the MP/NAT current strategy has been the elimination of documented cases of WNV transfusion transmission.

References

1 Peterson LR, Marfin AA: West Nile virus: a primer for the clinician. Ann Intern Med 2002; 137: 173-179.

2 Centers for Disease Control and Prevention. West Nile virus activity – United States, January 1-December 1, 2005. MMWR Morb Mortal Wkly Rep 2005; 54: 1253-1256.

3 Kreil TR, Berting A, Kistner O, Kindermann J: West Nile virus and the safety of plasma derviatives: verification of high safety margins, and the validity of predicitons based on model virus data. Transfusion 2003; 43: 1023-1028.

4 Petersen LR, Hayes EB: Westward ho? The spread of West Nile virus. N Engl J Med 2004; 351: 2257-2259.

5 Centers for Disease Control and Prevention. 2005 West Nile virus activity in the United States, February 23, 2006. http://www.cdc.gov/ncidod/dvbid/westnile/serv & control.htm.

6 Zucker JR: Changing patterns of autochthonous malaria transmission in the United States: a review of recent outbreaks. Emerg Inf Dis 1996; 2:37-43.

7 Hayes EB, Komar N, Nasci RS, Montgomery SP, O'Leary DR, Campbell GL: Epidemiology and transmission dynamics of West Nile virus disease. Emerg Infect Dis 2005; 11: 1167-1173.

8 Hayes EB, Sejvar JJ, Zaki SR, Lanciotti RS, Bode AV, Campbell GL: Virology, pathology, and clinical manifestations of West Nile virus disease. Emerg Infect Dis 2005; 11: 1174-1179.

9 Centers for Disease Control and Prevention. Update: investigations of West Nile virus infection in recipients of organ transplantation and blood transfusion. MMWR Morb Mortal Wkly Rep 2002; 51: 833-836.

10 Iwamoto M, Jernigan DB, Guasch A, Trepka MA, Blackmore CG, Hellinger WC, et al: Transmission of West Nile virus from an organ donor to four transplant recipients. N Engl J Med 2003; 348: 2196-2203.

11 Food and Drug Administration: Guidance for industry: assessing donor suitability and blood and blood product safety in cases of known or suspected West Nile virus infection. Rockville (MD): Center for Biologics Evaluation and Research (CBER), 2005 June.

12 Pealer LN, Marfin AA, Petersen LR, Lanciotti RS, Page PL, Stramer SL, et al: Transmission of West Nile virus through blood transfusion in the United States in 2002. N Engl J Med 2003; 349 (13): 1236-1245.

13 Mostashari F, Bunning M, Kitsutani PT, Singer DA, Nash D, Cooper MJ, et al: Epidemic West Nile encephalitis, New York, 1999: results of a household-based seroepidemiological survey. Lancet 2001; 358: 261-264.

14 Orton, SL, Stramer SL, Dodd RY: Self-reported symptoms associated with West Nile virus infection in RNA-positive blood donors. Transfusion 2006; 46: 272-277.

15 Busch, MP, Wright DJ, Tobler LH, Stramer SL, Kleinman SH, Prince HE, et al.: West Nile virus infections projected from blood donor screening data, United States, 2003. Emerg Infect Dis 2006; 12 (3): 395-402. www.cdc.gov/ncidod/EID/vol12no03/05-1287.htm.

16 Dodd RY: Emerging infections, transfusion safety, and epidemiology. N Engl J Med 2003; 349: 1205-1206.

17 Stramer SL, Fang CT, Foster GA, Wagner AG, Brodsky JP, Dodd RY: West Nile virus among blood donors in the United States, 2003 and 2004. N Engl J Med 2005; 353: 451-459.

18 Busch MP, Caglioti S, Robertson EF, McAuley JD, Tobler LH, Kamel H, et al: Screening the blood supply for West Nile virus RNA by nucleic acid amplification testing. N Engl J Med 2005; 353: 460-467.

19 Food and Drug Administration. Product Approval Information – Licensing Action. Dec 1, 2005. http://www.fda.gov/cber/approvltr/wnvgen120105L.htm.

20 Busch MP, Tobler L, Saldanha J, Caglioti S, Shyamala V, Linnen JM, et al: Analytical and clinical sensitivity of West Nile virus RNA screening and supplemental assays available in 2003. Transfusion 2005; 45: 492-499.

21 Gen-Probe, Inc. Gen-Probe submits regulatory application for use of Procleix® TIGRIS® system to screen donation blood for West Nile virus, April 24, 2006. http://biz.yahoo.com/prnews/060420/lath037.html?.v=49.

22 Hillyer CD, Lipton KS: Joint statement of AABB, America's Blood Centers and American Red Cross on testing for West Nile virus. AABB Bulletin No, 06-02. Bethesda, MD: AABB, 2006:1-2.

23 Biggerstaff BJ, Petersen LR: Estimated risk of transmission of the West Nile virus through blood transfusion in the US, 2002. Transfusion 2003; 43: 1007-1017.

24 Stramer SL, Beyers ML, Wagner AG, Dille, BJ, Dawson GJ, Schochetman G, et al: West Nile virus (WNV) RNA prevalence in blood donations during the 2002 US epidemic. Transfusion 2003; 43 (Suppl. 9S) 3A: S10.

25 Custer B, Tomasulo PA, Murphy EL, Caglioti S, Harpool D, McEvoy D, Busch MP. Triggers for switching from minipool testing by nucleic acid technology to individual-donation nucleic acid testing for West Nile virus: analysis of 2003 data to inform 2004 decision making. Transfusion 2004; 44 (11): 1547-1554.

26 Montgomery SP, Brown JA, Kuehnert M, Smith TL, Crall N, Lanciotti RS, et al: Transfusion-associated transmission of West Nile virus, United States 2003-2005. Transfusion 2006; 46: 2038-2046.

27 Centers for Disease Control and Prevention. Update: West Nile virus screening of blood donations and transfusion-associated transmission – United States, 2003. MMWR Morb Mortal Wkly Rep 2004; 53: 281-284.

28 Macedo de Oliveira A, Beecham BD, Montgomery SP, Lanciotti RS, Linnen JM, Giachetti C, Pietrelli LA, Stramer SL, Safranek TJ: West Nile virus blood transfusion-related infection despite nucleic acid testing. Transfusion 2004; 44: 1695-1699.

29 Centers for Disease Control and Prevention. Transfusion – associated transmission of West Nile virus – Arizona, 2004. MMWR Morb Mortal Wkly Rep 2004; 53: 842-844.

30 Centers for Disease Control and Prevention. West Nile virus infections in organ transplant recipient – New York and Pennsylvania, August-September, 2005. MMWR Morb Mortal Wkly Rep 2005; 54: 1021-1023.

31 Rios M, Daniel S, Stramer SL, Caglioti S, Wood O, Hewlett IK: West Nile virus NAT-positive human plasma containing WNV-IgM and IgG antibodies can infect Vero cells and human primary macrophages in culture. Transfusion 2005; 45 (Suppl. 3S): 3A.

32 Rios M, Daniel S, Wood O, Hewlett IK, Caglioti S, Stramer SL: Further studies of the infectivity of West Nile virus (WNV) in the presence of human specific antibodies. Abstract submitted 2006.

33 Stramer SL, Dodd RY, Caglioti S, Strong DM: Yield of minipool (MP) and individual donation (ID) nucleic acid amplification testing (NAT) for WNV RNA in United States blood donors, 2003-2005. 7th National Conference on West Nile virus, San Francisco, Calif., February, 2006.

34 Stramer SL, Brodsky JP, Dodd RY: Dynamics of WNV infection and resolution among blood donors. 6th National Conference on West Nile virus in the United States, San Jose, Calif., February, 2005.

35 Roehrig JT, Nash D, Maldin B, Labowitz A, Martin DA, Lanciotti RS, Campbell GL: Persistence of virus-reactive serum immunoglobulin M antibody in confirmed West Nile virus encephalitis cases. Emerg Infect Dis 2003; 9: 376-379.

36 Prince HE, Tobler LH, Lapé-Nixon M, Foster GA, Stramer SL, Busch MP: Development and persistence of West Nile virus-specific immunoglobulin M (IgM), IgA, and IgG in viremic blood donors. J Clin Microbiol 2005; 43: 4316-4320.

37 Food and Drug Administration. Guidance for industry: recommendations for the assessment of donor suitability and blood and blood product safety in cases of known or suspected West Nile virus infection. Rockville (MD): Center for Biologics Evaluation and Research (CBER), 2002 Oct.

38 Food and Drug Administration. Revised recommendations for the assessment of donor suitability of donor suitability and blood and blood product safety in cases of known or suspected Westn Nile virus infection. Rockville (MD): Center for Biologics Evaluation and Research (CBER), 2003 May.

39 Food and Drug Administration. Guidance for industry: revised recommendations for the assessment of donor suitability and blood and blood product safety in cases of known or suspected West Nile virus infection. Rockville (MD): Center for Biologics Evaluation and Research (CBER), 2005 April.

40 Stramer SL, Glynn SA, Kleinman SH, Strong DM, Caglioti S, Wright DJ, Dodd RY, Busch MP: Detection of HIV-1 and HCV infections among antibody-negative blood donors by nucleic acid-amplification testing. N Engl J Med 2004; 351: 760-768.

41 Custer B, Busch MP, Marfin AA, Petersen LR: The cost-effectiveness of screening the US blood supply for West Nile virus. Ann Intern Med. 2005; 143 (7): 486-492.

42 Korves CT, Goldie SJ, Murray MB: Cost-effectiveness of alternative blood-screening strategies for West Nile virus in the United States. PLoS Med. 2006; 3 (2) e21: 0211-0221.

43 Kuehn BM: Studies propose targeted screening of blood for West Nile virus. JAMA 2006; 295 (11): 1235-1236.

44 Aubuchon, JP: Meeting transfusion safety expectation. Ann Intern Med 2005; 143 (7) 537-538.

45 Stramer SL, Custer B, Busch MP, Dodd RY: Strategies for testing blood donors for West Nile virus. Transfusion 2006; 46: 2036-2037.

46 Ness PM, Lipton KS: Selective transfusion protocols: errors and accidents waiting to happen. Transfusion 2001; 41: 713-715.

Dr. S. L. Stramer, Scientific Support Office, American Red Cross Biomedical Services, 9315 Gaither Road, Gaithersburg, MD 20877, USA.
E-mail: stramers@usa.redcross.org

Dax EM, Farrugia A, Vyas G (eds): Advances in Transfusion Safety – Volume IV.
Dev Biol (Basel). Basel, Karger, 2007, vol 127, p 59.

SESSION III

Fitting New Techniques into the Safety Paradigm

Chairs: *J.-P. Allain and A. Heaton*

Dax EM, Farrugia A, Vyas G (eds): Advances in Transfusion Safety – Volume IV.
Dev Biol (Basel). Basel, Karger, 2007, vol 127, pp 61-70.

Fitting New Technologies into the Safety Paradigm: Use of Microarrays in Transfusion

C. Fournier-Wirth, J. Coste

Transfusion Transmitted Infectious Diseases R&D Unit, EFS Pyrénées Méditerranée, Montpellier, France

Key words: Blood testing, microarray, biosensor, biobarcode, nanotechnology.

Abstract: Until the late 1990s, mandatory blood screening for transmissible infectious agents depended entirely on antigen/antibody-based detection assays. The recent emergence of Nucleic acid Amplification Technologies (NAT) has revolutionised viral diagnosis, not only by increasing the level of sensitivity but also by facilitating the detection of several viruses in parallel by multiplexing specific primers. In more complex biological situations, when a broad spectrum of pathogens must be screened, the limitations of these first generation technologies became apparent. High throughput systems, such as DNA Arrays, permit a conceptually new approach. These miniaturised micro systems allow the detection of hundreds of different targets simultaneously, inducing a dramatic decrease in reagent consumption, a reduction in the number of confirmation tests and a simplification of data interpretation. However, the systems currently available require additional instrumentation and reagents for sample preparation and target amplification prior to detection on the DNA array. A major challenge in the area of DNA detection is the development of methods that do not rely on target amplification systems. Likewise, the advances of protein microarrays have lagged because of poor stability of proteins, complex coupling chemistry and weak detection signals. Emerging technologies like Biosensors and nano-particle based DNA or Protein Bio-Barcode Amplification Assays are promising diagnostic tools for a wide range of clinical applications, including blood donation screening.

Introduction

In line with the actively pursued zero risk policy for pathogen and immunological risk in the transfusion of blood components, scientific and technological innovation is constantly surveyed by Blood Transfusion Centers (BTCs). Until the late 1990s, mandatory blood screening, typing and diagnosis depended entirely on serological (antigen/antibody) techniques. Implementation of Nucleic acid Amplification Technologies (NAT) for use in routine screening for HIV and HCV a few years later posed a major problem [1,2]. Today, we are at the dawn of implementation of high throughput technologies in genomics and here speculate about their application in blood testing.

Nucleic Acid Amplification Technology

Historically, Nucleic acid Amplification Technologies were only used in fundamental research. Invention of Polymerase Chain Reaction (PCR) by K. Mullis [3], with the discovery of the Taq Polymerase, was a milestone in the application of these techniques to many fields of clinical biology such as genetics and preventive and forensic medicine.

Application to diagnosis developed more slowly because of the PCR patent bought by Roche. Eventually, this obstacle accelerated the development of alternative techniques. As a result, transcription-mediated amplification (TMA), nucleic acid sequence-based amplification (NASBA), ligase chain reaction (LCR) and branched DNA appeared, distributed by other manufacturers such as GenProbe-Chiron, Organon, Abbott, and Bayer, respectively. In infectious diseases, HCV was the first virus to be identified exclusively by molecular biology and subsequently the "hepatitis" G virus (HGV; also called GB virus) and the transfusion-transmitted virus (TTV). TTV has been found in 1-5% of eligible blood donors in developed countries and is still not associated with any disease. NAT extended into many fields of clinical biology and provided a new approach to blood testing through the genotyping of blood group antigens, human leukocyte antigens (HLA) and platelet-specific antigens (HPA). Concerning viral detection, safety of blood supply was improved by the introduction of NAT in parallel with serological tests in order to detect acute HIV and HCV infections in the window phase, which are not detected by current serological assays. These technologies are based on PCR for Roche and on TMA for Chiron. The first generation assays were at best semi-automated. The second generation of NAT technologies permit identification with increased automation of emerging pathogens such as West Nile Virus (WNV), parvovirus B19 and hepatitis A virus (HAV) and permit the detection of the three major viruses (HBV, HCV and HIV) of many different genotypes in one reaction. Indeed, the modular automated format for sample preparation, amplification and detection (Cobas s200 version, Roche, and Optiva system, Chiron) is leading to fully integrated systems (Cobas s400, Roche, and Tigris, Chiron). Thus, significant technical progress has been made in the field of viral NAT with increased multiplexing to detect two or three agents simultaneously. Nevertheless, as these assays represent additional, complementary and in some cases replacement assays, they do not change the fundamental aspects of blood testing and management. A chip capable of combining microbiology tests with blood and platelet typing would offer the opportunity for re-engineering blood bank operations.

DNA Microarrays

Microarrays are potential tools for simultaneous detection and quantification of multiple nucleotide sequences present in one sample [4]. The concept of microarray (or chip) technology is a miniaturised version of the classical reverse dot blot [5]. The chips consist of a small support of glass, plastic or silicon, on which probes are immobilized at a precise position. Practically, mixtures from nucleic targets isolated from biological source samples are labeled and hybridized to their probes. The targets are generally labeled with a fluorochrome during the amplification step. After washing, hybrids are usually detected by a system consisting of a laser and a confocal microscope interfaced with a computer, but many variations exist.

Because each probe occupies a known location on the chip, the identity of each labeled hybrid can be ascertained by the signal at each position of the array. DNA chip manufacturing is achieved either by "off-chip" technology, where DNA probes have been previously synthesized before being grafted onto the substrate, or by "on-chip" technology, where probes consisting of smaller oligonucleotides - ranging in size from 10-25 bases - are chemically synthesized in situ. The probes are grafted on the substrate using a number of different technologies such as mechanical, ink jet or electrochemical depositions [6]. Arrays can be divided into three groups according to their density and the material to be analyzed. Complexity of the array is adapted to the application requirements, i.e., low density chips (Nanogen, CEA,…) bearing 100 to 1000 probes are best for diagnostic tools, medium density chips (Stanford, Synteni,…) with 1000 to 10 000 probes are more appropriate for global gene expression analysis, and high density chips (Affimetrix, Protogene,…) of more than 100 000 probes are generally used for global polymorphism analysis. Thus, it is possible to analyze a considerable number of sequences at the same time.

Other than these planar formats, microparticle-based microarrays have emerged as powerful technologies in diagnostic applications [7]. Microparticules are functionalized with DNA, protein or small-molecule probes and identified by an optical detection method. Different microparticules can be mixed in one tube, allowing a simple multiplex approach of molecular analysis. Luminex (Austin, Texas, USA) developed a single tube system where up to 100 analytes can be analysed simultaneously using a "two-colour suspension array." Polystyrene beads are embedded with different ratios of red and infrared fluorescent dyes to yield 100 unique spectral addresses. A third fluorochrome coupled to a reporter molecule is used for reaction detection. Microparticles pass in single file through two separate laser beams, simultaneously identifying the particle (and the corresponding ligand) and the extent of the reaction [8].

Protein Microarrays

For DNA chips, designing capture molecules and developing read-out systems was relatively easy. Proteins pose a much more difficult challenge. Specific capture molecules must be designed for all proteins encoded by the genome and also for the modified forms produced by processes such as phosphorylation or glycosylation [9]. There are 40 000 to 70 000 genes in the human genome, encoding 250 000 to 1 million proteins whose synthesis is regulated by 10 000 transcription factors [10,11]. Furthermore, the concentrations of different proteins in a biological sample may vary over several orders of magnitude. For example, the plasma represents the largest and deepest version of the human proteome and has an extraordinary dynamic range of more than ten orders of magnitude in concentration (from 40 mg/ml to less than 1 pg/ml) [12,13]. As observed by Anderson et al [12], finding a molecule of an analyte present at 10 pg/ml among the albumin molecules is like finding one individual human being by searching through the population of the entire world. Capture molecules on a protein chip need to bind the target with high affinity because most proteins of interest in a biological sample are present at very low concentrations. Antibodies are the classical capture molecules for proteins because they have been demonstrated to capture with high specificity and sensitivity. The last ten years have also seen progress with microarrays printed with antigens that are used for the detection of circulating antibodies in clinical specimens [14]. In general, the protein-detecting microarrays are supported by three distinct technologies: surface chemistry, production of functional capture agents and development of high-throughput detection methods [15].

Applications

Progress in microarray technology has allowed the development of nucleic acid and protein assays. Arrays with the ability to detect in parallel antigens, antibodies or nucleic acids with different specificities have a wide range of potential applications in the field of gene expression and discovery, genotyping and pathogen detection.

DNA microarrays

Gene expression and discovery

We have compared the gene expression profiles of granulocytes taken from blood donors in two different situations - before and after administration of corticoids (dexamethazone) - in order to demarginate granulocytes prior to leukocyte donations [16]. Ghodsi et al [17] reported a correlation between administration of corticoids and an increased risk of sub-capsular cataracts, thus demonstrating that this treatment could have side effects for the donors. First, the transcriptome of the granulocyte was established by the Serial Analysis of Gene Expression (SAGE) method, which allowed the identification of more than 8500 genes for this cell [16,18]. The genes were classified according to their cell function. Then, 221 highly expressed genes were selected in the SAGE library as cDNA probes to be spotted on a microarray designed and produced by Memorec Biotec GmBH (Köln, Germany). Comparison of the two profiles showed that granulocytes of blood donors stimulated with dexamethazone presented major modifications essentially in the expression of the genes involved in cell viability and immune response. Thus, the physiological role of glucocorticoids was confirmed. The "Granulochip" could also contribute similarly to a better understanding of the mechanism involved in Transfusion-Related Lung Injury (TRALI).

Genotyping

In order to increase the direct availability of typed red blood cells (RBC) and platelet (PLT) antigens, Beiboer et al [19] developed a high throughput technique to type the whole donor population for clinically relevant RBC and PLT antigens. A multiplex PCR was set up to both amplify and fluorescently label 19 gene fragments of RBC and PLT antigens in one reaction. Specific genotyping was then performed by allele-specific oligonucleotide hybridisation of the PCR products on a microarray. Hashmi et al [20] reported the use of a bead array (Bead Chip, Illumina, San Diego, CA, USA) format for typing of alleles associated with blood group antigens in order to show the feasibility of the use of large scale DNA analysis in a microarray as a substitute for blood group typing. In Canada, a commercial genotyping platform (GenomeLab SNPstream, Beckman Coulter) was used to test, in blood donors, single-nucleotide polymorphisms (SNPs) related to RBC and PLT antigens [21,22]. The limiting step in high multiplexing is not the detection step but the PCR amplification [23]. Avent et al [24] have developed as an EC funded framework consortium a genechip that is capable of defining the major clinical blood group alleles in a single test format. Alleles of the ABO, RH, KEL, FY, JK, DI, MNS, DO and CO systems have been included on the BloodGen testing platform, which includes 96 blood group alleles and eventually will include all platelet and perhaps HLA alleles of clinical significance. The BloodGen project will become commercially available within the next two years as a product of Progenika SA (www.progenika.com). Concerning pathogen detection, a genomic approach was developed in order to detect multiple viruses [25]. The cornerstone of the approach was a long oligonucleotide (70-mer) DNA microarray capable of simultaneously detecting hundreds of viruses. Related viral serotypes could be distinguished by the unique pattern of hybridization generated by each virus. Furthermore, by selecting microarray elements derived from highly conserved regions within viral families, viruses that were not explicitly represented on the array were still detected. This raises the possibility that this approach could be used for virus discovery and identification of infectious diseases of unknown etiology, as well as in instances of bioterrorism. A recent study was published as a proof of concept demonstrating the potential to use a microarray to screen bioterror pathogens in blood [26].

Protein microarrays

Protein microarrays have the potential to impact diagnostics in transfusion. A Scottish group has recently shown that an antibody microarray technology can be used to phenotype erythrocytes by detecting complex mixtures of antigens on cell surfaces [27,28].

In the field of molecular diagnostics there is a constant need for new biomarkers with improved sensitivity and specificity [29]. Many aspects of HCV infection remain enigmatic. The findings from studies of HCV among blood donors and blood product recipients have yielded and should continue to provide important insights into HCV pathogenesis [30]. Understanding the virus-host interactions that enable approximately 15% of patients with acute HCV to clear their infection is probably an important key towards the development of more effective treatment and prevention strategies. We have developed a proteomic approach using a Protein Chip Technology (SELDI-TOF-MS, Ciphergen Biosystems [31]) to identify biomarkers for resolution of acute HCV infection. Expression profiling of plasma from donors who clear their infection versus those from chronic or negative donors have been compared. Protein profiles specific for viral clearance were obtained and identifications of biomarker candidates are in progress [32].

Microarray Technology: The Future of Blood Testing?

Potential targets

Petrick [33] of the Scottish National Blood Service in Edinburgh was the first to speculate about microarrays as the future of blood testing. Indeed, he predicts that the application of this technology may revolutionize blood testing, providing an integrated platform for comprehensive donation testing and replacing multiple individual assays. He listed candidate targets for a blood-testing chip. The number of probes for blood-group typing, platelet specific and granulocyte antigens, combined with a set of probes for microbiological screening, would not exceed 300-400 at present. Since the generic background of the majority of more than 240 antigens in 25 blood group systems is known, gradual transition to nucleic acid based testing is expected. Nevertheless, there is still a danger of erroneous genotyping with some phenotypic manifestations.

However, where pathogen detection is concerned, NAT assays are complementary to serological assays. For this reason, combination of a DNA-chip with a protein based chip for blood group typing and pathogen detection is therefore most probable.

Technological advances of DNA and protein – based Chips

The most promising and impressive DNA array data to date for use in diagnostic virology have been described by DeRisi and colleagues in detection and genotyping of viral pathogens [25]. This type of microarray was used in the identification of the SARS virus as a coronavirus [34]. However, it is complicated to develop and use this format of array.

Protein arrays are being prepared with antigens or antibodies bound to a solid phase. These are immunoassays in a microarray format [14]. Almost every sandwich-based microarray-assay that has been reported is directed at the analysis of human cytokines [35]. A protein array has been described for serodiagnosis of infectious diseases [36,37]. This format provides equivalent performance to ELISA tests and offers a significant advantage in convenience and cost when compared with traditional test formats. Nevertheless, antibodies have their drawbacks, as they tend to be denatured when heated or exposed to stress such as changes in pH. Furthermore, many key antibodies and antibody technologies are covered by patents. Given these limitations, alternative technologies are in progress to develop new capture molecules, such as protein scaffolds or aptamers (Affibody, Phylos, Somalogic) [9,15].

Sensitivity and specificity requirements

As for DNA microarrays, it seems likely that a signal amplification procedure will also be necessary to achieve biologically relevant sensitivities for most proteins in microarrays. Rolling circle amplification (RCA) has been reported to permit significant increases in sensitivity for multiplexed assays on antibody microarrays. In the adaptation of RCA used for protein signal amplification, the 5' end of an oligonucleotide primer is attached to an antibody. In the presence of a DNA circle, DNA polymerase and nucleotides, the RCA generates a concatemer of circle DNA sequence copies that remain attached to the antibody. The concatemer is then detected by the hybridization of fluorescent, complementary oligonucleotide probes. When utilised on microarrays of printed antibodies, a 100-1000 fold improvement over classical detection strategies using fluorescently labeled antibodies was observed [14]. Even though tremendous progress has been made in the quality of antibody-based microarrays, several limitations remain to be overcome. Multiplexing is limited by the availability of suitable antibodies that do not cross react or interfere with other proteins. Sensitivity remains a critically important limitation for many analyses, thus actual protein based microarrays may be more useful as screening rather than diagnostic tools [3].

Quality control

Aside from the costs and the difficulties associated with designing and making a suitable array, the most obvious problems with their use are ones relating to quality control.

The difficulties arise with the need for standardization and reproducibility in the large number of probes on an array and the large number of slides that need to be made [39,40]. Before the microarray technology can be applied in clinical practice and regulatory decision making, microarray standards, quality measures and consensus on data analysis methods need to be developed. The MicroArray Quality Control (MACQ) project, involving 51 organisations, was initiated by the FDA to address these concerns [41].

Routine use of antibody microarrays in diagnostic settings will require increased availability, inexpensive and robust platforms for microarray production and detection, as well as turn-key systems for running high-throughput assays [14].

Future Technologies

Lab-on-a-chip

One of the goals in microfluidic device development is the design of a true lab-on-a-chip platform. This goal has already been achieved in the area of nucleic acids, where a few commercial systems are available [23,42]. In the protein field, development is more difficult because proteins are much more diverse in nature and the challenge of analyzing them in their biological background at physiological levels is tremendous.

Biosensors

Biosensors are small devices that utilize biological reactions for detecting target analytes. Such devices intimately couple a biological recognition element (interacting with the target analyte) with a physical transducer. Common transducing elements, including optical, eletrochemical or mass-sensitive devices, generate light, current or frequency signals, respectively [43]. Microarrays constructed with microelectromechanical systems on a micron scale are related to micromanipulation, whereas nanotechnology-based chips are on a nanoscale and enable diagnosis at the single cell and molecule levels [44]. First generation DNA microarrays rely on the labeling of samples with a fluorescent tag, a procedure that is time consuming and expensive. Furthermore, molecular fluorophores have many significant drawbacks, including susceptibility to photobleaching and broad absorption and emission bands. Nanotechnologies offer new perspectives to circumvent target amplification and fluorescence labeling [45].

An attractive alternative to the target amplification method is to amplify the signal. A new detection technology for analyzing DNA arrays using oligonucleotide-modified gold nanoparticle probes and a conventional flatbed scanner has been described by Taton et al [46]. In addition, when coupled with a signal amplification method based on nanoparticle-promoted reduction of silver, the sensitivity of this scanometric array detection system exceeds that of the analogous fluorophore system by two orders of magnitude [46]. This technology, offering simplicity and sensitivity, could provide a useful approach for clinical diagnostic development with optical readout. Recently, Storhoff et al [47] demonstrated that specific DNA sequences within bacterial or human genomic DNA samples are detectable without target amplification or complexity reduction using this methodology.

Quantum Dots (QDs) have emerged as new class of fluorescent labels. These semiconductor nanocrystals with their broad excitation spectra and sharp emission spectra are potential candidates for replacing conventional fluorescent markers in biodetection assays [45,48,49]. QDs can be specifically attached to biological materials such as nucleic acids and proteins, making them powerful tagging agents [44]. Resonance Light Scattering (RLS) technology exploits submicroscopic gold or silver particles that scatter incident white light to generate monochromatic intense colored light viewed with the naked eye. This technology is up to 1 000 000 times more sensitive than current fluorescence signaling technology and does not require computer-enhanced imaging of data [44]. RLS technology can be applied to studies on microarrays.

Over the past 10 years, many important technological advances have been made in the development of biosensors using optical readout. Electrochemical transducers have received considerable recent attention to the detection of DNA hybridization. The electrochemical biosensors promise to provide simple, accurate and inexpensive platforms for diagnosis. The high sensitivity of such devices coupled to portability, low cost, and independence of sample turbidity or optical pathway make them excellent candidates for DNA diagnostics [43] or immuno-assays [50,51].

Biobarcode amplification assays

An innovative nanotech tool for ultra sensitive detection of detecting protein or DNA analytes has been developed by C. Mirkin and collaborators. Concerning DNA analytes, a PCR-less target DNA amplification method was developed that relies on novel two-component oligonucleotide-modified gold nanoparticles (NPs) and single-component oligonucleotide-modified microparticles, followed by detection of amplified DNA in the form of barcode DNA using a chip-based detection method [52]. Part of the technology's simplicity stems from its ability to detect targets without the use of enzymes [53,54]. The protein detection technique [55] uses barcode DNA as well, but antibodies against the target protein are tethered to the particle probes instead of complementary DNA. Because the nanoparticle probe carries with it a large number of oligonucleotide barcodes per protein binding event, there is substantial amplification, and antigen can be detected at 30 attomolar concentrations. This level of detection is 6 orders of magnitude more sensitive than conventional assays. A particular and promising application for the technique may be early detection of HIV in blood samples or assessment of patients taking antiretroviral drugs that suppress viral replication to levels undetectable by conventional tests. Recently, a multiplexed DNA detection with biobarcoded nanoparticle probes was published [56]. This feasibility study opens the way to high-throughput multiplexed DNA detection by avoiding a preliminar target amplification step.

Conclusion

Chip technology is rapidly advancing many fields, such as gene discovery, gene expression and genotyping. In blood testing, rather than continuing the trend of an ever increasing number of assays in the pursuit of zero risk policies, which results in a considerable cost increase, microarrays combined with nanomaterials will permit a conceptually new approach. Integrated platforms for pathogen detection, blood typing and platelet assays represent a real potential to revolutionize blood testing. However, complete, walk-away automation is years away !

References

1 Assal A, Coste J, Barlet V, et al: Application of molecular biology to blood transfusion safety: the nucleic acid testing. Transfus Clin Biol 2003; 10: 217-226.

2 Coste J, Levayer T, Izopet J, et al: Acute HCV infection detected in a blood donor by NAT. Transfusion 2003; 43: 116-118.

3 Mullis K, Faloona F, Scharf S, Saiki R, Horn G, Erlich H: Specific enzymatic amplification of DNA in vitro: the polymerase chain reaction. Cold Spring Harb Symp Quant Biol 1986; 51 Pt 1: 263-273.

4 Heller MJ: DNA microarray technology: devices, systems, and applications. Annu Rev Biomed Eng 2002; 4: 129-153.

5 Southern E, Mir K, Shchepinov M: Molecular interactions on microarrays. Nat Genet 1999; 21: 5-9.

6 Cuzin M: DNA chips: a new tool for genetic analysis and diagnostics. Transf Clin Biol 2001; 8: 291-296.

7 Petrik J: Diagnostic applications of microarrays. Transfus Med 2006; 16: 233-247.

8 Dunbar SA: Applications of Luminex xMAP technology for rapid, high-throughput multiplexed nucleic acid detection. Clin Chim Acta 2006; 363: 71-82.

9 Abbott A: Betting on tomorrow's chips. Nature 2002; 415: 112-114.

10 Harrison PM, Kumar A, Lang N, Snyder M, Gerstein M: A question of size: the eukaryotic proteome and the problems in defining it. Nucleic Acids Res 2002; 30: 1083-1090.

11 Kiechle FL, Holland-Staley CA: Genomics, transcriptomics, proteomics, and numbers. Arch Pathol Lab Med 2003; 127: 1089-1097.

12 Anderson NL, Anderson NG: The human plasma proteome: history, character, and diagnostic prospects. Mol Cell Proteomics 2002; 1: 845-867.

13 Lathrop JT, Hayes TK, Carrick K, Hammond DJ: Rarity gives a charm: evaluation of trace proteins in plasma and serum. Expert Rev Proteomics 2005; 2: 393-406.

14 Schweitzer B, Kingsmore SF: Measuring proteins on microarrays. Curr Opin Biotechnol 2002;13:14-19.

15 Tomizaki KY, Usui K, Mihara H Protein-detecting microarrays: current accomplishments and requirements. Chembiochem 2005; 6: 782-799.

16 Bertrand G, Coste J, Segarra C, Schved JF, Commes T, Marti J: Use of serial analysis of gene expression (SAGE) technology reveals new granulocytic markers. J Immunol Methods 2004; 292: 43-58.

17 Ghodsi Z, Strauss RG: Cataracts in neutrophil donors stimulated with adrenal corticosteroids. Transfusion 2001; 41: 1464-1468.

18 Bertrand G, Duprat E, Lefranc MP, Marti J, Coste J: Characterization of human FCGR3B*02 (HNA-1b, NA2) cDNAs and IMGT standardized description of FCGR3B alleles. Tissue Antigens 2004; 64: 119-131.

19 Beiboer SH, Wieringa-Jelsma T, Maaskant-Van Wijk PA, et al: Rapid genotyping of blood group antigens by multiplex polymerase chain reaction and DNA microarray hybridization. Transfusion 2005; 45: 667-679.

20 Hashmi G, Shariff T, Seul M, et al: A flexible array format for large-scale, rapid blood group DNA typing. Transfusion 2005; 45: 680-688.

21 Denomme GA, Van Oene M High-throughput multiplex single-nucleotide polymorphism analysis for red cell and platelet antigen genotypes. Transfusion 2005; 45: 660-666.

22 Montpetit A, Phillips MS, Mongrain I, Lemieux R, St-Louis M: High-throughput molecular profiling of blood donors for minor red blood cell and platelet antigens. Transfusion 2006; 46: 841-848.

23 Csako G: Present and future of rapid and/or high-throughput methods for nucleic acid testing. Clin Chim Acta 2006; 363: 6-31.

24 Avent D, Martinez A, Flegel W, et al: The bloodgen project : toward mass scale genotyping for human blood group antigens. Vox Sanguinis 2006; 91: 33.

25 Wang D, Coscoy L, Zylberberg M, et al: Microarray-based detection and genotyping of viral pathogens. Proc Natl Acad Sci U S A 2002; 99: 15687-15692.

26 Tomioka K, Peredelchuk M, Zhu X, et al: A multiplex polymerase chain reaction microarray assay to detect bioterror pathogens in blood. J Mol Diagn 2005; 7: 486-494.

27 Campbell CJ, O'Looney N, Chong Kwan M, et al: Cell interaction microarray for blood phenotyping. Anal Chem 2006; 78: 1930-1938.

28 Robb JS, Roy DJ, Ghazal P, Allan J, Petrik J: Development of non-agglutination microarray blood grouping. Transfus Med 2006; 16: 119-129.

29 Zolg JW, Langen H: How industry is approaching the search for new diagnostic markers and biomarkers. Mol Cell Proteomics 2004; 3: 345-354.

30 Busch MP: Insights into the epidemiology, natural history and pathogenesis of hepatitis C virus infection from studies of içnfected donors and blood product recipients. Transfus Clin Biol 2001; 8: 200-206.

31 Issaq HJ, Conrads TP, Prieto DA, Tirumalai R, Veenstra TD: SELDI-TOF MS for diagnostic proteomics. Anal Chem 2003; 75: 148A-155A.

32 Molina S, Maurel P, Coste J, Fournier-Wirth C: Recherche par une approche protéomique de biomarqueurs associés à la résolution de l'infection par le virus de lhépatite C. Transfus Clin Biol 2005; 12: S45.

33 Petrik J: Microarray technology: the future of blood testing? Vox Sang 2001; 80: 1-11.

34 Rota PA, Oberste MS, Monroe SS, et al: Characterization of a novel coronavirus associated with severe acute respiratory syndrome. Science 2003; 300: 1394-1399.

35 MacBeath G: Protein microarrays and proteomics. Nat Genet 2002; 32 Suppl: 526-532.

36 Mezzasoma L, Bacarese-Hamilton T, Di Cristina M, Rossi R, Bistoni F, Crisanti A: Antigen microarrays for serodiagnosis of infectious diseases. Clin Chem 2002; 48: 121-130.

37 Bacarese-Hamilton T, Mezzasoma L, Ardizzoni A, Bistoni F, Crisanti A: Serodiagnosis of infectious diseases with antigen microarrays. J Appl Microbiol 2004; 96: 10-17.

38 Kingsmore SF, Patel DD: Multiplexed protein profiling on antibody-based microarrays by rolling circle amplification. Curr Opin Biotechnol 2003; 14: 74-81.

39 Clewley JP: A role for arrays in clinical virology: fact or fiction? J Clin Virol 2004; 29: 2-12.

40 Loy A, Bodrossy L: Highly parallel microbial diagnostics using oligonucleotide microarrays. Clin Chim Acta 2006; 363: 106-119.

41 Shi L, Reid LH, Jones WD, et al: The MicroArray Quality Control (MAQC) project shows inter- and intraplatform reproducibility of gene expression measurements. Nat Biotechnol 2006; 24: 1151-1161.

42 Liu RH, Yang J, Lenigk R, Bonanno J, Grodzinski P: Self-contained, fully integrated biochip for sample preparation, polymerase chain reaction amplification, and DNA microarray detection. Anal Chem 2004; 76: 1824-1831.

43 Wang J: Electrochemical nucleic acid biosensors. Analytica Chimica Acta 2002; 469: 63-71.

44 Jain KK: Nanotechnology in clinical laboratory diagnostics. Clin Chim Acta 2005; 358: 37-54.

45 Rosi NL, Mirkin CA: Nanostructures in biodiagnostics. Chem Rev. 2005; 105: 1547-1562.

46 Taton TA, Mirkin CA, Letsinger RL. Scanometric DNA array detection with nanoparticle probes. Science 2000; 289: 1757-1760.

47 Storhoff JJ, Marla SS, Bao P, et al: Gold nanoparticle-based detection of genomic DNA targets on microarrays using a novel optical detection system. Biosens Bioelectron 2004; 19: 875-883.

48 Arya H, Kaul Z, Wadhwa R, Taira K, Hirano T, Kaul SC: Quantum dots in bio-imaging: Revolution by the small. Biochem Biophys Res Commun 2005; 329: 1173-1177.

49 Fortina P, Kricka LJ, Surrey S, Grodzinski P: Nanobiotechnology: the promise and reality of new approaches to molecular recognition. Trends Biotechnol 2005; 23: 168-173.

50 Helali S, Martelet C, Abdelghani A, Maaref MA, Jaffrezic-Renault N: A disposable immunomagnetic electrochemical sensor based on magnetic beads on gold surface for the detection of atrazine. Electrochemica Acta 2006; 51: 5181-5186.

51 Radke SM, Alocilja EC: A high density microelectrode array biosensor for detection of E. coli O157:H7. Biosens Bioelectron 2005; 20: 1662-1667.

52 Nam JM, Park SJ, Mirkin CA: Bio-barcodes based on oligonucleotide-modified nanoparticles. J Am Chem Soc 2002; 124: 3820-3821.

53 Hampton T: Nanotech group's "bio-barcode" test a promising diagnostic, research tool. Jama 2004;292:1291-1293.

54 Nam JM, Stoeva SI, Mirkin CA: Bio-bar-code-based DNA detection with PCR-like sensitivity. J Am Chem Soc 2004;126:5932-5933.

55 Nam JM, Thaxton CS, Mirkin CA: Nanoparticle-based bio-bar codes for the ultrasensitive detection of proteins. Science 2003;301:1884-1886.

56 Stoeva SI, Lee JS, Thaxton CS, Mirkin CA: Multiplexed DNA detection with biobarcoded nanoparticle probes. Angew Chem Int Ed Engl 2006;45:3303-3306.

Dr. J. Coste, Transfusion Transmitted Infectious Diseases R&D Unit, EFS Pyrénées Méditerranée, FR-34094 Montpellier, France. E-mail: joliette.coste@efs.sante.fr

Dax EM, Farrugia A, Vyas G (eds): Advances in Transfusion Safety – Volume IV.
Dev Biol (Basel). Basel, Karger, 2007, vol 127, pp 71-86.

The Utility of Multiplex NAT in Blood Screening

D. Candotti[1], *J.-P. Allain*[2]

[1] National Blood Service, Cambridge Blood Centre, Cambridge, UK
[2] Dept of Haematology, University of Cambridge, Cambridge, UK

Key words: NAT, bloodborne viruses, blood safety, multiplex

INTRODUCTION

Blood screening is characterized by large throughput of samples containing rare markers of infectious agents that compromise the safety of the recipients. In order to remain cost-effective, screening requires maximum sensitivity to identify low concentration of the targeted markers but also very high specificity in order to limit the deferral of units erroneously identified as infectious. With the considerable progresses made over the last 20 years in both of these critical parameters as well as in the automation of the screening process, the performance of serological assays detecting markers such as HBsAg, anti-HIV, and anti-HCV has reduced the risk of transmission by transfusion of the corresponding agents in a range of 1:50,000 to 1:1.5M. As a result, further risk reduction addressing the window period of infectivity preceding the detectability of serological markers or, in the case of HBV, following the disappearance of a detectable serological marker, has been characterized by an extremely low cost-effectiveness. Despite a situation in which the cost per Quality Adjusted Life Year (QALY) exceeded $ 1M instead of the generally accepted $ 50,000 threshold, the government and public willingness to pay for "no risk" blood encouraged transfusion scientists and diagnostic companies to develop genomic screening for the main infectious viral agents (HBV, HIV, HCV) and others such as human erythrovirus (HErV, formerly parvovirus B19), West Nile virus or Hepatitis A virus. The considerable cost of these new technologies, to a large extent related to patent charges, instigated the development of several options intended to reduce the cost of nucleic acid testing (NAT). Plasma pooling ranging between 8 and 500 samples had the disadvantage of reducing sensitivity, an inconvenience partially reduced in some cases by procedures aiming at concentrating the targeted agents. Multiplexing, a procedure enabling simultaneous screening for two-four nucleic acid targets, was developed. This approach reduces reagent costs, the volume of sample to process, and the time required to obtain results, but at the same time considerably complicates the already multi-step and delicate methods developed for single agent NAT. This review will describe the multiplexes currently available commercially or developed internally by a range of transfusion or regulatory establishments, as well as review the various technical problems attached to this type of methods and provide some examples of their clinical applications.

Multiplex Assays in Blood Screening

Over the past decade, several studies demonstrated the feasibility and efficiency of detecting and identifying viral pathogens in different clinical and epidemiological settings using multiplex NAT (Table 1). In the transfusion setting, multiplex NAT presents a practicable solution to the problem of rapid screening of large numbers of blood donations per day for multiple transfusion-transmitted viruses. NAT methodology proves to be sensitive enough to detect serologically silent viral infections, including human immunodeficiency virus (HIV), hepatitis C virus (HCV), hepatitis B virus (HBV) and human T-lymphotropic virus (HTLV). Most of the multiplex assays for blood borne virus described so far were diagnostic in-house assays; only a few were commercially developed for large-scale blood product screening. These assays are able to simultaneously detect two to four viral genomes (DNA and/or RNA). Few of them included an internal control of amplification. The viruses targeted were mainly HBV, HCV, and HIV-$1_{M, N, O}$, and to a lesser extent HIV-2, GBV-C and HTLV-I and HTLV-II (Table 2).

Multiplex assays relied on different methods for the amplification of viral DNA and/or RNA and the detection of the amplified sequences (amplicons) (Table 2). Multiplexing has been successfully applied to the most commonly used genomic amplification methods, including conventional polymerase chain reaction (PCR) or reverse transcription-polymerase chain reaction (RT-PCR) [1-4], real-time (RT)-PCR [5-10]; isothermal nucleic acid sequence-based amplification (NASBA) [11] and transcription-mediated amplification (TMA) assays [12,13].

Characteristics of the Different Multiplex Assays

In multiplex conventional (RT)-PCR assays, amplified products were detected and identified according to size differences after electrophoretic separation on agarose gel [1,14]. To increase sensitivity and specificity, nested-PCR that includes a second round of amplification was used, resulting in an increased risk of cross-contamination by the manipulation of amplified products [14]. To avoid the risk introduced by a second amplification step, specific oligonucleotide probes were used in association with different labelling and detection methods of the hybridized targets. Several methods have been described and can be classified in two groups according to the type of amplification signal generated.

The first group includes multiplex assays providing a single test signal. That is the case for assays using 5'-biotinylated probes and PCR ELISA DIG detection [4], LCx fluorometric detection [7], chemoluminescent probes to detect TMA-based amplification products [12,13], and fluorescent TaqMan probes in real-time PCR

Table 1 : Multiplex viral genome detection for blood screening.

Author	Year	Targeted genomes	Amplification system	Detection system	Internal control	Sample type & volume (µl)	Sensitivity/ml	Genotypes
Caudai	1998	HCV, GBV-C	RT-PCR	Gel	No	Plasma 100	7.8E2	
Vet	1999	HIV-1, HIV-2 HTLV-I, HTLV-II	QPCR	Multiple dyes	No	Whole blood 200	10 copies HIV-1 HIV-2 HTLV-II	A-G A, D, SD A, B
Mercier	1999	HCV, HBV	RT-QPCR	Multiple dyes	No	Plasma 200	50 copies	
Defoort	2000	HIV-1, HCV, HBV	RT-PCR	Flow cytometry	No	Plasma 100	0.4-1.2E5	
Meng	2001	HIV-1, HCV, HBV	RT-QPCR	Single signal	Yes	Plasma 200	HBV 22-60 IU HCV 61-112 IU HIV 33-66 IU	A-E 1-5 A-G
De Baar	2001	HIV-1 M, N, O	NASBA	Multiple dyes	No	Plasma 200	10 copies	
Abravaya	2001	HIV-1 M, O, HIV-2	LCR	Single signal	Yes	Plasma 1000	HIV-1 50 copies HIV-2 10 copies	A-G, O
Candotti	2003	HIV-1, HCV	TMA	Single signal	Yes	Plasma 500	HIV-1 15-20 IU HCV 16-18 IU	A-E 1-4
Adami	2004	HIV-1, HCV	RT-PCR	Single signal	No	Plasma 200	HIV-1 100 IU HCV 200 IU	
Candotti	2004	HIV-1, HCV, HBV	RT-QPCR	Multiple dyes	No	Plasma 200	HIV-1 680 IU HCV 167 IU HBV 30 IU	A-G 1-6 A-F
Koppelman	2005	HIV-1, HCV, HBV	TMA	Single signal	Yes	Plasma 500	HIV-1 26 IU HCV 4.6 IU HBV 11 IU	A-G
Dineva	2005	HIV-1, HIV-2, HBV	RT-QPCR	Specific bands	No	Plasma 200	HIV-1 HCV HBV	A-F 1-6 A-G

Table 2 : Clinical data collected by multiplex in plasma pools or single donations.

Author	**Country**	**Type sample**	**N samples**	**System**	**IR (%)**	**CR (%)**	**HCV RNA**		**HIV RNA**		**HBV DNA**		**Specificity (%)**
							Sero +	Sero -	Sero +	Sero -	Sero +	Sero -	
Candotti, 2003	UK	ID	50,000	Procleix	0.28	0.06	29	0	2	0	ND	ND	100
Ren, 2005	China	P16	80,791	Procleix		0.18	119	2	22	0			100
Fang, 2004	South Africa	ID	19,709	Procleix		0.83	2	0	159	2			
Mison, 2003	Australia	P24	1,1M 326,477	Procleix	0.37 0.09	0.33 0.01	149 41	4 0	0 0	2 2			100 100
Vargo, 2002	USA	P16	192,288	Procleix	1.46	1.14							> 99.7
Coste, 2005	Belgium	P8	596,052	Procleix		0.0003		2		0			99.97
	Hong Kong	P16	272,959			0.0004		0		1			> 99.9
Mine, 2001	Japan	P50	16M	AMPLINAT	0.28	0.10		46		6		308	99.8
Koppelman, 2005	Europe	P8	2192	Ultrio	0.55	0.38	5	0	0	0	0	6	99.8
Owusu-Ofori, 2005	Ghana	P10	517	In house	9.9	7.7	11	0	1	0	8	27	97.9

assay [8]. These assays are unable to discriminate between the viruses detected in the sample tested, and a secondary diagnostic step using virus-specific individual amplification is necessary to identify the origin of the initial test signal.

The second group includes assays that provide simultaneous detection and direct identification of multiplex-amplified DNA/RNA. These assays have been developed using conventional RT-PCR, NASBA, and, more frequently, real-time (RT)-PCR. Direct identification of amplified products has been obtained using flow cytometer microsphere-based hybridization assay [2]. However, the whole process involves separate amplification and detection steps that are labour-intensive and time-consuming. Recently, Dineva et al described a rapid, simple, and instrument-independent method for the visual detection and identification of multiple nucleic acid amplicons by probe-mediated hybridization on a dipstick membrane [10]. Real-time (RT)-PCR and NASBA methods present the benefits of single-step 'closed' systems that do not require post-amplification detection procedures, minimizing the risk of carry-over contamination, and have an increased speed due to reduced cycle time and the use of fluorogenic labels associated to sensitive signal detection [5,6,9,11]. Initially, the transfer of real-time amplification to a multiplex format was limited by the number of fluorophores available due to the common use of a monochromatic energising light source. Excitation by a single wavelength restricts the number of fluorophores that can be included in the reaction and the ability to directly distinguish different amplified targets [8,15]. However, the development of real-time multiplex PCR assays that provide direct, single step identification of viral genomes was achieved by taking advantage of two recent technical improvements: first, the development of dark or "black-hole" non-fluorescent quenchers that increase the number of fluorophores available with minimum overlap between emission spectra, and second, the recent introduction of real-time PCR platforms that incorporate either multiple light-emitting diodes to span the entire visible spectrum or a tungsten light source emitting light over a broad range of wavelengths (350-750 nm) associated to photomultiplier tubes with a detection range of 350-830 nm [16]. Taking advantage of these innovations, it is possible to include in a reaction up to four spectrally discernable fluorescent oligoprobes to achieve immediate identification of different amplified targets [6,9,11]. Continuous improvements to the design and chemistry of oligoprobes enhance the ability to discriminate an increasing number of targets. Ultimately, by combining fluorescence emission spectra and temperature melting (T_m) curve analysis, the number of distinguishable products might in theory be equal to the number of discernable dyes times the number of separable oligoprobe T_ms [17].

Real-Time Multiplex (RT)-PCR

Most of the multiplex assays for viral nucleic acid screening reported in the literature are based on real-time (RT)-PCR (Table 1). Real-time amplification seems to be widely accepted due to its sensitivity, improved rapidity and reduced result turnaround, and the reduced risk of carry-over contamination as mentioned above. The increased speed of real-time PCR is essentially due to reduced cycle times sufficient to amplify short size products (60-120 nucleotides), removal of post-amplification detection procedures, and the use of fluorogenic labels and sensitive methods to detect light emissions. Five major chemistries based on amplicon specific or non-specific methods are currently used for real-time PCR detection [18]. One of the most commonly used real-time methods relies upon 5' endonuclease oligoprobe and fluorescence resonance energy transfer (FRET) [18,19]. This technology has been extensively used for single qualitative and quantitative detection of viral genomes, but its transfer to a multiplex format may be problematic. Ideally, in a multiplex reaction, each target should be amplified with similar efficiency. Primers and probes design, selection of fluorophores, the use of a hot-start DNA polymerase, and assay optimization are important factors to consider. A trial-and-error approach appears to be the only way to optimize the different parameters when developing a multiplex assay.

The presence of several primer pairs and probes in a multiplex assay increases the possibility of synthesizing spurious amplification products due to unspecific priming and primer-primer and primer-probe interactions that may result in poor sensitivity or specificity and/or preferential amplification of specific targets. To limit this risk, primers and probes should be designed to avoid self-complementarity, hairpin formation, and significant homology to one another. In contrast, they should have nearly identical optimum annealing temperatures (59° C - 68° C), length between 18 and 30 bp, and GC content of 30-60 %. These requirements may be difficult to combine with the need of targeting conserved sequences when designing primers/probes for the detection of hypervariable RNA viruses such as retroviruses and flaviviruses. Despite the increasing number of softwares available for primer and oligoprobe design, there is no sure means to predict the performance of primers/probes other than testing them. In addition, it may be valuable to adjust the concentration of each primer set and probe for each locus to compensate for differences in annealing efficiency during the critical first cycles of PCR, which may result in a preferential amplification, consuming reaction components and producing impaired rates for the other reactions.

The choice of the fluorophores may also be critical to limit interference in the detection of the different amplified targets. The fluorophore emission spectra should be discernable from each other with minimum overlapping. As mentioned above, this is now easily achievable according to the recent development of multiplex PCR platforms using a light source that emits over a broad range of wavelengths.

The utilization of hot start polymerases, which are activated by heating the reaction at ~ 95°C for 10 min, proved to be an efficient solution to eliminate non-specific reactions caused by primer annealing at low temperature before the first denaturation step. In addition, it has been reported that increasing the amount of enzyme in the reaction could enhance multiplex amplification efficiency [20,21]. It may also be necessary to optimize other essential PCR components, including deoxyribonucleoside triphosphates (dNTPs), divalent ions (Mg^{2+}), and PCR buffer constituents, even if it has been rarely reported to significantly improve the efficiency of multiplexing [22,23].

Despite accurate optimization of multiplexing conditions, the ability of a multiplex assay to detect low concentrations of a viral genome in the presence of another abundant viral genome may still be affected. In a previous study using a multiplex HBV/HCV/HIV-1 assay, we reported that detection of low HBV DNA load was not affected by the co-amplification of high load of either HCV or HIV-1 RNA and vice-versa [9]. In contrast, there was evidence of competition between the two viral RNA amplifications that mainly affected the yield of HIV-1 amplification. In that case, HIV-1 detection was delayed rather than inhibited. However, using an optimized real-time multiplex HBV/HHV-8/HErV PCR assay to test individual plasma samples, we observed that HErV DNA detection (~10^3 IU/ml) was inhibited by the rapid and efficient co-amplification of a high load of HBV DNA (~10^7 IU/ml), showing that competition within a multiplex assay might produce a false-negative result (unpublished data). Consequently, in the presence of high viral load, it is recommended to test for eventual multiple infections using separate single PCR.

Real-time PCR using 5' nuclease oligoprobe may generate non-reproducible low fluorescence signals with generally no confirmation of specific amplicons in the corresponding sample [9]. Using different multiplex assays for viral DNA and/or RNA detection, these low signals are observed randomly above 38 cycles of amplification and are not related to a specific combination of fluorophore and quencher, nor to a specific viral sequence as shown in Figure 1. Apparently, such a signal results from background fluorescence due to the unspecific degradation of the probe. Consequently, specificity of the real-time PCR decreases with an increasing risk of a false-positive result above 38-40 cycles of amplification depending on the assay as reported by several groups [9,24,25]. To limit this risk of a false-positive result, it is useful to define a virus-specific amplification cycle cut-off providing a predictive value > 95 % by analyzing the ratio between confirmed positive and false positive results beyond a certain number of amplification cycles [9]. In addition, it is necessary to use a specific and sensitive confirmatory assay to differentiate between false positive and low positive results obtained with the real-time assay.

Internal Control

Negative amplification test results do not necessary indicate absence of infection unless the effectiveness of every step during the assay process has been controlled. Relatively simple commercial procedures provide viral nucleic acids of reasonable purity from plasma, serum and whole blood. Both viral DNA and RNA can be efficiently extracted simultaneously using their ability to bind specifically to the surface of glass fibers or silica-gel membranes in the presence of a chaotropic salt [26], or using magnetic microsphere particules coated with specific capture probes [27]. Nevertheless, extracted specimens may still contain impurities that inhibit reverse transcription and/or nucleic acid amplification. The inclusion of an internal control in the assay is an essential approach to achieving a higher degree of confidence in negative results. The internal control should be added prior to sample processing to control for nucleic acid recovery, presence of inhibitors in the extracted samples, and technical errors [28]. Interestingly, an internal control is included in all commercial multiplex NAT assays [12,13,29], but in only a few in-house developed assays [7,14]. The more usual approach consists of adding small quantities of cloned DNA or in vitro RNA transcripts unrelated to the multiplex targets. DNA internal controls are generally used because of their stability in plasma compared to exogenous RNA sequences. However, their use for RNA virus PCR fails to validate the effectiveness of cDNA synthesis, which is one critical step to be affected by inhibitors carried over during the extraction process. The use of RNA transcripts can be also problematic due to the difficulty of quantifying and purifying them from contaminating DNA sequences from which they are transcribed. Long-term storage in the ubiquitous presence of RNAses may also be a problem and affect the reproducibility of the

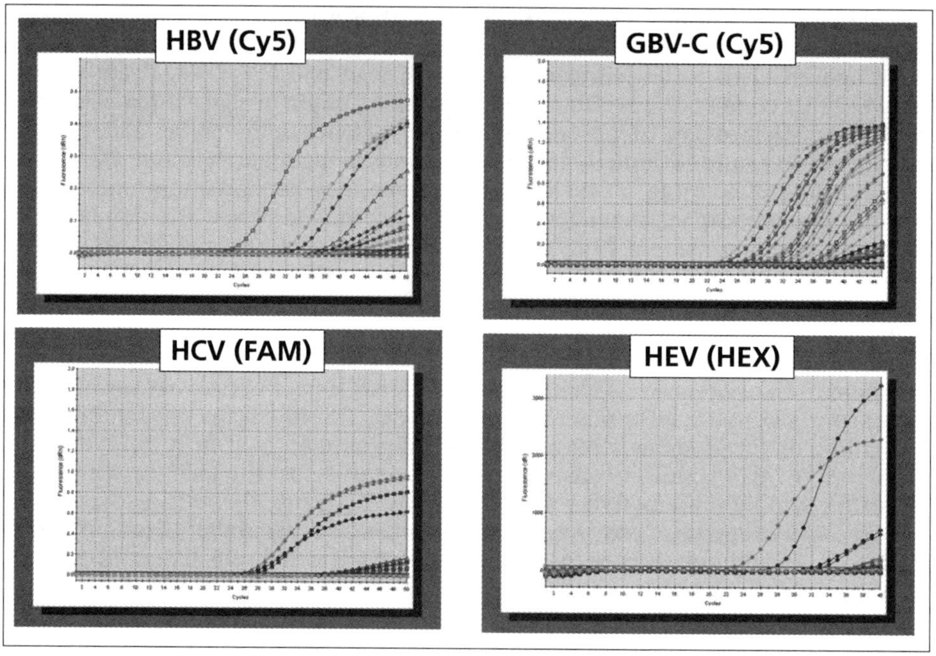

Fig. 1: Amplification plots generated with different multiplex (RT)-PCR assays from different samples containing HBV DNA, HCV RNA, GBV-C RNA, or human erythrovirus (HEV) DNA. HBV (Cy5 signal) and HCV (FAM signal) amplification signals were obtained using a multiplex HBV/HCV/HIV-1 real-time RT-PCR assay; GBV-C (Cy5 signal) and HEV (HEX signal) amplification signals were obtained using a multiplex GBV-C/West Nile virus/Dengue virus real-time RT-PCR and a HBV/HHV-8/HEV real-time PCR, respectively; the x-axis is the time from the initiation of the amplification; the y-axis is the increase in fluorescence (dRn); threshold fluorescence is shown as the horizontal line.

assays. To overcome this difficulty, armoured RNA technology was successfully developed to produce homogeneous and non-infectious ribonuclease-resistant viral RNA controls [30,31]. The sequence of most internal controls is generally similar to that of the amplification target and may share some of the primer-binding regions but show an altered sequence between these regions. Virus and control amplicons can then be differentiated by hybridization with specific probes [27,28,32]. However, amplification of homologous internal control may compete with target amplification and affect the test sensitivity. A more relevant approach is to add an unrelated DNA or RNA virus as internal control during sample processing. Human or non-infectious non-human virus packaged into virions can be selected to have similar physicochemical properties than the target viruses but no sequence similarity to avoid PCR competition. In addition, virions can be easily produced in in vitro culture and viral stocks can be accurately quantified. This strategy has been successfully applied by some authors using bovine viral diarrhoea virus [3], lambda phage [33], chimeric swine fever virus [34] (Hofmann, 2003) or HTLV-I (Candotti et al, unpublished data).

Application of Multiplex NAT to Large-Scale Blood Donation Screening

HBV, HCV and HIV-1 infections constitute the main residual risk of transfusion-transmitted viral infections due to the pre-seroconversion window period, infection with immunovariant viruses, immunosilent carriage, or occult carriage in the case of HBV infection [35-39]. NAT methods have been successfully developed to reduce these risks and their feasibility, and high level of performance in screening blood donations have been demonstrated. Consequently, large-scale screening of donated blood for transfusion-transmitted viruses is increasingly implemented in Western countries despite the fact that it remains controversial considering an extremely poor cost-effectiveness related to the very low prevalence of these viruses in Western blood donor populations [40]. As mentioned above, multiplex assays have the potential not only to improve cost-effectiveness but also to save time and effort without compromising the test efficiency and feasibility [23]. However, only a limited number of studies have reported on commercial or in-house multiplex NAT assays routinely used to detect and identify HBV, HCV and HIV-1 in blood donations. These are summarized below and in Table 3.

The commercial semi-automated Duplex HIV-1/HCV TMA Procleix assay is actually used for routine blood screening in several European countries (Belgium, England, France, Germany, Greece, Italy, Spain), USA, Australia, Hong Kong, and South Africa [41], and is currently under evaluation in China [42]. Clinical evaluations performed by testing individual donations and plasma mini-pools of various sizes (8, 16 and 24 plasmas per pool) showed optimal specificity (> 99%) and high sensitivity for HIV-$1_{M,O}$ (~30 IU/ml) and HCV genotypes 1-6 (~ 10 IU/ml) [12, 41-45]. When mini-pool testing is performed, these limits of detection decrease by a factor equivalent to the number of plasmas included in the pool [46]. However, the comparison of the performance of mini-pool testing (46,387 24-plasma pools) with individual testing (326,477 plasmas) showed only minor differences that did not significantly impact the overall efficiency of the multiplex testing or the timely release of the products [45]. This unexpectedly low difference in efficacy for detecting these two viruses is related to the fact that yield cases are almost exclusively limited to the pre-seroconversion window period. For HIV and HCV, the viral load during the window period ranges between 10^4 and 10^7, a level detected in pools of 24 or below (detection limit $5x10^3$ IU/ml). The 'ramp-up' period during which the viral load increases from undetectable to a plateau is brief (doubling times < 24h) so that the period of time during which single unit testing is more sensitive than mini pool is reduced to one or two days [47]. Several studies reported a test failure rate between < 1 % and 4.7 % related to human error, minute contaminations, and equipment malfunction at the nucleic acid extraction stage [12,41,45]. Implementation of mini-pool NAT (multiplex and single) has been reported to reduce the residual risk of HIV-1 and HCV transmission to 0.5 per million [48]. Overall large-scale clinical studies conducted in Western countries and Hong Kong indicate a rate of HIV-1 and HCV RNA positive/antibody negative samples of 0-0.0006 % and 0-0.0004 %, respectively. In contrast, a significantly higher yield of NAT-only reactive samples (0.01-0.04 % HIV and/or HCV positive) was observed in high endemic areas such as South Africa and Ghana [44,49]. Preliminary data from China obtained by screening 16-plasma pools identified two HCV and no HIV-1 yield cases among 80,259 seronegative donations [42].

Table 3 : Multiplex for virologic diagnostic.

Author	System	Viral target	Internal control	Samples	Equipment
Druce, 2002	Nested QPCR	HSV1, HSV 2, VZV, CMV	No		
Kirschberg, 2004	PCR	HBV genotype A-F	No	Serum	
Safronetz, 2003	QPCR, melting curve	HHV-6A, HHV-6B, HHV-7	No	Tissue	Lightcycler
Del Mar, 2002	RT-PCR	MeV, RUBV, B19V	No	Clinical samples	Promega
Templeton, 2004	QPCR	Influenza A, Influenza B, RSV PIV1, PIV2, PIV3, PIV4	No No	Clinical respiratory samples	iCycler IQ
Tucker, 2001	QPCR	PPV6, PPV11, PPV16, PPV18	No	Cervical fluid	ABI Prism 7700
Klein, 2001	RT-QPCR	FIV subtypes	No	Plasma	ABI Prism 7700
O'Neill, 2003	QPCR, melting curve	HSV1, HSV2, VZV	No	Clinical samples	Lightcycler
Beuret, 2004	QPCR, melting curve	NV1, NV2, enterovirus, astrovirus	No	Clinical samples	Lightcycler
Boivin, 2004	QPCR, melting curve	Influenza A, Influenza B, HRSV	No	Respiratory tract	Lightcycler
Scheltinga, 2005	QPCR	HMPV, RRSV	Yes	Respiratory tract	iCycler IQ

From February 2000, HBV, HCV and HIV-1 multiplex NAT screening of pools of 500 then 50 serologically negative plasmas was implemented by the Japanese Red Cross blood transfusion services with results reported within one day after donation [26]. The assay used, AMPLINAT MPX, consisted of virus extraction and target sequence-specific probe capture and multiplex amplification and detection by TaqMan PCR with inclusion of an internal control. The 95 % detection limits are 22-60 copies/ml for HBV DNA, 61-112 copies/ml for HCV RNA, and 33-66 copies/ml for HIV-1 RNA using a specimen input volume of 0.2 ml. This assay detected a broad range of genotypes or subtypes for all three viruses with a specificity of 99.6 %. Using seroconversion panels, Meng et al reported that the AMPLINAT MPX assay detected HBV DNA 24 days before the detection of HBsAg, HCV RNA 31 days before HCV antibodies, and HIV-1 RNA 14 days before HIV antibodies and 9 days before p24 antigen. The screening results obtained with the same assay in 50 plasma pools from over 16 million serologically negative blood donations yielded 308 (0.002 %), 46 (0.0003 %) and 6 (0.00004 %) units with HBV DNA, HCV RNA and HIV-1 RNA, respectively [29]. The proportion of invalid run was 2 %, and the false positive and internal control failure rates were 0.2 % and 0.17 %, respectively. This study demonstrated the feasibility and efficiency of large-scale blood donation testing with an HCV/HIV/HBV triplex NAT assay.

Despite these Japanese data, the relatively uncontroversial situation of NAT screening of donated blood in plasma pools might well be considerably challenged by the recent addition of HBV DNA NAT to the existing HIV and HCV in a triplex format. Recently, a new generation triplex TMA assay was launched (Procleix Ultrio assay, Chiron/Gen-Probe), which is a modified version of the Procleix HIV-1 and HCV assay that also includes HBV amplification and detection. HBV DNA testing is expected to decrease the residual risk for HBV transfusion-transmission two to fivefold when used with mini-pools with prior virus enrichment, less than 8-plasma pool size, or in single donations [50]. The 95 percent detection limits of this multiplex assay on WHO International Standards were 16-58 IU/ml for HIV-1 RNA, 3.7-6.5 IU/ml for HCV RNA and 7.3-22 IU/ml for HBV DNA [13]. Comparing this data with previous studies using the HIV-1/HCV Procleix showed that the detection limits for HIV-1 and HCV were not affected by the addition of the HBV detection. Robustness and specificity were assessed in a multicenter study by testing 2,912 pools of eight donations [13]. No cross-contamination was observed. Sixteen pools were initially reactive and 11 were confirmed after resolution (6 HBV DNA- and 5 HCV RNA-reactive). The specificity after initial testing and rate of invalid results were 99.8 % and 0.48 %, respectively. Invalid results were attributed to failure of internal control amplification, errors by pipetting robot, or operational failures. The ability of the Procleix Ultrio assay to reduce the HBV window period was assessed by testing seroconversion panels and comparing the results to different HBsAg tests. The results showed that the reduction of the HBV window period decreased with sample dilutions. Window period reductions of 14, 6, and 3 days were observed when samples were tested neat, diluted 1-in-8, and diluted 1-in-16, respectively. These data were in agreement with a previous study using two single PCR- and TMA-based methods [51]. Overall data indicate that pooling blood donations will affect the sensitivity of HBV DNA testing whether using a single or a multiplex amplification assay. Ultrio has been implemented in blood centers in several European countries since early 2005. Southern European countries such as Italy and Spain, where the prevalence of HBV infection in blood donors is above 5 %, which prevents them from screening for anti-HBc, were among the first to utilize this assay in single donations. Unpublished data suggest that the yield of confirmed HBV DNA is considerably higher than obtained in Japan and consists of relatively few window period cases but a considerable number of occult HBV infections [52]. A majority of samples contain either anti-HBc and anti-HBs or anti-HBc only, while a few do not reveal any serological markers. This preliminary data confirms what was described in a West African high endemicity area [53] where the yield of HBV DNA was considerably higher in single unit than in pools of 10 plasmas. Two questions are then raised: (i) what is the infectivity of these "occult" HBV DNA positive units in immunocompetent and immunodeficient recipients? And (ii) should the current strategy of pooling be revised, particularly if occult HBV proves infectious in the various serological scenarios and in the different categories of patient susceptibility?

In addition to the commercial semi-automated multiplex assays described above, an in-house HBV/HCV/HIV-1 multiplex real-time RT-PCR assay has been developed for blood screening [9]. Preliminary data showed that genomic amplification of one virus was unaffected by the amplification of the other two. However, competition between HCV and HIV-1 amplification slightly affected the yield of HIV-1 amplification. The assay detected with similar efficiency strains of HBV genotypes A-F, HCV genotypes 1-6, and HIV-1 subtypes A-G and circulating recombinant forms. The 95 % detection limits were 30, 167, and 680 IU/ml for HBV DNA, HCV RNA, and HIV-1 RNA, respectively. Compared to Procleix Ultrio and AMPLINAT MPX assays, the multiplex real-time RT-PCR assay showed a lower analytical sensitivity, especially for HIV-1. The difference of sensitivity between these assays can be in part related to the difference in the volume of plasma used for nucleic acid purification and the final amount of target molecules loaded in each amplification reaction. The Procleix Ultrio and AMPLINAT MPX assays are performed with 500 and 200 µl of plasma, respectively, and the totality of the purified nucleic acids is used in the amplification reaction. In the RT-PCR assay, nucleic acids are extracted from 200 µl of plasma, but only one fifth of the purified nucleic acids are used in the amplification reaction. Consequently, the amount of target molecules loaded in each amplification reaction is 12.5 and 5 times higher in the Procleix Ultrio and AMPLINAT MPX, respectively, than in this RT-PCR assay. In a preliminary study conducted in Ghanaian blood donors, this multiplex assay has been evaluated as part of a novel strategy for blood safety in high endemic, resource-poor settings that associates pre-donation serological screening of blood donors with rapid tests and multiplex NAT screening of pools of 10 plasma samples from serologically negative donated units [53]. The multiplex screening of 517 pools containing 5,109 individual plasmas negative by pre-donation rapid testing showed that no HIV-1 or HCV RNA-containing samples remained undetected by rapid tests and were included in the pools unless a human testing error was involved. In contrast, 1.7 % of these pre-screened samples contained occult HBV undetected by both rapid tests and standard enzyme immunoassays but detected in individual donations with genomic amplification. However, half of these HBV DNA-containing units remained undetected when HBV DNA screening was performed in pools of 10 plasmas. Most of these HBV-containing samples undetected in the pools (81.3 %) contained less than 100 IU of HBV DNA per ml [53]. These data clearly indicate that HBV DNA testing efficiency is impaired in pools of 10 or more as reported by others [13,51]. This study also provides elements to support the new strategy associating pre-donation serologic screening with rapid tests and post-donation multiplex NAT that might make the blood supply in high-prevalence, resource-poor areas as safe as in affluent, low prevalence areas. However, field evaluation and careful economic assessment are still required and are currently in progress in Ghana as a collaborative pilot study.

Other multiplexes than the most needed HIV/HCV/HBV currently available can be developed for exploratory purposes and applied to blood donor or other populations. In our hands, RT-PCR technology proves to be particularly suitable for multiplexing due to its flexibility. Recently, the real time QPCR methodology was used to rapidly develop two other triplex assays potentially suitable for blood screening. The first triplex assay was intended for the simultaneous detection and identification of three flaviviruses: GB virus C (GBV-C), West Nile virus (WNV), and Dengue virus. This assay was used to screen plasma samples from 795 Ghanaian candidate blood donors, pregnant women and HIV-1-infected patients (41 % and 38 % of the selected candidate blood donors and pregnant women selected for this study, respectively, were HIV-1 infected) [54]. No WNV or Dengue virus RNA were detected in these samples. The prevalence of GBV-C RNA was significantly lower in HIV-1 non-infected blood donors (12.9 %) than in HIV-1 infected individuals (23.5 %) and HIV-1 non-infected pregnant women (25 %). Further analysis of GBV-C and HIV-1 RNA loads showed a moderate impact of GBV-C on HIV-1 viremia that is unlikely to entirely account for a favorable clinical outcome of replicating co-infections.

The second multiplex real-time PCR assay was designed for HBV, HHV-8, and HErV DNA detection. In a preliminary study, assay performance was assessed by testing 885 plasmas from Ghanaian pregnant women (unpublished data). The prevalence observed was 13, 0.6, and 1.8 % for HBV DNA, HHV-8 DNA and HErV DNA, respectively. Occult HBV infection and chronic HErV infection, characterized by low viral load and specific IgG, were observed in 8.9 % of HBV DNA-positive and HErV DNA-positive women, respectively.

Conclusions

Recent developments in genomic amplification technology have enhanced the development of multiplex NAT assays for detection and possibly direct identification of viral genomes. Optimization of multiplex assays may prove difficult, and particular attention should be devoted to selection of optimal primer pairs to be combined in a multiplex format. The main limitations to overcome are the risk of false-negative results due to amplification competition, as well as specificity issues according to the methodology used, and a confirmatory NAT assay may be needed. Despite these limitations, multiplex NAT has been successfully applied to large-scale screening of blood products for HBV, HCV and HIV-1 that constitute the main residual risk of transfusion-transmitted viral infection. Several studies demonstrated that commercial and in-house multiplex assays were suitable and efficient, showing high sensitivity and specificity, and had the potential to decrease operating costs and testing turnaround time. In addition, multiplexing has the potential to improve blood safety in resource-limited high endemic areas in a cost-effective way when associated with other cost-reducing procedures such as plasma pooling and pre-donation serological screening. Considering the advantages already demonstrated by the use of multiplex assays along with the recent advances in this technology, commercial development of multiple detection systems for clinically and epidemiologically relevant viruses should be expected in the future.

References

1 Caudai C, Padula MG, Bettini V, Valensin PE: Detection of HCV and GBV-C/HGV infection by multiplex PCR in plasma samples of transfused subjects. J Virol Methods 1998; 70: 79-83.

2 Defoort J-P, Martin M, Casano B, Prato S, Camilla C, Fert V: Simultaneous detection of multiplex-amplified human immunodeficiency virus type 1 RNA, hepatitis C virus RNA, and hepatitis B virus DNA using a flow cytometer microsphere-based hybridization assay. J Clin Microbiol 2000; 38: 1066-1071.

3 Cleland A, Davis C, Adams N, Lycett C, Jarvis LM, Holmes H, Simmonds P: Development of multiplexed nucleic acid testing for human immunodeficiency virus type 1 and hepatitis C virus. Vox Sang 2001; 81: 93-101.

4 Adami V, Falasca E, Dorotea L, Malangone W, Astori G, Marini L, Biffoni F, Rinaldi C, Degrassi A, Pipan C: Qualitative multiplex RT-PCR for simultaneous detection of hepatitis C virus and human immunodeficiency virus in plasma samples. Clin Microbiol Infect 2004; 10: 1075-1080.

5 Mercier B, Burlot L, Ferec C: Simultaneous screening for HBV DNA and HCV RNA genomes in blood donations using a novel TaqMan PCR assay. J Virol Methods 1999; 77: 1-9.

6 Vet JAM, Majithia AR, Marras SAE, Tyagi S, Dube S, Poiesz BJ, Kramer FR: Multiplex detection of four pathogenic retroviruses using molecular beacons. Proc Natl Acad Sci USA 1999; 96: 6394-6399.

7 Abravaya K, Esping C, Hoenle R, Gorzowski J, Perry R, Kroeger P, Robinson J, Flanders R: Performance of a multiplex qualitative PCR LCx assay for detection of human immunodeficiency virus type 1 (HIV-1) group M subtypes, group O, and HIV-2. J Clin Microbiol 2000; 38: 716-723.

8 Meng Q, Wong C, Rangachari A, Tamatsukuri S, Sasaki M, Fiss E, Cheng L, Ramankutty T, Clarke D, Yawata H, Sakakura Y, Hirose T, Impraim C: Automated multiplex assay system for simultaneous detection of hepatitis B virus DNA, hepatitis C virus RNA, and human immunodeficiency virus type 1 RNA. J Clin Mcrobiol 2001; 39: 2937-2947.

9 Candotti D, Temple J, Owusu-Ofori S, Allain J-P: Multiplex real-time quantitative RT-PCR assay for hepatitis B virus, hepatitis C virus, and human immunodeficiency virus type 1. J Virol Methods 2004; 118: 39-47.

10 Dineva MA, Candotti D, Fletcher-Brown F, Allain J-P, Lee H: Simultaneous visual detection of multiple viral amplicons by dipstick assay. J Clin Microbiol 2005; 43: 4015-4021.

11 de Baar MP, van Dooren MW, de Rooij E, Bakker M, van Gemen B, Goudsmit J, de Ronde A: Single rapid real-time monitored isothermal RNA amplification assay for quantification of human immunodeficiency virus type 1 isolates from groups M, N, and O. J Clin Microbiol 2001; 39: 1378-1384.

12 Candotti D, Richetin A, Cant B, Temple J, Sims C, Reeves I, Barbara JAJ, Allain J-P: Evaluation of a transcription-mediated amplification-based HCV and HIV-1 RNA duplex assay for screening individual blood donations: a comparison with a minipool testing system. Transfusion 2003; 43: 215-225.

13 Koppelman HGM, Assal A, Chudy M, Torres P, Garcia de Villaescusa R, Reesink HW, Lelie PN, Cuypers HTM: Multicenter performance evaluation of a transcription-mediated amplification assay for screening of human immunodeficiency virus-1 RNA, hepatitis C virus RNA, and hepatitis B virus DNA in blood donations. Transfusion 2005; 45: 1258-1266.

14 Cleland A, Nettleton P, Jarvis LM, Simmonds P: Use of bovine viral diarrhoea virus as an internal control for amplification of hepatitis C virus. Vox Sang 1999; 76: 170-174.

15 Tucker RA, Unger ER, Holloway BP, Swan DC: Real-time PCR-based fluorescent assay for quantitation of human papillomavirus types 6, 11, 16, and 18. Molecular Diagnosis 2001; 6:39-47.

16 Bustin SA: Quantification of mRNA using real-time reverse transcription PCR (RT-PCR): trends and problems. J Mol Endocrin 2002; 29: 23-39.

17 Wittwer CT, Herrmann MG, Gundry CN, Elenitoba-Johnson KSJ: Real-time multiplex PCR assays. Methods 2001; 25: 430-442.

18 Mackay IM, Arden KE, Nitsche A: Real-time PCR in virology. Nucl Acids Res 2002; 30: 1292-1305.

19 Holland PM, Abramson RD, Watson R, Gelfand DH: Detection of specific polymerase chain reaction product by utilizing the 5' → 3' exonuclease activity of Thermus aquaticus DNA polymerase. Proc Natl Acad Sci USA 1991; 88: 7276-7280.

20 Exner MM, Lewinski MA: Sensitivity of multiplex real-time PCR reactions, using the LighyCycler and the ABI PRISM 7700 Sequence Detection System, is dependent on the concentration of the DNA polymerase. Molecular & Cellular Probes 2002; 16: 351-357.

21 Persson K, Hamby K, Ugozzoli LA: Four-color multiplex reverse transcription polymerase chain reaction – overcoming its limitations. Anal Biochem 2005; 344: 33-42.

22 Henegariu O, Heerema NA, Dlouhy SR, Vance GH, Vogt PH: Multiplex PCR: critical parameters and step-by-step protocol. BioTechniques 1997; 23: 504-511.

23 Elnifro EM, Ashshi A, Cooper RJ, Klapper PE: Multiplex PCR: optimization and application in diagnostic virology. Clin Microbiol Rev 2000; 13: 559-570.

24 Schutten M, van den Hoogen B, van der Ende ME, Gruters RA, Osterhaus ADME, Niesters HGM: Development of a real-time quantitative RT-PCR for the detection of HIV-2 RNA in plasma. J Virol Methods 2000; 88: 81-87.

25 Lanciotti RS, Kerst AJ: Nucleic acid sequence-based amplification assays for rapid detection of West Nile and St. Louis Encephalitis viruses. J Clin Microbiol 2001; 39: 4506-4513.

26 Vogelstein B, Gillespie D: Preparative and analytical purification of DNA from agarose. Proc Natl Acad Sci USA 1979; 76: 615-619.

27 Giachetti C, Linnen JM, Kolk DP, Dockter J, Gillotte-Taylor K, Park M, Ho-Sing-Loy M, McCormick MK, Mimms LT, McDonough SH: Highly sensitive multiplex assay for detection of human immunodeficiency virus type 1 and hepatitis C virus RNA. J Clin Microbiol 2002; 40: 2408-2419.

28 Rosenstraus M, Wang Z, Chang S-Y, DeBonville D, Spadoro JP: An internal control for routine diagnostic PCR: design, properties, and effect on clinical performance. J Clin Microbiol 1998; 36: 191-197.

29 Mine H, Emura H, Miyamoto M, Tomono T, Minegishi K, Murokawa H, Yamanaka R, Yoshikawa A, Nishioka K, Japanese Red Cross NAT Research Group: High throughput screening of 16 million serologically negative blood donors for hepatitis B virus, hepatitis C virus, and human immunodeficiency virus type 1 by nucleic acid amplification testing with specific and sensitive multiplex reagents in Japan. J Virol Methods 2003; 112: 145-151.

30 Pasloske BL, Walkerpeach CR, Obermoeller RD, Winkler M, DuBois DB: Armored RNA technology for production of ribonuclease-resistant viral RNA controls and standards. J Clin Microbiol 1998; 36: 3590-3594.

31 Drosten C, Seifried E, Roth WK: TaqMan 5'-nuclease human immunodeficiency virus type 1 PCR assay with phage-packaged competitive internal control for high-throughput blood donor screening. J Clin Microbiol 2001; 39: 4302-4308.

32 Eisler DL, McNabb A, Jorgensen DR, Isaac-Renton JL: Use of an internal positive control in a multiplex reverse transcription-PCR to detect West Nile virus RNA in mosquito pools. J Clin Microbiol 2004; 42: 841-843.

33 Aubin J-T, Defer C, Vidaud M, Maniez Montreuil M, Flan B: Large-scale screening for human parvovirus B19 DNA by PCR: application to the quality control of plasma for fractionation. Vox Sang 2000; 78: 7-12.

34 Hofmann MA: Construction of an infectious chimeric classical swine fever virus containing the 5'UTR of bovine viral diarrhea virus, and its application as a universal internal positive control in real-time RT-PCR. J Virol Methods 2003; 114: 77-90.

35 Loussert-Ajaka I, Ly TD, Chaix ML, Ingrand D, Saragosti S, Courouce AM, Brun-Vezinet F, Simon F: HIV-1/HIV-2 seronegativity in HIV-1 subtype O infected patients. Lancet 1994; 343: 1393-1394.

36 Widell A, Elmud H, Persson MH, Jonsson M: Transmission of hepatitis C via both erythrocyte and platelet transfusions from a single donor in serological window-phase of hepatitis C. Vox sang 1996; 71: 55-57.

37 Allain J-P, Hewitt PE, Tedder RS, Williamson LM: Evidence that anti-HBc but not HBV DNA testing may prevent some HBV transmission by transfusion. Br J Haematol 1999; 107: 186-195.

38 Candotti D, Adu-Sarkodie Y, Davies F, Baldrich-Rubio E, Stirrups K, Lee H, Allain J-P: AIDS in an HIV-seronegative Ghanaian woman with intersubtype A/G recombinant HIV-1 infection. J Med Virol 2000; 62: 1-8.

39 Soldan K, Barbara JA, Ramsay ME, Hall AJ: Estimation of the risk of hepatitis B virus, hepatitis C virus, and human immunodeficiency virus infectious donations entering the blood supply in England. Vox sang 2003; 84: 274-286.

40 Jackson BR, Busch MP, Stramer SL, AuBuchon JP: The cost-effectiveness of NAT for HIV, HCV, and HBV in whole-blood donations. Transfusion 2003; 43: 721-729.

41 Coste J, Reesink HW, Laperche S: International Forum. Implementation of donor screening for infectious agents transmitted by blood by nucleic acid technology: update to 2003. Vox Sang 2005; 88: 289-303.

42 Ren F, Wang J, Lu S, Yao F, Zhao H, Zhu F, Bai X, Zheng Y, Gong X, Liu C, Yu L, Shan H: Nucleic amplification testing (NAT) for HIV and HCV among Chinese blood donors. Transfusion 2005; 45 Supp: 91A.

43 Vargo J, Smith K, Knott C, Wang S, Fang C, McDonough S, Giachetti C, Caglioti S, Gammon R, Gilbert D, Jackson JB, Richards W, Stramer S, Mimms L: Clinical specificity and sensitivity of blood screening assay for detection of HIV-1 and HCV RNA. Transfusion 2002; 42: 876-885.

44 Fang CT, Field SP, Busch MP, du P Heyns A: Human immunodeficiency virus-1 and hepatitis C virus RNA among South African blood donors: estimation of residual transfusion risk and yield of nucleic acid testing. Vox Sang 2003; 85: 9-19.

45 Mison L, Seed CR, Margaritis AR, Hyland C, the ARCBS NAT Study Group: Nucleic acid technology screening of Australian blood donors for hepatitis C and human immunodeficiency virus-1 RNA: comparison of two high-throughput testing strategies. Vox Sang 2003; 84: 11-19.

46 Busch MP, Stramer SL, Strong DM, Hewlett IK, Epstein JS: International forum letter. Vox sang 2005; 88: 298-301.

47 Busch MP: Closing the windows on viral transmission by blood transfusion. In: Stramer SL, editor. Blood safety in the new millennium. AABB 2000 Emily Cooley Seminar Book. Bethesda: American Association of Blood Banks 2001:33-54.

48 Stramer SL, Glynn SA. Kleinman SH, Strong DM, Caglioti S, Wright DJ, Dodd RY, Busch MP for the National Heart, Lung, and Blood Institute Nucleic Acid Test Study Group: Detection of HIV-1 and HCV infections among antibody-negative blood donors by nucleic acid amplification testing. N Engl J Med 2004; 351: 760-768.

49 Candotti D, Sarkodie F, Allain J-P: Residual risk of transfusion in Ghana. Brit J Haematol 2001; 113: 37-39.

50 Weusten JJ, van Drimmelen HA, Lelie PN: Mathematic modeling of the risk of HBV, HCV, and HIV transmission by window-phase donations not detected by NAT. Transfusion 2002; 42: 537-548.

51 Biswas R, Tabor E, Hsia CC, Wright DJ, Laycock ME, Fiebig EW, Peddada L, Smith R, Schreiber GB, Epstein JS, Nemo GJ, Busch MP: Comparative sensitivity of HBV NATs and HBsAg assays for detection of acute HBV infection. Transfusion 2003; 43: 788-798.

52 Allain J-P: Occult hepatitis B virus infection: implications in transfusion. Vox sang 2004; 86: 83-91.

53 Owusu-Ofori S, Temple J, Sarkodie F, Anokwa M, Candotti D, Allain J-P: predonation screening of blood donors with rapid tests: implementation and efficacy of a novel approach to blood safety in resource-poor settings. Transfusion 2005; 45: 133-140.

54 Li C, Collini P, Danso K, Owusu-Ofori S, Dompreh A, Candotti D, Opare-Sem O, Allain JP: GB virus C and HIV-1 RNA load in single virus and co-infected West African individuals. AIDS 2006; 20: 379-386.

Prof. J.-P. Allain, Cambridge Blood Centre, Long Road, Cambridge, CB2 2PT, U.K.
E-mail: jpa1000@cam.ac.uk

Dax EM, Farrugia A, Vyas G (eds): Advances in Transfusion Safety – Volume IV.
Dev Biol (Basel). Basel, Karger, 2007, vol 127, pp 87-112.

Evolving Approaches to Estimate Risks of Transfusion-Transmitted Viral Infections: Incidence-Window Period Model after Ten Years

M.P. Busch

Blood Systems Research Institute, San Francisco, CA, USA

Key words: Blood transfusion, human immunodeficiency virus (HIV), hepatitis B virus (HBV), hepatitis C virus (HCV), nucleic-acid amplification testing (NAT).

INTRODUCTION

Concern over transmission of viral infections by blood transfusions has existed since cases of post-transfusion hepatitis were first observed during World War II, when blood and plasma use dramatically increased. However, studies to accurately measure risks of transfusion-transmitted viral infections (TTVIs) were not initiated for several decades since they required epidemiological approaches and laboratory tools that only became available in the 1970s. Even then, the challenge of measuring transfusion risks of previously uncharacterized agents like Hepatitis C Virus (HCV) and emerging viruses like Human Immunodeficiency Virus (HIV) was daunting.

Discovery of novel agents and quantitation of associated transfusion risks depended on basic research in viral discovery, translational and commercial research in diagnostic assay development, and government funding of large-scale donor-recipient cohort studies. Such studies were first launched in the late 1970s, and the Era of Prospective/Retrospective Cohort Studies began (Fig. 1). In addition to prospective donor and recipient enrollment and follow-up, these cohort studies established large-scale frozen specimen repositories. These repositories enabled investigation of clinically overt as well as asymptomatic infections by retrospective application of increasingly sophisticated laboratory methods, including immunoassays and nucleic acid based tests.

As the major TTVI agents were discovered and interventions implemented, it was initially possible to directly measure residual TTVI risks by quantifying rates of infection in screened donors or rates of breakthrough transmissions to recipients.

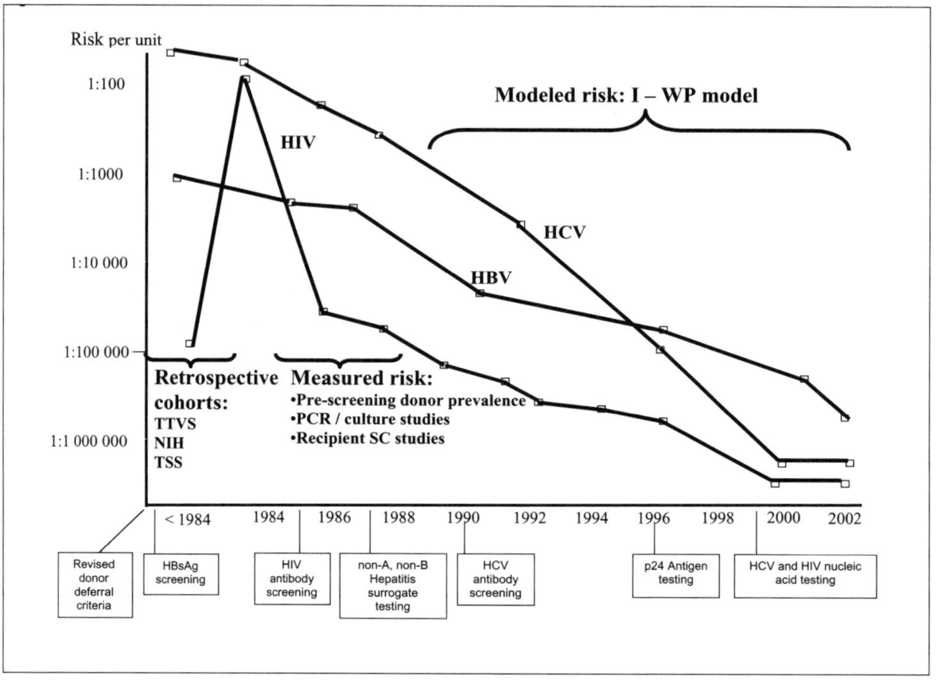

Fig. 1: Evolution of approaches to estimating the risks of transmission by blood transfusion, for HIV, HBV, and HCV.

This Era of Direct Risk Measurement was, unfortunately, short-lived as refined donor risk factor screening and increasingly sensitive laboratory testing reduced risks to such low levels that direct measurement was no longer possible.

Novel approaches were needed to meet this challenge, most notably the development and refinement of the incidence-window period (I-WP) model, but also other modeling strategies that are employed in the current Era of Risk Modeling. This chapter will review the evolution of approaches to TTVI risk estimation, with particular emphasis on the development, enhancement and widespread implementation of the I-WP model over the past 10 years.

Era of Retrospective and Prospective Cohort Studies: 1960s-1985 (Table 1)

Early studies of post-transfusion hepatitis

Development of methods to identify etiological agents and measure risks of their transmission by blood transfusion can be traced to the earliest studies of post-transfusion hepatitis (PTH). PTH was first reported in the US by Beeson in 1943 who described 7 cases of icteric hepatitis that occurred in soldiers 1-4 months after

Table 1: Era of retrospective and prospective cohort studies (1960s-1985).

HIV	HCV	HBV
		Retrospective studies to establish incidence of post-transfusion (PT) hepatitis and association with paid donors
	Exclusion of HAV as cause of PTH and distinct definition of non-A, non-B hepatitis (NANBH)	Discovery of HBV and implementation of HBsAg screening
Risk of transfusion HIV prior to screening estimated using Transfusion Safety Study (TSS) and gay cohort HIV prevalence and AIDS-case donor lookback data	Rates of NANBH established using TTVS and NIH cohorts	Rates of PT-HBV established using TTVS and NIH cohorts
TSS repository used to define transmission rates by seropositive units and correlates of transmission		
Progressive decrease in infected donations following early HIV Ab screening	Retrospective testing of repositories to estimate HCV risk prior to anti-HCV screening, and document impact of anti-HBc & ALT on HCV risk	Retrospective testing of repositories to estimate impact of improved HBsAg, anti-HBc, and HBV DNA on HBV risk

transfusion of plasma [1]. In 1964, Grady and Chalmers reported the results of a 10 year retrospective study of PTH in nine Boston teaching hospitals [2]. In one of the hospitals, 29 % of transfused blood was from commercial (paid donor) sources, while in the other eight hospitals only volunteer donor blood was transfused. The incidence of clinically overt (i.e., symptomatic or icteric) PTH in recipients of blood products from volunteer blood donors was 0.6 cases/1000 units, compared with 2.8 cases/1000 units in recipients of blood products from a mixture of volunteer and commercial blood donors.

In 1970, scientists at the National Institutes of Health (NIH) reported the results of the first prospective study to determine the incidence of icteric and anicteric hepatitis in patients undergoing open-heart surgery [3]. Icteric and anicteric hepatitis developed in 51 % of the recipients of commercial blood, whereas no hepatitis occurred in patients who received blood from volunteer donors. These authors estimated the hepatitis carrier rate for commercial blood donors to be 6.3 %, while among volunteer donors the rate was < 0.6 %. By 1971, the association between a paid blood donor and an increased risk of PTH was accepted, and in 1975 the Food and Drug Administration (FDA) mandated an all-voluntary blood donor system (Fig. 2) [4].

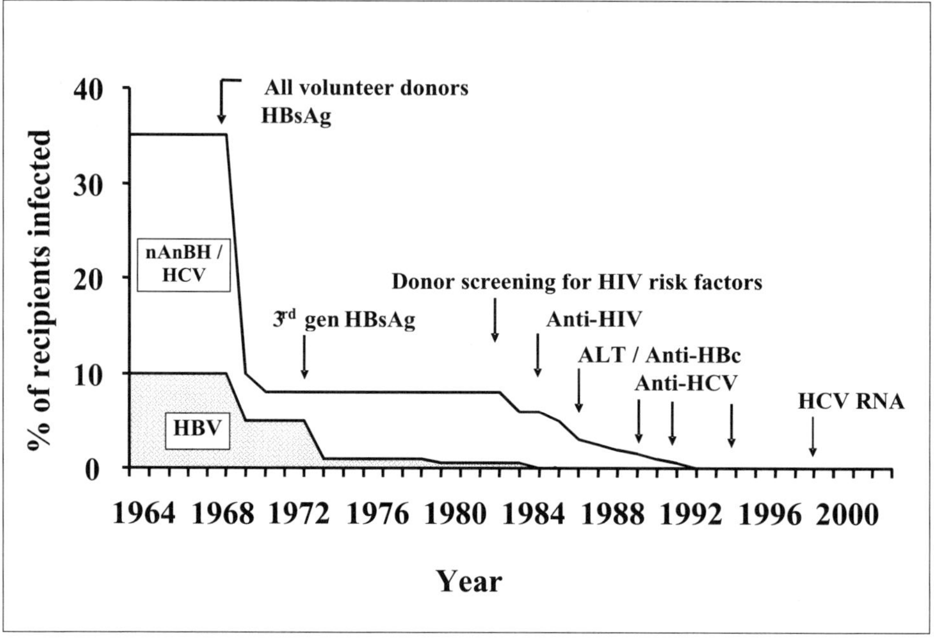

Fig. 2: The declining risk of transfusion-associated hepatitis.

Discovery of HBV and its role in PTH

A viral etiology for PTH was long suspected but difficult to establish. In 1965, Blumberg et al [5] first described the Australia antigen (subsequently renamed hepatitis B surface antigen, HBsAg) and stated that this antigen could be identified in the sera of many hemophiliacs who had received multiple transfusions. Subsequently, retrospective studies of specimens from the NIH cohort and other small specimen banks demonstrated that HBsAg in donor blood was clearly associated with the occurrence of PTH [6]. In 1970, Gocke et al [7], using retrospective studies, estimated that exclusion of HBsAg-positive blood donors through either first- or second-generation assays (e.g., agar gel diffusion or counterelectrophoresis) would decrease the rate of PTH by ~ 25 %. Results of a prospective study on the effectiveness of exclusion of commercial donors and HBsAg-positive blood on the incidence of PTH was reported in 1972 [8]. The exclusion of HBsAg-positive blood resulted in a 25 % reduction in the PTH rate as predicted, while the elimination of commercial donors resulted in a 70 % reduction in the PTH rate. With the simultaneous exclusion of commercial and HBsAg-positive donors, the PTH rate was reduced to 7.1 % of the prior rate (Fig. 2).

On the basis of these studies, routine screening of blood donations for HBsAg was initiated in 1971. The initial methods used to detect HBsAg were relatively insensitive, and transfusion-associated HBV cases continued to occur. In 1975, regulations were implemented requiring the screening of all donor blood for HBsAg by one of the third-generation tests (i.e., radioimmunoassay [RIA] or enzyme-linked immunoassay [EIA]), as well as the labeling of blood components with respect to the volunteer or paid status of the donor. Although this led to further reduction in HBV-related cases, PTH continued to be observed, particularly subclinical cases manifested only by persistent hepatic enzyme elevations.

Studies of non-A, non-B hepatitis and surrogate markers

In 1973, the causative agent of hepatitis A was detected by immune electron microscopy on stools from patients with acute food-borne hepatitis [9]. Hepatitis A virus (HAV) was quickly determined to be associated with acute resolving hepatitis without a chronic carrier state. Retrospective studies demonstrated that multiply transfused thalassemia patients were at no greater risk of HAV infection than non-transfused children [10]. Similarly, analysis of donor and recipient samples from cases of PTH not associated with HBV showed no evidence of involvement by HAV [11].

When it became clear that PTH cases continued to occur that were not caused by infections with HAV, HBV or other known viral agents (e.g., Epstein Barr virus and cytomegalovirus), the term non-A, non-B hepatitis (NANBH) was coined by Dr. Harvey Alter at NIH. Retrospective analysis of NIH cohort data suggested that NANBH represented 90 % of residual PTH cases in the US in the late 1970s and early1980s, with rates in multiply transfused patients as high as 10 %. Several large studies were launched at that time to establish the incidence, correlates, and clinical consequences of NANBH, as well as to help identify the etiological agent. The initial results of the multi-center Transfusion-Transmitted Viruses Study (TTVS) were published in 1981 [12]. This report showed a substantial association between recipients with NANBH and donor alanine aminotransferase (ALT) concentrations, which was quickly confirmed by the NIH group and others [13]. TTVS subsequently reported an association between occurrence of NANBH in recipients of blood that tested positive for antibody to the core protein of HBV (anti-HBc) [14]. The research group at NIH also confirmed this observation and showed that anti-HBc testing of donors, in concert with ALT testing, would eliminate 30-50 % of recipient NANBH [15]. On the basis of these studies, in the late 1980s blood collection agencies in the U.S. began screening donated blood for anti-HBc and ALT as surrogate markers of NANBH [16]. The rate of PTH among recipients followed at the NIH subsequently dropped to 2 % (Fig. 2) [17].

Studies establishing the role of HCV as the etiological agent of NANBH

Extensive research was conducted in the 1970s and 1980s to identify the etiological agent(s) of NANBH. More than 25 preliminary reports of associated agents were determined to be false. Then, in 1988, the hepatitis C virus (HCV) was identified using then-novel molecular biology techniques by scientists at Chiron Corporation in collaboration with investigators at the Centers for Disease Control (CDC) and NIH [18]. The process of virus discovery involved construction of a cDNA expression library in a bacteriophage using high-titer plasma from a chimpanzee inoculated with PTH plasma. The library was then screened for rare clones expressing viral antigen with serum from a recipient with chronic NANBH as a presumed source of viral antibodies. Screening over 10,000 clones from this library led to the identification of a positive cDNA clone expressing what was termed 5-1-1 antigen [19]. The entire viral genome was sequenced within 1 year, and antigens were expressed for development of antibody detection assays. Early studies established that HCV was the etiological agent of at least 80 % of residual NANBH [17]. The era of molecular discovery of TTVI had been launched.

Subsequent studies by TTVS and NIH investigators, as well as many groups from around the world, quickly established the prevalence of HCV infection in donor and recipient populations and the rates and correlates of transmission of the virus by seropositive transfusions and plasma derivatives [20,21]. Studies of HCV infection in donor and recipient populations also contributed substantially to our understanding of the natural history, virology, immunology and pathogenesis of liver disease in HCV infection [22-24]. Investigations of PTH, thus, were critical to the discovery of HCV and have continued to yield important scientific insights for the field to this day.

Emergence of the Acquired Immunodeficiency Syndrome (AIDS) and Human Immunodeficiency Virus (HIV)

The success with virtual eradication of PTH in the 1980s was, unfortunately, obscured by the concurrent emergence of transfusion-associated AIDS. AIDS cases were reported in transfusion recipients and hemophiliacs in 1982 and 1983, spawning global concern over the safety of the blood supply. In the U.S., the Transfusion Safety Study (TSS) was launched by the National Heart, Lung and Blood Institute (NHLBI) in 1983 to investigate the etiology of transfusion-associated AIDS, establish the magnitude of risk, and identify possible deferral policies, tests or other measures to reduce the risk. One component of TSS was establishment of a repository of 200,000 donation specimens collected in late 1984 in 5 high AIDS prevalence cities [25]. Subsequent testing of these specimens for anti-HIV (and later for antibodies to Human T-lymphotropic Viruses (HTLV-I/II) and HIV-1 p24 antigen) allowed for determination of the prevalence of HIV infection in the donor pool at that critical time and subsequently led to studies that established rates of transmission to recipients and course of infection in donors, recipient and hemophiliacs (see below).

A major contribution of TSS was estimation of the risk of HIV from transfusions over the decade prior to implementation of serological screening in 1985 [26]. This was achieved by combining data from the TSS donor repository collected in late 1984 with HIV-1 seroincidence data among homosexual men and data from lookback investigations that traced recipients of prior donations from donors who later developed AIDS. Using a model developed to integrate these data sources, it was possible to piece together an accurate picture of the risk of HIV-1 transmission by transfusion in the San Francisco bay area between 1978 and 1985 (Fig. 3). The analysis showed that the risk of transfusion-associated (TA) HIV-1 infection rose rapidly from its first occurrence in 1978 to a peak risk of approximately 1.1 percent per transfused unit in late 1982. Beginning in early 1983 and continuing through implementation of anti-HIV-1 screening, there was a marked, progressive decline in risk as a result of declining numbers of blood donations from at-risk individuals. This decline was directly attributable to increasing awareness of the infectious nature of AIDS in the homosexual community and to implementation of donor education and deferral measures by blood banks [26,27]. These data illustrate the effectiveness of donor education and self-deferral measures at safeguarding the blood supply in the absence of specific testing options.

This temporal profile for the risk of HIV from blood components and derivatives was corroborated in a report from the Centers for Disease Control and Pre-

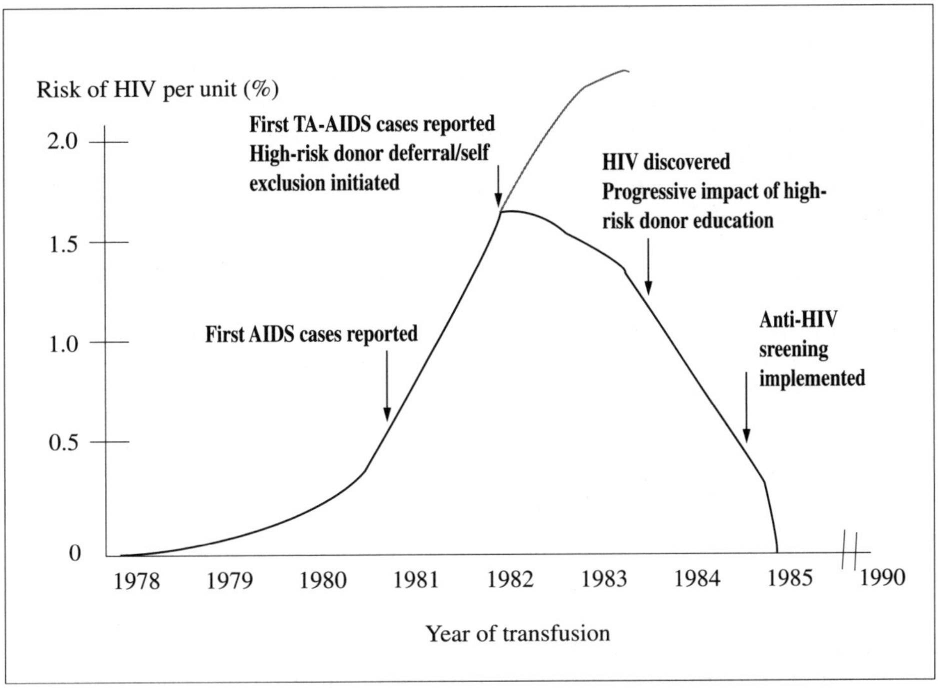

Fig. 3: Risk of HIV transmission by blood transfusion before the implementation of HIV-1 antibody screening.

vention (CDC), in which 4,619 TA AIDS cases reported from 1982 through 1991 were reviewed [28]. When plotted by year of implicated transfusion that led to HIV infection, the number of cases rose from 56 in 1978 to 714 in 1984, then dropped sharply to 288 by 1985 when screening for antibody began, falling to a mean of 20 per year from 1986 through 1991. Over 95 percent of AIDS cases diagnosed subsequent to screening were attributable to transfusions received before implementation of anti-HIV screening in early 1985. Upon further investigation, the patients in most of the cases diagnosed from post-1985 transfusions were found to be infected from sources other than HIV seronegative blood transfusions [28].

The TSS was unique in being the only study that traced and enrolled recipients of known seropositive units, which allowed for direct measurement of HIV transmission rates and correlates of transmission by seropositive blood. In the TSS, 111 (89.5 percent) of 124 enrolled recipients transfused with anti-HIV-1 positive blood components seroconverted to anti-HIV-1 positivity [29]. Variables initially identified to correlate with likelihood of HIV-1 transmission were type of blood component transfused and its duration of storage [30,31]. With subsequent development of viral load assays in the early 1990s, the TSS repository was further studied to establish the importance of the level of viremia for HIV transmission in cases of transfusion-acquired infection [32], as well as for heterosexual transmissions from persons infected through transfusion to their sexual partners [33].

TSS enrolled infected donors, recipients and hemophiliacs into prospective follow-up in order to establish the rate of progression to clinical disease and clinical and laboratory correlates of progression. The rate of AIDS in recipients was found to be faster than the rate of progression among infected donors and hemophiliacs followed in parallel [34,35]. However, once age and underlying disease were controlled for, progression rates to clinical AIDS were virtually identical for TSS donors, recipients and hemophiliacs [36]. This suggests that factors such as route of infection, inoculum size, and proposed co-factors such as other viral infections (e.g., cytomegalovirus or hepatitis B virus), are not highly significant in determining the course of HIV disease.

Archived samples from the TSS also served to investigate the role of the beta-chemokine CCR5, a co-receptor for non-syncytium-inducing (NSI) strains of HIV-1, in parenteral transmission of virus [37]. Recipients of HIV seropositive blood units and coagulation factor concentrates who had a 32 base pair deletion in the CCR5 gene were less susceptible to infection, although those that were infected progressed at the same rate as recipients with a normal CCR5 gene. TSS samples were also critical for the demonstration of rare cases of dual strain HIV infection and subsequent recombination and to understanding the rate and determinants of molecular evolution of the same strain of virus in multiple donors and recipients in transmission clusters [38-40]. The significance of a virulence gene, nef, was demonstrated in an Australian cohort of a blood donor and eight transfusion recipients who were infected with an HIV-1 viral strain lacking a functioning nef gene and had markedly prolonged disease-free survival without therapy [41]. Thus, as with HBV and HCV, studies of HIV infected blood donors and recipients resulted in significant contributions to our understanding of viral transmission and pathogenesis.

Interestingly, transfusions not only proved to be an efficient mode of transmission for HIV, but, according to some evidence, may also affect the course of disease in patients with AIDS. Observations from retrospective studies and small prospective studies suggest that allogeneic transfusions from non-infected donors might accelerate disease progression in HIV-infected patients [42]. In vitro experiments provided evidence that transfusion of allogeneic leukocytes, presumably through immunological activation of lymphocytes and macrophages, cause greater replication of HIV, whereas transfusion of autologous leukocytes and allogeneic red cells, platelets and plasma did not show this effect [43]. The Viral Activation [by] Transfusion Study (VATS), a multi-center US clinical trial, addressed this issue and investigated the benefits of providing leukoreduced blood to patients in late-stage HIV infection. The study found no evidence of significant activation of HIV replication or accelerated disease progression in recipients of either leukoreduced or non-leukoreduced transfusions [44].

Era of Direct Risk Measurement: 1985-1990 (Table 2)

Direct measurement of HIV risk from antibody screened transfusions

After introduction of HIV antibody screening in 1985, rates of infected donations declined markedly as seropositive donors were identified and deferred, and risk factor screening criteria were enhanced based on findings from interviews of infected donors (Fig. 4). These data led to initial optimism that the problem of transfusion-transmitted HIV had been solved. However, cases of AIDS linked to screened blood

Table 2: Era of direct risk measurement (1985-1990).

HIV	HCV	HBV
Recipients of screened units enrolled into FACTS with documentation of breakthrough transmission rates	Recipients of screened units tested to document rates of HCV infection in FACTS and impact of surrogate tests and HCV EIA 1.0	Recipients of screened units tested to document rates of HBV infection in FACTS
Pooled PBMC HIV culture & DNA PCR performed on antibody screened units to document rate of viremic seronegative donations		
Transfusion AIDS case reports and lookback transmission data used to derive risk projections		
Large-scale studies of p24 Ag yield using prospective donations and TSS repository		

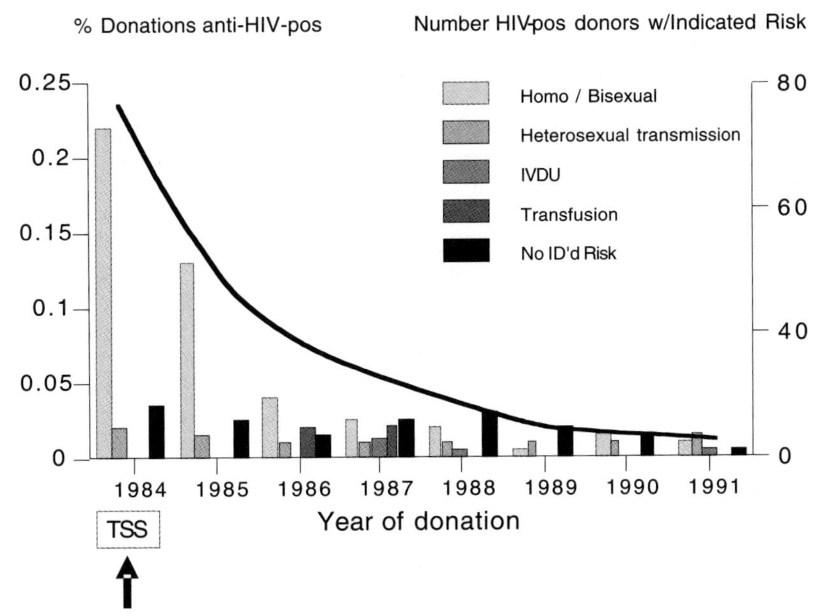

Fig. 4: Rates and risk factors of HIV-infected blood donors in San Francisco, California, through 1991.

transfusions continued to be observed. One early study in the U.S. found that 14 of 106 cases (13 %) initially reported to CDC as possible infections from screened blood transfusions were confirmed as transfusion transmissions by linkage to donors who later seroconverted [45]. After adjustment for non-investigated cases, CDC estimated that at least 10 TA-AIDS cases had occurred annually from 1986 through 1991 due to anti-HIV-screened blood transfusions [28]. This was no doubt an underestimate of the national recipient infection rate, given underlying recipient mortality and the long incubation period from infection to clinical AIDS resulting in poor case ascertainment.

Two prospective studies in the U.S. were launched in 1986 to specifically measure residual HIV risk from antibody screened units. The first study (the Frequency of Agents Communicated by Transfusions Study [FACTS]) was carried out in Baltimore and Houston hospitals, involving testing patients for anti-HIV-1 before and after cardiac surgery [46]. Cases of recipient seroconversion were investigated to rule out other risk factors, and donors were traced to document the source of infection. Two cases of HIV-1 infection were documented after transfusion of 120,000 units of blood; seroconverting donors were identified in both cases. In the other study, viral culture and polymerase chain reaction (PCR) methods were used to detect HIV-1 in pooled peripheral blood mononuclear cells derived from 200,000 anti-HIV-negative donations given in the San Francisco Bay Area from 1987-1990 (a prelude to subsequent introduction of mini-pool nucleic acid amplification testing (MP-NAT) a decade later) [47]. A single seronegative donation collected in 1987 was identified as infected by both PCR and culture. After adjusting for assay sensitivity and the pooled analyses, a risk estimate of 1 : 160,000 donations was calculated.

In the late 1980s, a more practical approach for estimating the risk of HIV infection from transfusions on an ongoing basis was beginning to evolve. This approach involved using data from "lookback" investigations to estimate the rate of HIV-1 transmissions that occur from donors who donate in the "window period" preceding detectable antibody. This approach was first used by CDC investigators and collaborating U.S. blood bankers who traced previous recipients of 701 blood donors who had seroconverted to anti-HIV positivity prior to 1991 [48]. Recipients of pre-seroconversion donations were identified and tested for 179 of the seroconverting donors, and the most recent seronegative donation resulted in infection in 36 (20 %) of the cases. Infection rates correlated indirectly with the time interval between the seropositive and seronegative donations (i.e., intervals < 90 days, 76 % transmission; 91-180 days, 28 % transmission; > 180 days, 11 % transmission). Mathematical modeling of these data indicated a median 45-day infectious window period (95 % CI: 34-55 days) for the overall period (1985-1990). Separate analysis of donations given prior and subsequent to March 1987 (when improved sensitivity EIAs were implemented in U.S. donor centers) indicated a reduction in the median infectious seronegative window from 55 days to 42 days. The results of this study represent the earliest germ of the incidence-window period model discussed later.

The p24 antigen controversy

Documentation of significant residual risk of HIV-1 transmission by window period donations fueled political and regulatory concerns over blood safety that had been ignited by widening appreciation of the extent of infections that had occurred among hemophiliacs and component recipients in the U.S. and elsewhere prior to antibody screening. This led to consideration of the need to introduce additional screening measures to interdict window phase donations. Seminal studies of serial plasma donor specimens (seroconversion panels) by scientists at Abbott Laboratories were reported in 1989 that documented detection of HIV-1 p24 antigen by screening EIAs 1-2 weeks prior to antibody seroconversion, leading to recommendations that this test be implemented into donor screening [49]. Two large studies were launched in the U.S. to directly evaluate the utility of p24 antigen screening. The first was a prospective, multi-center study that tested 500,000 donations for p24 antigen in parallel with antibody testing [50]. The second study involved p24 antigen EIA screening of 8,597 specimens selected from the TSS repository based on the corresponding donors being male, less than 45 years old, and who reside in high HIV prevalence ZIP codes; based on the 1.5 % seroprevalence in the selected donation subset, these samples were equivalent to over 2 million contemporary donations [51]. Both studies failed to detect p24 antigen-positive, antibody-negative donation, indicating very low potential yield. Furthermore, concerns were also raised over a possible magnet effect, related to high-risk persons going to blood banks to get a more sensitive HIV assay, which could lead to increased rather than decreased risk were antigen screening introduced [52]. Although these data led to an initial decision against p24 antigen screening, political pressure continued to mount, and eventually the FDA mandated p24 antigen screening in the U.S. Subsequent results from 5 years of national p24 antigen screening confirmed the findings of the earlier studies, with only 1 antigen-positive, antibody-negative donation detected per 6 million donations [53]. This experience highlighted the dilemma of trying to directly measure extremely low-level residual risk or the yield of new assays in the context of a growing public expectation for a zero risk blood supply.

Direct measurement of transfusion risk of other viruses in the late 1980s

The FACTS repository discussed above was also used to directly measure risks of hepatitis viruses and human T cell leukemia viruses in the late 1980s [46,54,55]. The data were particularly informative for HCV, since the study was conducted during the time period when NANBH surrogate markers and HCV antibody testing were first implemented. These researchers found that the risk of HCV infection was 0.45 % per unit prior to the implementation of any testing. After the implementation of testing for ALT and anti-HBc, the rate of infection dropped to 0.19 % per unit. Finally, once the version 1.0 EIA test for anti-HCV was implemented the rate dropped to 0.03 %, or 1 per 3,300 units [54]. A subsequent reevaluation using the more sensitive 2.0 EIA on blood recipients indicated that the risk was closer to 1 in 1700 [55]. Once the version 2.0 test was implemented for blood donor screening, the frequency of residual infection declined precipitously, such that transmission cases could no longer be documented by prospective follow-up studies.

Era of Risk Modeling: 1991 – present (Table 3)

The studies reviewed above designed to directly measure risk were discontinued in the early 1990s because of their high cost and the realization that they were too insensitive to assess residual risks of viral transmission from screened transfusions (with the exception of ongoing enrollment and follow-up of ~500 recipients per

Table 3: Era of risk modeling (1991 – present).

HIV	HCV	HBV
1991-1995 Development of incidence – Window Period Model		
REDS and ARC/CDC measure IR based on seroconversions (SC) among repeat donors	REDS measures IR based on SC among repeat donors	IR derived using HBsAg SC rate and HBV incidence conversion factor
Lookback dataset used to to model infectious WP	WP estimated using serial samples from recipients in TTVS and other NANBH cohorts	WP estimated from recipients in TTVS cohort
SC plasma donor panels used to estimate WP closure by RNA, Ag, & improved Ab tests	SC plasma donor panel studies to estimate WP closure by RNA & improved Ab tests	SC plasma donor panel studies to estimate WP closure by HBV DNA, HBsAg and anti-HBc
I-WP model applied to estimate risk, & project yield of p24 Ag and NAT	I-WP model applied to estimate risk, & project yield of NAT	I-WP model applied to estimate risk, & project yield of NAT
1996-1999 Refinement of incidence – Window Period Model		
WP stages and viral load dynamics defined based on plasma donor panels	WP stages and viral load dynamics defined based on plasma donor panels	WP stages and viral load dynamics defined based on plasma donor panels
Correlates of infectivity established using TSS repository	Correlates of infectivity established using TTVS repository	
Chimp infectivity studies	Chimp infectivity studies	Chimp infectivity studies
Sensitive/Less-sensitive ("detuned")-EIA developed and used to estimate HIV incidence in FT donors		
2000-2002 Global application of incidence – Window Period Model		
International application of I-WP model to project risk	International application of I-WP model to project risk	International application of I-WP model to project risk
MP-NAT yield data confirms model predictions	MP-NAT yield data confirms model predictions	I-WP model and empirical screening data indicate limited yield of MP-NAT →

Table 3: continued.

HIV	HCV	HBV
2000-2002 Global application of incidence – Window Period Model		
Modification of IR based on First-Time/Repeat NAT yield ratio	Modification of IR based on First-Time/Repeat NAT yield ratio	
Cost-effectiveness analyses performed based on I-WP model projections	Cost-effectiveness analyses performed based on I-WP model projections	Cost-effectiveness analyses performed based on I-WP model projections
2003-2005 Refined understanding of infectious Window Periods		
Characterization of "blip" viremia	Characterization of "blip" viremia	Possible "blip" viremia
Calculation of infectious WP by extrapolation using doubling time model	Calculation of infectious WP by extrapolation using doubling time model	Calculation of infectious WP by extrapolation using doubling time model
New strategy of applying MP-NAT yield to deriving risk estimates	New strategy of applying MP-NAT yield to deriving risk estimates	New strategy of applying MP-NAT yield to deriving risk estimates
	Chimp experiments to further define infectious WP	Chimp experiments to further define infectious WP

year at the NIH Clinical Center). Since then, an alternative approach has been developed for estimating risk, now known as the incidence rate – window period (IR-WP) model [56]. The remainder of this chapter will discuss the development and subsequent refinement of this new approach for risk monitoring.

Principles and initial application of Incidence Rate – Window Period Model

Prevalence and incidence have commonly been used to measure risks in the blood supply. Prevalence measures the percentage of donations that test positive on a screening and confirmatory test, including old and new infections, while incidence measures the rate at which new infections develop in a population at risk. Since donations that have positive screening tests are discarded, the greatest threat to the safety of the blood supply is the donation of blood in the infectious window period (WP), the time between infection, or more precisely infectivity, and detectability by screening tests. Additional sources of transfusion-risk attributable to variant viral strains, immunosilent carriers, and testing errors [57-64] contribute only minimally to risk, especially when dual testing systems are in place, i.e., serology tests targeting antibodies and antigen or nucleic acid amplification tests to detect viremia.

The IR-WP model was developed in parallel by investigators from the National Heart, Lung, and Blood Institute-sponsored Retrovirus Epidemiology Donor Study (REDS) [56,65] and the CDC and American National Red Cross [66] and has been used in the United States to estimate the probability of a WP donation for each TTVI since the early 1990s [67]. The model estimates the probability of a potentially infectious donation being released into the blood supply, or residual risk, by multiplying the IR by the number of days during which an infection may be present but not detectable by current screening assays (i.e. the length of the WP). This modeling approach can be implemented without the need to fund special research projects and can be used to generate risk estimates for multiple agents using the same dataset.

The IR-WP model requires that two parameters, the IR and the WP, are known with accuracy. IRs are classically derived by dividing the numbers of known confirmed incident cases (detected by serological or NAT screening) by the number of person-years or the sum of the periods of time during which donors are at risk (i.e. are not infected yet). This derivation is usually confined to repeat donors since this population is followed for a certain period of time, allowing evaluation of how many donors are incident, i.e. first tested negative on all assays and then tested positive for a particular marker on a subsequent donation. The minimum statistics required for IR calculations are the number of incident cases (the numerator), the total number of repeat donations, and the mean inter-donation interval length (multiplication of the last two entities provides the number of person-years or denominator). Alternatively, if donation histories are available for all repeat donors, we can derive person-years by summing up the length of all inter-donation intervals. The interested reader should refer to the commentaries by Kleinman et al [56,67] and Glynn et al [68] for detailed discussions of adjustments, derivation of confidence intervals and other factors impacting the accuracy of IR estimates.

The second key statistic needed to estimate residual risk is the length of the WP for each test. WP estimates for HCV and HBV initially used in the IR-WP model were based on analyses of repository specimens from post-transfusion hepatitis cases [64-66]. Serial samples from HBV and HCV infected recipients were tested, and the time from transfusion to development of a positive test was calculated. Multiple studies involving testing of serial post-transfusion samples from over 200 HCV cases demonstrated that the WP from transfusion to HCV antibody detection ranged from 60 to 80 days, depending on sampling interval and whether EIA-2 or EIA-3 was used to detect seroconversion [69-73]. The WP for HBV was much less well defined, since the commonly cited estimate of 59 days from transfusion to HBsAg conversion was based on a series of only seven evaluable TTVS cases [74]. By combining these WP estimates with IR estimates from 1990 through 1993, the REDS group derived residual risk estimates for HCV of 1 in 103,000 and for HBV of 1 in 63,000 [65].

The WP estimate used for HIV in the initial IR-WP models was derived from the mathematical modeling of transfusion-transmitted infections occurring from HIV seronegative units donated by persons who subsequently seroconverted, as discussed above [48,64]. Further analysis indicated that the HIV-1 WP was reduced from a median of 45 days for the period from 1985 to 1990, derived from the look-back data, to approximately 22 to 25 days with introduction in 1992 of new format anti-HIV-1/HIV-2 EIAs which detect HIV-specific IgM antibody 10 to 15 days earlier than previously available assays [75]. By combining the 25-day window period estimate with HIV IRs derived from repeat donors in large US donor populations, two independent studies derived point estimates for the risk for HIV transmission during the 1992-1995 period of 1 : 450,000 [66] and 1 : 495,000, [65] respectively.

Although the early models used these WP estimates, what we are really interested in is the period of time during which a donation is infectious; this infectivity period may or may not be the same as the length of the WP commonly used to estimate residual risks. For example, it is unclear whether donations given in the early stages after exposure, i.e. during the so-called eclipse (RNA-negative), pre-ramp-up intermittent RNA-positive, and very early ramp-up viremia phases of infection, contain enough virus to be infectious [64]. In particular, the significance and infectivity of the low-level intermittent "blips" of RNA/DNA recently detected in plasma donor seroconversion panels in the pre-ramp-up phase are uncertain (Fig. 5a-b) [76-78]. Further studies, including animal transmission experiments in appropriate model systems [79], donor lookback studies (where prior units from sero- or NAT-positive RPT donors are traced and recipients of these units tested) [80,81] and recipient traceback studies (investigation by recall or testing of stored donation specimens of donors whose blood products were transfused to recipients who subsequently acquired an infection post-transfusion) [82] are clearly needed to answer these questions and permit better estimation of risks. For example, Weusten et al [83] used minimum chimpanzee infectious doses data to statistically predict human infectivity, relative to viral load and NAT assay performance, in a recently published mathematical model of WP risk. While this is a clear conceptual advance and seems like a reasonable approach, the animal infectivity data employed in the model were very limited and it is unclear whether the animal data are directly transferable to humans. Further work in this area is now in progress to define the minimal infectious dose and infectivity of "blip" viremia for each of the major agents.

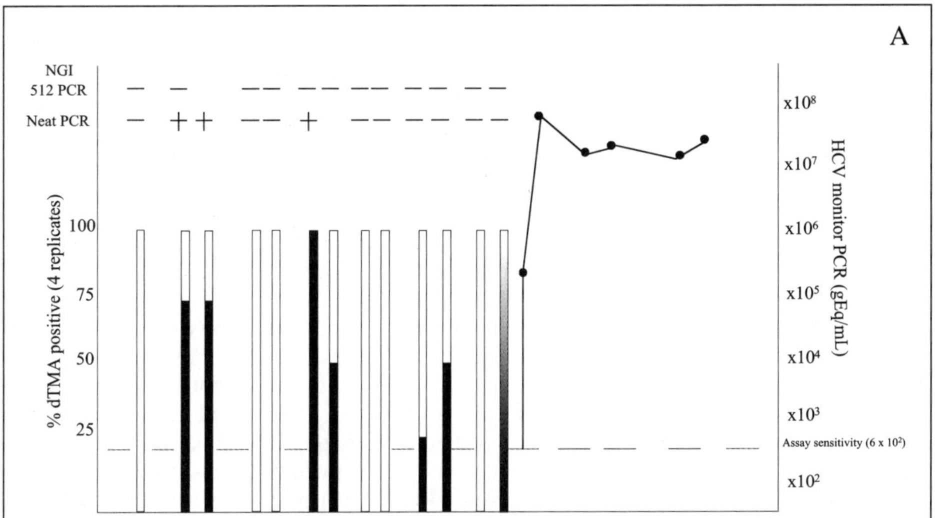

Fig. 5a: Dynamics of early HCV infection. Panel A: Low-level intermittent viremia preceding "ramp-up" phase. Panel B: Viral load in early HCV infection. (N = 55 donors).

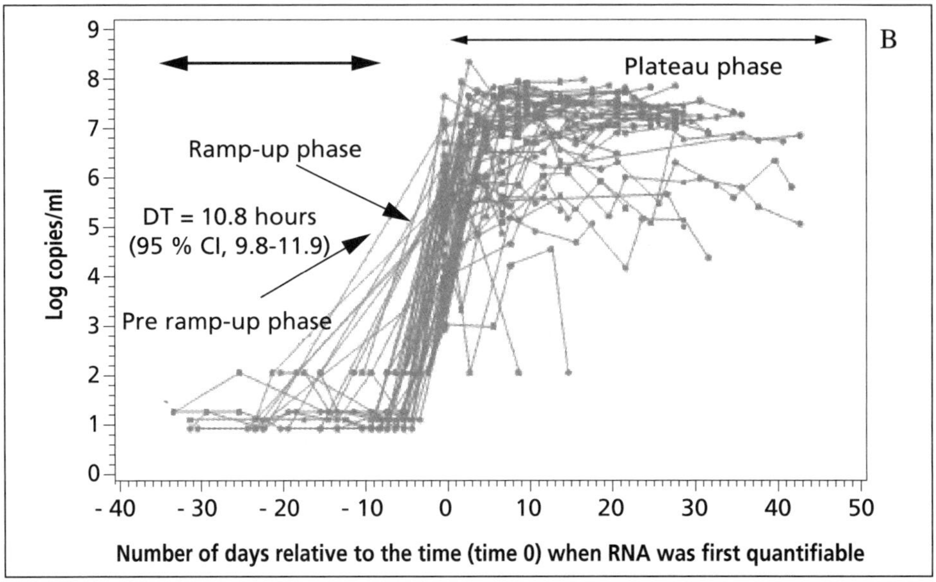

Fig. 5b: Dynamics of early HCV infection. Panel A: Low-level intermittent viremia preceding "ramp-up" phase. Panel B: Viral load in early HCV infection. (N = 55 donors).

International application of IR-WP model

The IR-WP model has now been applied successfully worldwide to provide country specific viral-TTI estimates [84-92]. In developed countries in Europe, North America and the Asia-Pacific regions, the residual risk estimates are uniformly low and suggest that the donor selection process (self-selection, behavioral screening) and test screening adopted over the past several decades were very effective. More importantly, reports using the model clearly demonstrate that HIV and HCV residual risks have been further reduced to extremely low levels after mini-pool NAT implementation. For HIV, the estimated probability of having a potentially infectious donation being released in the blood supply varied from about 1 in 450,000 (Italy) to 1 in 3 million (Australia) donations pre-NAT, whereas residual risks post-NAT varied between 1 in 900,000 (Italy) and 1 in 5 million (Australia). Even more marked was the reduction for HCV, with risks decreasing from about 1 in 120,000 (Australia, Italy) to 1 in 800,000 (France) donations pre-NAT (EIA 3.0), to approximately 1 in 1 million (Australia, Italy) to 1 in 10 million (France) post-NAT. Although HBV risk estimates need to be evaluated with some caution (see below), data from most reports suggest that of the major viral TTIs evaluated, HBV remains most likely to be transmissible by transfusion, with residual risks of 1 in 75,000 (Spain) to 1 in 500,000 (France) donations. Mini-pool HBV NAT testing only reduces the WP by about 10 days [93] since the ramp-up viremia phase for HBV is characterized by a much slower doubling time (2.6 days) than for HIV (20.5 hours) [94] or HCV (14.9 hours) [76,77]. The difficulty in decreasing HBV risks also stems from the fact that no risk factor can be identified in 30-40 % of HBV cases [95] and consequent inability to develop donor screening criteria that are sensitive enough to effectively screen out HBV-infected donors and specific enough to avoid unnecessary deferral of healthy donors. Widespread implementation of HBV immunization programs should, in the future, help reduce risks of HBV transfusion-transmission by decreasing the number of infectious donors and susceptible transfusion recipients.

Several groups have recently applied the IR-WP model to estimate residual risk and project the yield of NAT or p24 antigen screening in developing country settings, documenting substantially greater risk than exists in developed countries. For example, HIV risk in Brazil has been estimated at 1 in 66,000 [96,97], while HIV risk in the Republic of South Africa was 1 in 38,000 in the context of screening for both HIV antibody and p24 antigen [98,99]. Given the relatively high HIV incidence and residual risk levels in such countries, the yield and safety impact of NAT screening would be relatively greater than in developed countries [97,99]. Unfortunately, the financial resources to support NAT screening in developing country settings are limited, although screening has recently been implemented in the Republic of South Africa as a result of criticism and consequent discontinuation of their previous blood safety strategy that included use of race as an eligibility criterion [99].

Assumptions, limitations and refinement of IR-WP Model

The basic assumptions of the IR-WP model are: i) WP donations represent the most dominant source of risk, ii) overall IR in repeat donors (RPT) is constant throughout the time period of the study, iii) a recently infected donor is as likely to donate in the early interval after infection as he or she is to donate subsequently, and iv) if no further adjustment is made, first-time (FT) donors have the same IR as RPT donors. The first assumption appears valid for HIV and HCV with WP-risk probably accounting for 90 % or more of the total risk and other sources of risk (viral variants, chronic seronegative carriers, and testing error) for 10 % or less [64]. This is also the case for HBV in countries performing anti-HBc screening, whereas HBsAg-negative/anti-HBc reactive chronic carriers may contribute a level of risk equal or greater to WP risk in the absence of anti-HBc screening [81,100]. We have no reason to doubt the validity of the second assumption if the time period of the study is short (or for longer periods, if there does not appear to be changes in rates through time that can result from changes in the epidemiology of the agent in the population or revision of screening criteria).

The third assumption may be more problematic since more recent studies have noted that the seroconversion interval may be longer than expected for HIV [101] or HCV incident cases [102,103]. This would imply that some donors delay their return around time of infection and suggests that the model (which assumes a steady state rate of donation) may tend to overestimate the yield of tests that detect infection earlier (i.e. NAT or HIV p24Ag). Consistent with this concern, Seed et al [102] reported that the duration of the seroconversion interval for HCV seroconverters in Australia was much longer than for the other viruses, and consequently the IR-WP model predicted three times the yield of HCV NAT-only donations than were observed. Similarly, an apparent difference in observed vs. expected HCV yield was noted for several countries in Central Europe [89,104]. In contrast, no significant difference has been found in predicted vs. observed HCV yield data in France or the US, compatible with the finding of no delay in return for HCV seroconverters in the US [101]. Furthermore, no significant differences were found in any study between observed (0.0-0.6 per 10^6 donations) and predicted (0.2-0.4 per 10^6 donations) yields for HIV [89]. Thus, the model seems to predict the yield of new assays reasonably well unless donors significantly delay their return around the time of infection/seroconversion.

Regarding the fourth assumption, the recent development of a sensitive/less-sensitive ("detuned") HIV-1 assay [106] and evaluation of NAT-yield data [105] have recently permitted direct assessment of the relative IRs in FT vs. repeat donors. Janssen et al [106] reported a 2.4 fold higher IR in FT donors (7.18 per 100,000 person-years) than in repeat donors (2.95 per 100,000 person-years) in the US using the sensitive/less-sensitive HIV-testing strategy. Using NAT-yield data, Dodd et al [87] and Stramer et al [88] have confirmed this 2-fold differential in IRs between FT and repeat donors for HIV and extended this finding to HCV where the IR ratio was 2.4. It is therefore now possible to estimate IRs in all donors if the relative proportion of FT and repeat donors is known and repeat donor IR are measured. This approach works well in developed countries where 70 %-80 % of donations are from repeat donors. In contrast, in many developing countries a very high proportion of donations are from FT donors, and hence new approaches such as the sensitive/less-sensitive EIA method are particularly useful to estimate FT donor incidence and derive risk estimates [96-99].

"New Strategy" for estimating risk based on viral dynamics and rates of detection of donors with incident infections

A new strategy for risk estimation has recently been developed that employs more accurate estimates of infectious and marker positive window periods for HIV, HCV, and HBV, and then uses window period ratios and rates of detection of donors with incident infections to project risk [107]. The first component of this approach is based on back extrapolation of data documenting increasing concentrations of viral nucleic acids in plasma during the ramp-up phase of primary viremia. The approach involves several steps. The first step is testing of plasma or blood donor seroconversion panels to determine the exponential viral growth rate during the ramp-up phase preceding serological marker reactivity; this is expressed as the number of days for the viral load to double (i.e. HBV doubling time) [76,77,94]. The second step is to determine the number of viral nucleic acid copies present at the time that the relevant donor screening assays become positive. In the case of an HBsAg assay, this is defined as the number of HBV DNA copies present when the HBsAg signal-to-cutoff (S/CO) ratio is 1.0 [108,109]. For a NAT assay, this is defined as the reported 50 % limit of detection [107-109]. These viral load parameters are derived by regression or probit analyses and are dependent upon the sensitivity of the particular HBsAg or NAT donor screening assay used in each country or screening program. Then, based on an assumption that infectivity first occurs when HBV is present at a specified concentration (e.g., one viral copy per 20 mL of plasma, which is the amount of plasma assumed to be in additive-solution red cell concentrate), an extrapolation (using the doubling time) is performed from the copy number at the HBsAg or NAT threshold of detection to the time at which the minimal infectious dose of virus would be present. This is the imputed length of the infectious window period. Figure 6 summarizes the estimated lengths of relevant WPs for each agent.

The second component of the new strategy is monitoring NAT screening data and/or HIV-1 detuned EIA data to determine the rate that donations are given by donors in the early stages of infection detected by these assays. Table 4 summarizes representative NAT yield data from the US and uses ratios of the pre-NAT infectious WP relative to the NAT yield WP for each agent to transform the NAT yield rates

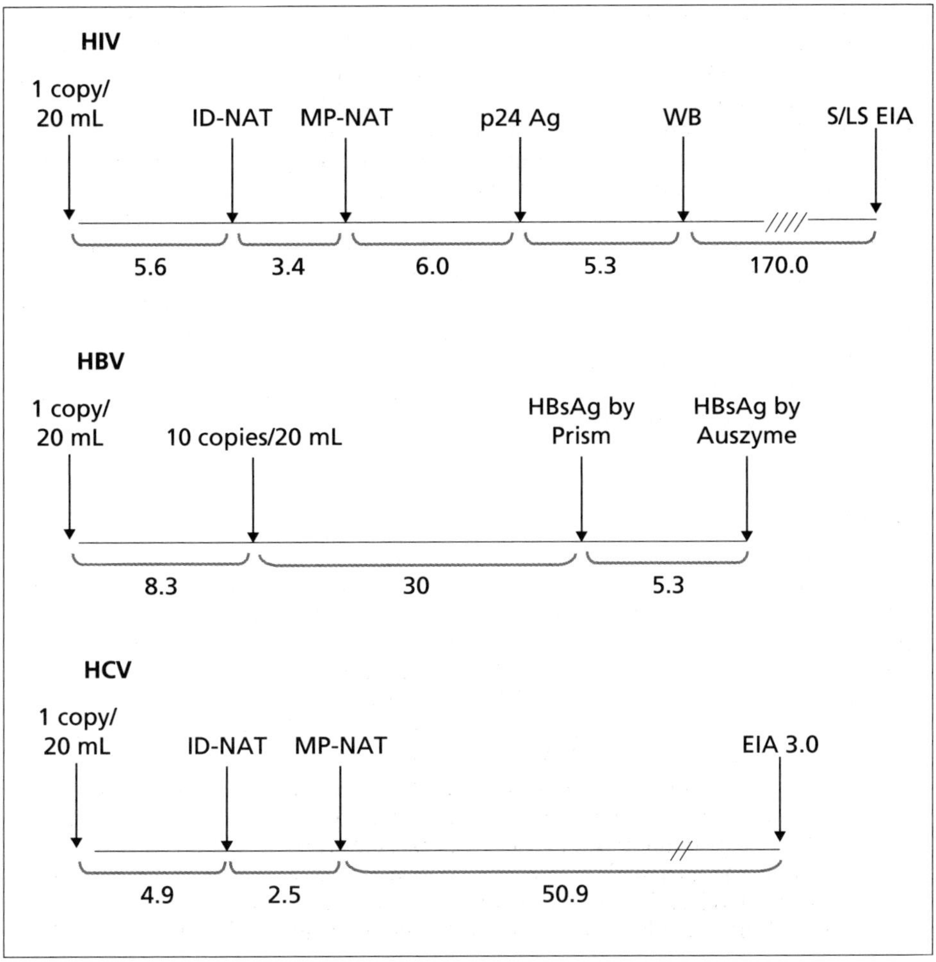

Fig. 6: Time points of earliest detectability of HIV, HBV, and HCV by different means, and resulting window periods.

Table 4: Use of 'New Strategy" based on NAT yield data and window period ratios to project risks of transfusion HCV, HIV and HBV, and comparison with risks derived from classic IR-WP model.

Virus	No. cases	No. units screened	MP-NAT yield	Risk derived from MP-NAT yield	Risk from IR-WP Model
HCV	145	37.5 x 106	1 in 2.6 x 105	1 in 1.55 x 106	1 in 1.61 x 106
HIV	10	36.7 x 106	1 in 3.7 x 106	1 in 1.67 x 106	1 in 1.78 x 106
HBV	4	1.4 x 106	1 in 352,000	1 in 174,000	1 in 269,000

into residual risk rates (see ref. 107 for details on derivation of these ratios). The table demonstrates that these rates projected from NAT yield data are very similar to those derived using the now classical IR-WP model. This approach can also be used to project that conversion from MP- to ID-NAT would detect only 2-3 additional HIV-1 and HCV infectious units annually in the US, whereas for HBV ID NAT would yield 25-30 infectious donations missed by HBsAg and MP NAT [107-109].

The new strategy approach for risk and yield projection is attractive because it: i) does not require discrimination of FT from repeat donations and therefore does not require adjustment factors to account for differential incidence, ii) avoids biases discussed above related to the assumption that infected donors donate at a steady state during the pre-seroconversion WP, and iii) employs more accurate yet still conservative estimates for the infectious WPs. A collaborative project is now under way, under the auspices of the Infectious Diseases Working Party of the International Society of Blood Transfusion, to apply the new strategy approach to global NAT yield data and LS-EIA data.

Conclusions

Our ability to understand, measure and consequently reduce infectious risks from transfusions has evolved dramatically over the past 50 years. The rate of recent progress in developing modeling approaches for estimating risk is particularly noteworthy. The IR-WP model and its derivatives are now accepted as accurate by blood bankers and regulators around the world. In addition to establishing risk estimates, the estimates of test utility from IR-WP models have been widely used in cost-effectiveness analyses to inform policy debates over the merits of implementing NAT screening, converting from MP-NAT to ID-NAT or introduction of pathogen inactivation [110-112]. They have also been used to inform discussions over donor recruitment and deferral policies such as acceptance of male donors who have had sex with other males in the past [113,114], or policies related to eligibility of donors from racial-ethic groups with different risk profiles [99]. Modified IR-WP model approaches can also be adapted to quickly understand and estimate risk from emerging agents such as West Nile, Dengue, and pandemic influenza viruses [115,116].

References

1 Beeson PB: Jaundice occurring one to four months after transfusion of blood or plasma. Report of seven cases. JAMA 1943; 121: 1332-1334.

2 Grady GF, Chalmers TC: Risk of post-transfusion viral hepatitis. N Engl J Med 1964; 271: 337-342.

3 Walsh JH, Purcell RH, Morrow AG, Chanock RM, Schmidt PJ: Posttransfusion hepatitis after open-heart operations. Incidence after the administration of blood from commercial and volunteer donor populations. JAMA 1970; 211: 261-265.

4 Domen RE: Paid-versus-volunteer blood donation in the United States: a historical review. Transfus Med Rev 1995; 9:53-59.

5 Blumberg BS, Alter HJ, Visnich S: A "new" antigen in leukemia sera. JAMA 1965; 191: 541-546.

6 Gocke DJ, Greenberg HB, Kavey NB: Hepatitis antigen. Detection of infectious blood donors. Lancet 1969; ii: 248-249.

7 Gocke DJ, Greenberg HB, Kavey NB: Correlation of Australia antigen with posttrasfusion hepatitis. JAMA 1970; 77: 877-879.

8 Alter HJ, Holland PV, Purcell RH, Lander JJ, Feinstone SM Morrow AG, Schmidt PJ: Posttransfusion hepatitis after exclusion of commercial and hepatitis-B antigen-positive donors. Ann Intern Med 1972; 77: 691-699.

9 Feinstone SM, Kapikian AZ, Purcell RH: Hepatitis A: detection by immune electron microscopy of a virus-like antigen associated with acute illness. Science 1973; 182: 1026-1028.

10 Stevens CE, Silbert JA, Miller DR, Dienstag JL, Purcell RH, Szmuness W: Serologic evidence of hepatitis A and B virus infections in thalassemia patients: a retrospective study. Transfusion 1978; 18: 356-360.

11 Dienstag JL, Feinstone SM, Purcell RH, Feinstone SM, Wong DC, Holland PV: Non-A, non-B post-transfusion hepatitis. Lancet 1977; i: 560-562.

12 Aach RD, Szmuness W, Mosley JW, Hollinger FB, Kahn RA, Stevens CE, et al; Serum alanine aminotransferase of donors in relation to the risk of non-A, non-B hepatitis in recipients. The Transfusion-Transmitted Viruses Study. N Engl J Med 1981; 04: 989-994.

13 Alter HJ, Purcell RH, Holland PV, Alling DW, Koziol DE: Donor transaminase and recipient hepatitis. JAMA 1981; 246: 630-634.

14 Stevens CE, Aach RD, Hollinger FB, Mosley JW, Szmuness W, Kahn R, Werch J, et al: Hepatitis B virus antibody in blood donors and the occurrence of non-A, non-B hepatitis in transfusion recipients. An analysis of the Transfusion-Transmitted Viruses Study. Ann Int Med 1984; 101: 733-738.

15 Koziol DE, Holland PV, Alling DW, Melpolder JC, Solomon RE, Purcell RH, et al: Antibody to Hepatitis B core Antigen as a Paradoxical Marker for Non-A, Non-B Hepatitis Agents in Donated Blood. Ann Int Med 1986; 104: 488-495.

16 Infectious disease testing for blood transfusions. NIH Consensus Statement 1995 Jan 9-11; 13 (1): 1-27.

17 Alter HJ: To C or not to C: these are the questions. Blood 1995; 85: 1681-1695.

18 Ezzell C: Candidate cause identified of non-A, non-B hepatitis. [news] Nature 1988; 333: 195.

19 Choo QL, Kuo G, Weiner AJ, Overby LR, Bradley DW, Houghton M: Isolation of a cDNA clone derived from a blood-borne non-A, non-B viral hepatitis genome. Science 1989; 244: 359-361.

20 Operskalski EA, Mosley JW, Tobler LH, Fiebig EW, Nowicki MJ, Mimms LT, Gallarda J, Phelps BH, Busch MP, for the Transfusion-Transmitted Viruses Study (TTVS) and the Retrovirus Epidemiology Donor Study (REDS): HCV Viral Load in anti-HCV-Reactive Donors and Infectivity for Their Recipients. Transfusion 2003; 43: 1433-1441.

21 Mimms LT, Mosley JW, Hollinger FB, et al: Transfusion-transmitted co-infection with human hepatitis B and hepatitis C viruses. Br Med J 1993; 307: 1095-1097.

22 Mosley JW, Operskalski EA, Tobler LH, Andrews WW, Phelps B, Dockter J, Giachetti C, Busch MP: Viral and Host Factors in Early Hepatitis C Virus Infection. Hepatology 2005; 42: 86-92.

23 Seeff LB, et al: Long-term mortality and morbidity of transfusion-associated non-A, non-B, and type C hepatitis: A National Heart, Lung, and Blood Institute collaborative study. Hepatology 2001; 33 (2): 455-463.

24 Busch MP: Insights into the Epidemiology. Natural History and Pathogenesis of Hepatitis C Virus Infection from Studies of Infected Donors and Blood Product Recipients. State of the Art Lecture, presented at 7th European Congress of the International Society of Blood Transfusion, Paris, July 2001. Transfusion Clinique et Biologique 2001; 8: 200-206.

25 Kleinman SH, Niland JC, Azen SP, Operskalski EA, Barbosa LH, Chernoff AI, Edwards VM, Lenes BA, Marshall GJ, Nemo GJ, et al: Prevalence of antibodies to human immunodeficiency virus type 1 among blood donors prior to screening. The Transfusion Safety Study/NHLBI Donor Repository. Transfusion 1989; 29 (7): 572-580.

26 Busch MP, Young MJ, Samson SM et al and the Transfusion Safety Study Group: Risk of human immunodeficiency virus transmission by blood transfusions prior to the implementation of HIV antibody screening in the San Francisco Bay Area. Transfusion 1991; 31: 4.

27 Perkins HA, Samson S, Busch MP: How well has self-exclusion worked? Transfusion 1988; 28: 601.

28 Selik RM, Ward JW, Buehler JW: Trends in transfusion-associated acquired immune deficiency syndrome in the United States, 1982 through 1991. Transfusion 1993; 33: 890.

29 Donegan E, Stuart M, Niland JC et al and the Transfusion Safety Study Group: Infection with human immunodeficiency virus type I (HIV-1) among recipients of antibody-positive blood donations. Ann Intern Med 1990; 113: 733.

30 Busch M, Donegan E, Stuart M, Mosley JW, for theTransfusion Safety Study Group: Donor HIV-1 p24 antigenaemia and course of infection in recipients. Lancet 1990; i: 1342.

31 Donegan E, Lenes BA, Tomasulo RA, Mosley JW and the Transfusion Safety Study Group: Transmission of HIV-l by components type and duration of shelf storage before transfusion. Transfusion 1990; 30: 851.

32 Busch MP, Operskalski EA, Mosley JW, Lee TH, Henrard D, Herman S, Sachs DH, Harris M, Huang W, Stram DO: Factors influencing human immunodeficiency virus type 1 transmission by blood transfusion. Transfusion Safety Study Group. J Infect Dis 1996; 174: 26.

33 Operskalski EA, Stram DO, Busch MP, Huang W, Harris M, Dietrich SL, Schiff ER, Donegan E, Mosley JW: Role of viral load in heterosexual transmission of human immunodeficiency virus type 1 by blood transfusion recipients. Transfusion Safety Study Group. Am J Epidemiol 1997; 146: 655.

34 Operskalski EA, Stram DO, Lee H, Zhou Y, Donegan E, Busch MP, Stevens CE, Schiff ER, Dietrich SL, Mosley JW: Human immunodeficiency virus type 1 infection: relationship of risk group and age to rate of progression to AIDS. Transfusion Safety Study Group. J Infect Dis 1995; 172: 648.

35 Busch MP, Operskalski EA, Mosley JW et al and the Transfusion Safety Study Group: Epidemiologic background and long-term course of disease in human immunodeficiency virus type 1-infected blood donors identified before routine laboratory screening. Transfusion 1994; 34: 858.

36 Operskalski EA, Busch MP, Mosley JW, Stram DO: Comparative rates of disease progression among persons infected with the same or different HIV-1 strains. The Transfusion Safety Study Group. J Acquir Immune Defic Syndr Hum Retrovirol 1997; 15: 145.

37 Wilkinson DA, Operskalski EA, Busch MP, Mosley JW, Koup RA: A 32-bp deletion within the CCR5 locus protects against transmission of parenterally acquired human immunodeficiency virus but does not affect progression to AIDS-defining illness. J Infect Dis 1998; 178: 1163.

38 Diaz R, Sabino EC, Mayer A, Mosley JW, Busch MP: Dual Human Immunodeficiency Virus Type 1 Infection and Recombination in a Dually Exposed Transfusion Recipient. J Virol 1995; 69: 3273-3281.

39 Diaz RS, Zhang L-Q, Busch MP, Mosley JW, Mayer A: Divergence of HIV 1 Quasispecies in an Epidemiologic Cluster. AIDS 1997; 11: 415-422.

40 Zhang LQ, Diaz RS, Ho DD, Mosley JW, Busch MP, Mayer A: Host-Specific Driving Force in HIV-1 Evolution in vivo. J Virol 1997; 71: 2555-2561.

41 Learmont JC, Geczy AF, Mills J, Ashton LJ, Raynes-Greenow CH, Garsia RJ, Dyer WB, McIntyre L, Oelrichs RB, Rhodes DI, Deacon NJ, Sullivan JS: Immunologic and virologic status after 14 to 18 years of infection with an attenuated strain of HIV-1. A report from the Sydney Blood Bank Cohort. N Engl J Med 1999; 340: 1715.

42 Busch MP, Collier A, Gernsheimer T, Carrington JD, Flanigan TP, Kashkari M, Kennedy M, Kumar PN, Lane TA, Mellors JW, Mohandas K, Pollard RB, Viele M, Yomtovian R, Holland PV, McCurdy PR: The Viral Activation Transfusion Study VATS: rationale, objectives, and design overview: Transfusion 1996; 36: 854.

43 Busch MP, Lee TH, Heitman J: Allogeneic leukocytes but not therapeutic blood elements induce reactivation and dissemination of latent human immunodeficiency virus type 1 infection: implications for transfusion support of infected patients. Blood 1992; 80: 2128.

44 Collier AC, Kalish LA, Busch MP, Gernsheimer T, Assmann SF, Lane TA, Asmuth DM, Lederman MM, Murphy EL, Kumar P, Kelley M, Flanigan TP, McMahon DK, Sacks HS, Kennedy MS, Holland PV, for the Viral Activation Transfusion Study Group: Leukocyte-Reduced Red Blood Cell Transfusions in Patients with Anemia and Human Immunodeficiency Virus Infection. The Viral Activation Transfusion Study: A Randomized Controlled Trial. JAMA 2001; 285: 1592-1601.

45 Ward JW, Holmberg SD, Allen JR et al: Transmission of human immunodeficiency virus (HIV) by blood transfusions screened as negative for HIV antibody. N Engl J Med 1988; 318: 473.

46 Nelson KE, Donahue JG, Muñoz A, Cohen ND, Ness PM, Teague A, Stambolis VA, Yawn DH, Callicott B, McAllister H, Reitz BA, Lee H, Farzadegan H, Hollingsworth CG. Transmission of retroviruses from seronegative donors by transfusion during cardiac surgery. A multicenter study of HIV-1 and HTLV-I/II infections. [see comments]. Ann Intern Med 1992; 117 (7): 554-559.

47 Busch MP, Eble BE, Khayam-Bashi H, Murphy EL, Heilbron D, Kwok S, Sninsky JJ, Perkins HA, Vyas GN: Evaluation of Screened Blood Donations for Human Immunodeficiency Virus Type 1 Infection by Culture and DNA Amplification of Pooled Cells. N Engl J Med 1991; 325: 1-5.

48 Petersen LR, Satten GA, Dodd R, Busch M, Kleinman S, Grindon A, Lenes B, and the HIV Seroconversion Study Group: Duration of Time from Onset of Human Immunodeficiency Virus Type 1 Infectiousness to Development of Detectable Antibody. Transfusion 1994; 34: 283-289.

49 Stramer SL, Heller JS, Coombs RW, Parry JV, Ho DD, Allain JP: Markers of HIV infection prior to IgG antibody seropositivity. Jama 1989; 262: 64-69

50 Alter HJ, Epstein JS, Swenson SG, VanRaden MJ, Ward JW, Kaslow RA, Menitove JE, Klein HG, Sandler SG, Sayers MH: Prevalence of human immunodeficiency virus type 1 p24 antigen in U.S. blood donors – an assessment of the efficacy of testing in donor screening. The HIV-Antigen Study Group. N Engl J Med 1990; 323 (19): 1312-1317.

51 Busch MP, Taylor PE, Lenes BA, Kleinman SH, Stuart M, Stevens CE, Tomasulo PA, Allain J-P, Hollingsworth CG, Mosley JW, and the Transfusion Safety Study Group: Screening of Selected Male Blood Donors for p24 Antigen of Human Immunodeficiency Virus Type 1. N Engl J Med 1990; 323: 1308-1312.

52 Korelitz JJ, Busch MP, Williams AE, and the Retrovirus Epidemiology Donor Study: Antigen Testing for Human Immunodeficiency Virus (HIV) and the Magnet Effect: Will the Benefit of a New HIV Test be Offset by the Numbers of Higher-Risk, Test-Seeking Donors Attracted to Blood Centers? Transfusion 1996; 36: 203-208.

53 Busch MP, Stramer SL: The Efficiency of HIV p24 Antigen Screening of US Blood Donors: Projections versus Reality. Infusionther Transfusionmed 1998; 25 (2): 5-8.

54 Donahue JG, Munoz A, Ness PM, Brown DE, Yawn DH, McAllister HA, et al: The declining risk of post-transfusion hepatitis C virus infection. N Engl J Med 1992; 327: 369-373.

55 Nelson KE, Ahmed F, Ness P, Donahue JG: The incidence of post-transfusion hepatitis: Reply. New Engl J Med 1993; 328: 1280-1281.

56 Kleinman S, Busch MP, Korelitz JJ, Schreiber GB: The incidence/window period model and its use to assess the risk of transfusion-transmitted human immunodeficiency virus and hepatitis C virus infection. Transfus Med Rev 1997; 11: 155.

57 Centers for Disease Control and Prevention. Persistent Lack of detectable HIV-1 antibody in a person with HIV infection – Utah, 1995. MMWR 1996; 45: 181-185.

58 Delwart EL, Orton S, Parekh B, Dobbs T, Clark K, Busch MP: Two Percent of HIV-Positive U.S. Blood Donors are Infected with Non-Subtype-B Strains. AIDS Res & Hum Retrovir 2003; 19: 1065-1070.

59 Delwart E, Kuhns MC, Busch MP: Surveillance of the Genetic Variation in Incident HIV, HCV, and HBV Infections in Blood and Plasma Donors: Implications for Blood Safety, Diagnostics, Treatment, and Molecular Epidemiology. J Med Virol, (Suppl) 2006 (in press).

60 Jongerius JM, Wester M, Cuypers HTM, van Oostendorp WR, Lelie PN, van der Poel CL, van Leeuwen EF: New hepatitis B virus mutant form in a blood donor that is undetectable in several hepatitis B surface antigen screening assays. Transfusion 1998; 38: 56-65.

61 Loussert-Ajaka I, Ly TD, Chaix ML, Ingrand D, Saragosti S, Courouce AM, Brun-Vezinet F Simon F: HIV-1/HIV-2 seronegativity in HIV-1 subtype O infected patients [see comments]. Lancet 1994; 343 (8910): 1393-1394.

62 Alter MJ, Margolis HS, Krawczynski K, et al, for The Sentinel Counties Chronic Non-A, Non-B Hepatitis Study Team: The natural history of community-acquired hepatitis C in the United States. N Engl J Med 1992; 327: 1899-1905.

63 Busch MP, Watanabe KK, Smith JW, Hermansen SW, Thomson RA, for the Retrovirus Epidemiology Donor Study: False-Negative Testing Errors in Routine Viral Marker Screening of Blood Donors. Transfusion 2000; 40: 585-589.

64 Busch MP: Closing the Windows on Viral Transmission by Blood Transfusion, in Stramer SL (ed): Blood Safety in the New Millennium. AABB 2000 Emily Cooley Seminar Book. Bethesda MD, AABB Press, 2001, pp 33-54.

65 Schreiber GB, Busch MP, Kleinman SH, Korelitz JJ: The risk of transfusion-transmitted viral infections. N Engl J Med 1996; 334: 1685-1690.

66 Lackritz EM, Satten GA, Aberle-Grasse J, Dodd RY, Raimondi VP, Janssen RS, Lewis WF, Notari EP 4th, Petersen LR; Estimated risk of transmission of the human immunodeficiency virus by screened blood in the United States [see comments]. New England Journal of Medicine 1995; 333 (26): 1721-1725.

67 Kleinman SH, Busch MP: Risks of Transfusion Transmitted Infection: Direct Estimation and Mathematical Modeling, in Contreras M (ed): New Aspects of Blood Transfusion, in Bailliere's Best Practice and Research in Clinical Haematology. London, Bailliere-Tindall, 2000, vol 13 (4), pp 631-649.

68 Glynn SA, Kleinman SH, Wright DJ, Busch MP, for the NHLBI Retrovirus Epidemiology Donor Study. International Application of the Incidence Rate/Window Period Model. Transfusion 2002; 42: 966-972.

69 Kleinman S, Alter H, Busch M, Holland P, Tegtmeier G, Nelles M, Lee S, et al: Increased detection of hepatitis C virus (HCV)- infected blood donors by a multiple-antigen HCV enzyme immunoassay. Transfusion 1992; 32: 805-813.

70 Alter H: Transfusion-transmitted non-A, non-B and hepatitis C virus infections, in Rossi EC, Simon TL, Moss GS, Gould SA (eds): Principles of Transfusion Medicine. Baltimore, Williams & Wilkins, 1996, pp 687-698.

71 Busch MP, Korelitz JJ, Kleinman SH, Lee SR, AuBuchon JP, Schreiber GB: Declining value of alanine aminotransferase in screening of blood donors to prevent posttransfusion hepatitis B and C virus infection. Transfusion 1995; 35: 903-910.

72 Barrera JM, Francis B, Ercilla G, Nelles M, Achord D, Darner J, Lee SR: Improved detection of anti-HCV in post-transfusion hepatitis by a third-generation ELISA. Vox Sang 1995; 68: 15-18.

73 Courouce AM, Le Marrec N, Girault A, Ducamp S, Simon N: Anti-hepatitis C virus (anti-HCV) seroconversion in patients undergoing hemodialysis: comparison of second- and third-generation anti-HCV assays. Transfusion 1994; 34: 790-795.

74 Mimms LT, Mosley JW, Hollinger FB, Aach RD, Stevens CE, Cunningham M, Vallari DV, Barbosa LH, Nemo GJ: Effect of concurrent acute infection with hepatitis C virus on acute hepatitis B virus infection. Brit Med J 1993; 307 (6912): 1095-1097.

75 Busch MP, Lee LLL, Satten GA, Henrard DR, Farzadegan H, Nelson KE, Read S, Dodd RY, Petersen LR: Time Course of Detection of Viral and Serological Markers Preceding HIV-1 Seroconversion; Implications for Blood and Tissue Donor Screening. Transfusion 1995; 35: 91-97.

76 Nübling CM, Unger G, Chudy M, Raia S, Löwer J: Sensitivity of HCV core antigen and RNA detection in the early infection phase. Transfusion 2002; 42: 1037-1045.

77 Glynn SA, Wright DJ, Kleinman SH, Hirschkorn D, Tu Y, Heldebrant C, Smith R Giachetti C, Gallarda J, Busch MP: Dynamics of Viremia in Early Hepatitis C Virus Infection. Transfusion 2005; 45: 994-1002.

78 Fiebig EW, Heldebrant C, Smith RIF, Conrad A, Delwart EL, Busch MP: Intermittent Low-Level Viremia in Very Early Primary HIV-1 Infection. J AIDS 2005; 39: 133-137.

79 Murthy KK, Henrard DR, Eichberg JW, et al: Redefining the HIV-infectious window period in the chimpanzee model: evidence to suggest that viral nucleic acid testing can prevent blood-borne transmission. Transfusion 1999; 39: 688-693.

80 Roth WK, Weber M, Buhr S, et al: Yield of HCV and HIV-1 NAT after screening of 3.6 million blood donations in Central Europe. Transfusion 2002; 42: 862-868.

81 Roth WK, Weber M, Petersen D, et al: Nucleic Acid Testing (NAT) for hepatitis B virus and anti-HBc testing increase blood safety. Transfusion 2002; 42: 869-875.

82 Matsumoto C, Tadokoro K, Fujimura K, et al: Analysis of HBV infection after blood transfusion in Japan through investigation of a comprehensive donor specimen repository. Transfusion 2001; 41: 878-884.

83 Weusten JJ, van Drimmelen AA, Lelie PN: Mathematical modeling of the risk of HBV, HCV, and HIV transmission by window phase donations not detected by NAT. Transfusion 2002; 42: 537-548.

84 Alvarez M, Oyonarte S, Rodriguez PM, Hernandez JM: Estimated risk of transfusion-transmitted viral infection in Spain. Transfusion 2002; 42: 994-998.

85 Pillonel J, Laperche S, Saura C, Desenclos JC, Courouce AM: Trends in residual risk of transfusion-transmitted viral infection in France between 1992 and 2000. Transfusion 2002; 42: 980-988.

86 Velati C, Romano L, Baruffi L, et al: Residual risk of transfusion-transmitted HCV and HIV infections by antibody-screened blood in Italy. Transfusion 2002; 42: 989-993.

87 Dodd RY, Notari EP, Stramer SL: Current prevalence and incidence of infectious disease markers and estimated window-period risk in the American Red Cross blood donor population. Transfusion 2002; 42: 975-979.

88 Stramer SL, Glynn SA, Kleinman SH, Strong DM, Caglioti S, Wright DJ, Dodd RY, Busch MP, for the NHLBI Nucleic Acid Test Study Group: Detection of HIV-1 and HCV Infections Among Antibody-Negative Blood Donors by Nucleic Acid-Amplification Testing. N Engl J Med 2004; 351: 760-768.

89 Coste J, Reesink HW, Engelfriet CP, Laperche S, et al: ISBT International Forum: Implementation of Donor Screening for Infectious Agents Transmitted by Blood by Nucleic Acid Technology: Update to 2003. Vox Sang 2005; 88: 289-303.

90 Laperche S: Blood Safety and nucleic acid testing in Europe. Euro Surveill 2005; 10: 3-4.

91 Velati C, Fomiatti l, Baruffi L, Zanetti A: Impact of NAT in Italy in the three years following implementation (2001-2003). Euro Surveill 2005; 10:12-14.

92 Pilonel J, Laperche S: Trends in risk of transfusion-transmitted viral infections (HIV, HCV, HBV) in France between 1992 and 2003 and impact of nucleic acid testing (NAT). Euro Surveill 2005; 10: 5-8.

93 Biswas R, Tabor E, Hsia CC, Wright DJ, Laycock ME, Fiebig EW, Peddada L, Smith R, Schreiber GB, Epstein JS, Nemo GJ, Busch MP: Comparative Sensitivity of HBV NATs and HBsAg Assays for Detection of Acute HBV Infection. Transfusion 2003; 43: 788-798.

94 Fiebig EW, Wright DJ, Rawal BD, Garrett PE, Schumacher RT, Peddada L, Heldebrant C, Smith R, Conrad A, Kleinman SH, Busch MP: Dynamics of HIV Viremia and Antibody Seroconversion in Plasma Donors: Implications for Diagnosis and Staging of Primary HIV Infection. AIDS 2003; 17: 1871-1879.

95 Alter MJ, Mast EE: The epidemiology of viral hepatitis in the Untied States. Gastroenterol Clin North Amer 1994:23: 437-455.

96 Sabino EC, Salles N, Saez-Alquezar A, Ribeiro-dos-Santos G, Busch MP, Chamone DF: Estimated Risk of Transfusion Transmitted HIV Infection in a Public Blood Bank in Sao Paulo, Brazil. Transfusion 1999; 39: 1152-1153.

97 Barreto CC, Sabino EC, Goncales TT, Laycock ME, Pappalardo BL, Salles NA, Wright DJ, Chamone DF, Busch MP: Prevalence, Incidence and Residual Risk of Human Immunodeficiency Virus among Community and Replacement First-Time Blood Donors in São Paulo, Brazil. Transfusion 2005; 45: 1709-1714.

98 Fang CT, Field SP, Busch MP, Heyns AduP: HIV-1 and HCV RNA Among South African Blood Donors: Estimation of Residual Transfusion Risk and Yield of Nucleic Acid Testing. Vox Sang 2003; 85: 9-19.

99 Heyns AduP, Benjamin RJ, Swanelvelder JPR, Laycock ME, Pappalardo BL, Crookes RL, Wright DJ, Busch MP: The Impact of a Structured Blood Safety Policy on HIV-1 Transfusion Transmission Risk in South Africa. JAMA 2006; 295: 519-526.

100 Kleinman SH, Busch MP: HBV: Amplified and Back in the Blood Safety Spotlight. [editorial] Transfusion 2001; 41: 1081-1085.

101 Schreiber GB, Glynn SA, Satten GA, Kong F, Wright DJ, Busch MP, Tu Y, Kleinman SH, for the Retrovirus Epidemiology Donor Study (REDS): HIV Seroconverting Donors Delay Their Return: Screening Test Implications. Transfusion 2002; 42: 414-421.

102 Seed CR, Cheng A, Ismay SL, et al: Assessing the accuracy of three viral risk models in predicting the outcome of implementing HIV and HCV NAT donor screening in Australia and the implications for future HBV NAT. Transfusion 2002; 42: 1365-1372.

103 Müller-Breitkreutz K: Results of viral marker screening of unpaid blood donations and probability of window period donations in 1997. Vox Sang 2000; 78: 149-157.

104 Koerner K, Cardoso M, Dengler Th, Kerowgan M, Kubanek B: Estimated risk of transmission of hepatitis C virus by blood transfusion. Vox Sang 1998; 74: 213-216.

105 International Forum: Implementation of donor screening for infectious agents transmitted by blood b nucleic acid technology. Vox Sang 2001; 82; 87-111.

106 Janssen RS, Satten GA, Stramer SL, Rawal BD, O'Brien TR, Weiblen BJ, Hecht FM, Jack N, Cleghorn FR, Kahn JO, Chesney MA, Busch MP: New Testing Strategy to Detect Early HIV-1 Infection for Use in Incidence Estimates and for Clinical and Prevention Purposes. Jama 1998; 280: 42-48.

107 Busch MP, Glynn SA, Stramer SL, et al: A new strategy for estimating risks of transfusion-transmitted viral infections based on rates of detection of recently infected donors. Transfusion 2005; 45: 254-264.

108 Yoshikawa A, Gotanda Y, Itabashi M, et al: Hepatitis B NAT virus-positive blood donors in the early and late stages of HBV infection: analyses of the window period and kinetics of HBV DNA. Vox Sang 2005; 88: 77-86.

109 Busch MP, Kleinman SK: Assessing the Impact of HBV NAT on Window Period Reduction and Residual Risk. J Med Virol (in press).

110 AuBuchon JP, Birkmeyer JD, Busch MP: Cost-effectiveness of expanded human immunodeficiency virus-testing protocols for donated blood. Transfusion 1997; 37: 45-51.

111 Jackson BR, Busch MP, Stramer SL, AuBuchon JP: The cost-effectiveness of NAT for HIV, HCV, and HBV in whole-blood donations. Transfusion 2003; 43: 721-729.

112 Marshall DA, Kleinman SH, Wong JB, AuBuchon JP, Grima DT, Kulin NA et al: Cost-effectiveness of nucleic acid test screening of volunteer blood donations for hepatitis B, hepatitis C and human immunodeficiency virus in the United States. Vox Sang 2004; 86: 28-40.

113 Sanchez AM, Schreiber GB, Nass CC, Glynn SA, Kessler D, Hirschler N, Fridey J, Bethel J, Murphy EL, Busch MP, for the Retrovirus Epidemiology Donor Study (REDS): The Impact of Male-to-Male Sexual Experience on Risk Profiles of Blood Donors. Transfusion 2005; 45: 404-413.

114 Soldan K, Sinka K: Evaluation of de-selection of men who have had sex with men from blood donation in England. Vox Sang 2003; 84: 265-273.

115 Busch MP, Caglioti S, Robertson EF, McAuley JD, Tobler LH, Kamel H, Linnen JM, Shyamala V, Tomasulo PA, Kleinman SH: Screening the Blood Supply for West Nile Virus RNA by Nucleic Acid Amplification Testing. N Engl J Med 2005; 353: 460-467.

116 Busch MP, Wright DJ, Tobler LH, Stramer SL, Custer B, Kleinman SH, Prince HE, Bianco C, Foster G, Petersen LR, Nemo G, Glynn SA: Estimated Proportion of the U.S. Population Infected with West Nile Virus during the 2003 Epidemic Based on National Blood Donor Screening Data. Emerg Infect Dis, 2005.

Dr. M.P. Busch, Blood Systems Research Institute, 270 Masonic Avenue, San Francisco, CA 94118, USA.
E-mail: mbusch@bloodsystems.org

Dax EM, Farrugia A, Vyas G (eds): Advances in Transfusion Safety – Volume IV.
Dev Biol (Basel). Basel, Karger, 2007, vol 127, pp 113-121.

Value of HCV Antigen-Antibody Combined HCV Assay in Hepatitis C Diagnosis

N. Lambert

Bio-Rad Laboratories, R & D Blood Virus Division, Marnes-la-Coquette, France

Key words: HCV, core antigen, RNA, window period, NAT.

Abstract: Reduction of the window period of hepatitis C virus (HCV) infection represents an important goal in the transfusional and diagnostic settings. Currently, the detection of HCV infection relies on the use of immunoassays to detect viral antibodies. A new enzyme immunoassay (Monolisa HCV Ag-Ab ULTRA) designed to simultaneously detect circulating HCV antigen and anti-HCV antibodies has been developed by Bio-Rad and registered by the European Authorities. Several evaluations have been conducted in Europe to determine whether this new assay can improve early detection of HCV infection. Sensitivity studies included 130 HCV RNA positive/anti-HCV negative samples, 21 well documented seroconversion panels and 430 anti-HCV genotyped samples from France and Italy. Specificity has also been assessed in 15,302 non-selected blood donations and hospital samples. Studies have shown that Monolisa HCV Ag-Ab ULTRA assay has been able to detect 40-90 % of HCV RNA positive/anti-HCV negative samples collected in the window period, improving early detection of HCV when antibodies may be undetectable. The mean delay in detecting HCV infection between HCV-RNA and this new test was found to be 5 days, reducing the window period by an average of 37 days. All samples collected after seroconversion were detected with the HCV Ag-Ab ULTRA assay. The specificity analyzed in 15,302 random blood donations and hospital samples was estimated at 99.86 %. Although less sensitive than NAT (71 % of HCV RNA positive/anti-HCV negative in window period), this assay could be a reasonable alternative when NAT cannot be used for reasons such as cost, organization, emergency or logistic difficulties.

INTRODUCTION

Hepatitis C virus (HCV) is a common cause of worldwide liver infection. It is estimated that more than 170 million people, 3 % of the world's population, are infected with HCV and are at risk of developing liver cirrhosis and/or liver cancer. Approximately 3 to 4 million new infections occur each year globally [1].

Historically, HCV screening of blood donations has been based on the use of immunoassays to detect viral antibodies (Ab). Three generations of enzyme-linked immunosorbant assay (EIA) testing have been developed since 1989 [2]. Significant reduction of the serological window has been accomplished with the third generation kits, which can detect antibodies within 4-10 weeks [3,4], compared with 82 days [5] for the second generation and 150 days for the first generation kits.

To prevent transmission of HCV during the window period before seroconversion, nucleic acid testing (NAT) for HCV RNA has been implemented in some countries [6-10] (USA in March 1999, European countries and Japan, Canada and Australia). For logistical and cost reasons, most of these NAT screening programs test pools of plasma that are typically composed of 16 to 128 blood-donor specimens per pool. A huge reduction of the window period was observed with implementation of NAT. HCV RNA is detected by NAT an average of 12 days after infection [11]. However, studies demonstrating that low-level HCV viremia detected only stochastically by individual HCV NAT was infectious pointed out that NAT cannot totally prevent HCV transmission, and anti-HCV screening must be continued [12-15]. An alternative approach to NAT in reducing the window period is the detection of circulating HCV core antigen (Ag) by ELISA [16-17]. The HCV core Ag assays have sensitivities close to that of NAT, with mean detection differences of 1 to 2 days in the window period [16]. Consequently, an assay combining the detection of HCV Ag and anti-HCV Ab into a single test could speed up the diagnosis of infection, simplify the flow-charts in transfusion and minimize the cost of blood safety improvement, especially in countries which have not yet introduced direct viral detection methods [18-19]. A new assay based on the simultaneous detection of HCV core antigen and anti-HCV (Monolisa HCV Ag-Ab ULTRA, Bio-Rad, Marnes-la-Coquette, France) has been developed and was registered by the European authorities in February 2005.

In order to assess the sensitivity and specificity of this assay in the early detection of HCV infection, we have reported here the evaluations performed in Europe. The overall objective was to determine if this combined test could constitute an alternative to NAT for the diagnosis of HCV infection during the window period in blood donations.

Design of the Test

The design of this assay is more complicated than HIV assay because the same region (capsid) is involved for detecting Ag and Ab. This innovative patented feature was achieved by the use of anti-core monoclonal antibodies for antigen detection and a mutated peptide from the core (or capsid) for anti-HCV antibody detection.

This mutated core peptide is able to react with the anti-HCV capsid antibodies from the patient sample but, due to the peptide's mutations, not with the anti-capsid monoclonal antibody used for the detection of HCV core Ag.

The selection of monoclonal antibodies was based on epitope mapping and detection of all genotypes.

Method

Monolisa HCV Ag-Ab ULTRA assay is based on the combination of an indirect test for antibody detection (core, NS3, NS4) and a sandwich test for core antigen detection. The assay format is illustrated in Figure 1. The main steps of the procedure are the following: 50 µL of each sample and controls are incubated at 37°C for 90 minutes, with 100 µL of conjugate 1 (biotinylated anti-HCV core monoclonal antibody) in microwells coated with a monoclonal antibody specific for HCV capsid protein, NS3 (genotypes 1 and 3) and NS4 purified recombinant HCV proteins and a specific mutated capsid peptide. After a cycle of washing steps, 100 µL of conjugate 2 (peroxidase-labelled antibodies to human IgG and streptavidin-peroxidase) is added

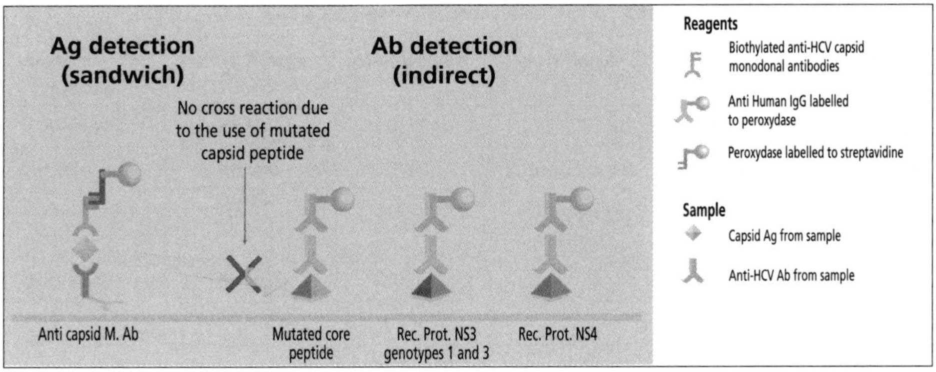

Fig. 1 : Monolisa HCV Ag-Ab ULTRA assay format.

to each well and incubated for 30 minutes at 37° C. After a second cycle washing, the antigen-antibody complex is revealed by the addition of substrate and the reaction is stopped after 30 minutes incubation at room temperature by addition of 100 µL of a 1 N sulfuric acid solution to each well. The absorbance is measured at 450 nm with a 620 nm reference wavelength. A sample is considered as positive when its optical density (OD) is greater or equal to cut-off (CO) value (determined by the mean of positive control OD divided by 4). A 10 % grey zone is recommended.

Monolisa HCV Ag-Ab Ultra Evaluations

Protocol

Two different types of evaluations have been conducted in Europe : prospective studies that evaluate the specificity of the assay and retrospective studies to assess the sensitivity. The results have been compared with NAT individual donation or minipool (MP) and commercial anti-HCV assays.

Prospective studies (Table 1)

In the first study done by Lambert et al., 12,401 random blood donations were tested in four French Blood Banks (Marseille, Montpellier, Rungis, Bordeaux) [20]. Among the 12,401 samples tested, 12,399 were negative with anti-HCV and HCV-MP-NAT assays routinely used in blood centers. Two samples were true positive. Nineteen samples were found repeatedly positive. The specificity was estimated at 99.85 % (95 % IC : 99.76 %-99.91 %).

In the second study, the specificity was analyzed in 2,503 random blood donations [21]. The results have been compared to those obtained with the routinely used EIA screening assay (Prism HCV, Abbott). The 2,503 random blood donations were negative with anti-HCV and HCV-MP-NAT assays that are routinely used in blood centers. Three samples were repeatedly positive, with ratios between 1.5 and 1.9, and 2 samples were in the grey zone. Figure 2 shows the distribution of the ratios of the 2,503 negative samples. Excluding samples in the grey zone, the specificity was estimated at 99.88 % (95 % IC : 99.65 %-99.98 %).

Table 1 : Prospective evaluations of Monolisa HCV Ag-Ab ULTRA assay : specificity.

Evaluation	Sample types	Number tested	Specificity (%)	95% confidence interval
Lambert et al (2005) [20]	Blood donors	12,399	99.85	99.76-99.91
Laperche et al (2005) [21]	Blood donors	2,503	99.88	99.65-99.98
Ansaldi et al (2006) [22]	Hospital routine	400	100	99.25-100
Total		15,302	99.86	99.78-99.91

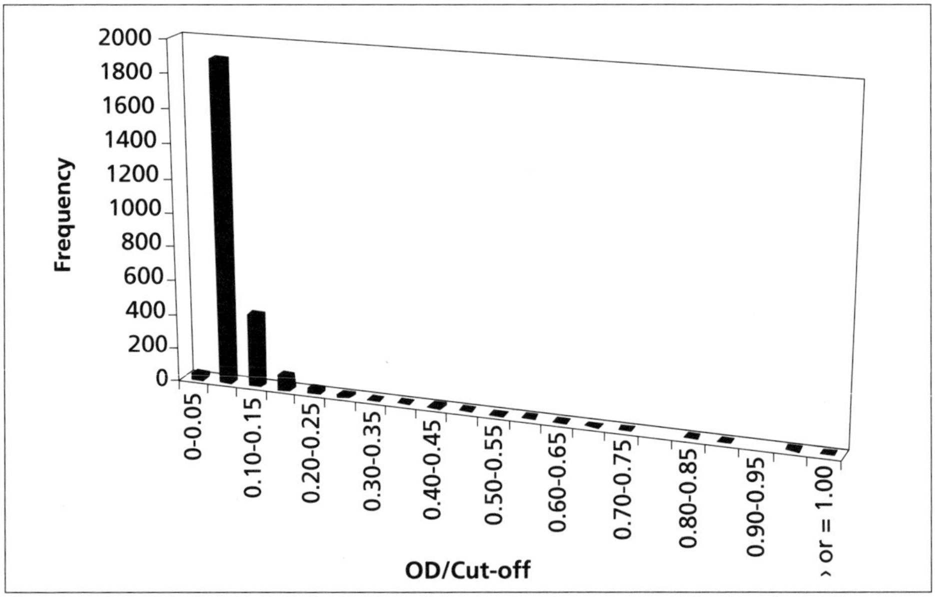

Fig. 2 : Distribution of the results (optical density/cut-off) obtained in 2,503 random anti-HCV (Prism HCV, Abbott) negative blood donations.

The third specificity study was carried out by Ansaldi et al, on samples from the general population (hospital routine in Italy) [22]. The 400 samples tested were negative with Monolisa HCV Ag-Ab ULTRA assay, corresponding to a specificity of 100 % (95 % IC : 99.25 %-100 %)

Finally, the combined assays had a repeatedly reactive rate of 0.14 percent or an apparent specificity of 99.86 % (95 % IC : 99.78 %-99.91 %) based on testing a population of 15,302 specimens from blood donors and hospital routine.

Retrospective studies (Table 2)

107 sequential samples from 10 HCV seroconversion commercial panels were tested in the first study (Laperche et al, 2005) [21] 8 from Bioclinical Partners (BCP 6211, BCP 6213, BCP 6222, BCP 6225, BCP 6227, BCP 9041, BCP 9054, BCP

Table 2: Retrospective evaluations of Monolisa HCV Ag-Ab ULTRA assay: sensitivity.

Evaluation	Samples Ab neg/NAT pos collected in WP	Reduction of the Ab WP (day)	Mean delay between HCV NAT/Ag-Ab (day)
Laperche et al (2005) [21]	70.5 % (31/44)	26.8	5.1
Laperche et al (2005) [23]	40.8 % (29/71)	30.1	–
Ansaldi et al (2006) [22]	91.4 % (85/93)	24	–
Lambert et al (2005) [20]	87.7 % (43/49)	33.3	4.4
Schnuriger et al (2005) [24]	–	49	–
Average		37	

9055) and 2 from Boston Biomedica Inc (BBI 917, BBI 919). All panels began with at least one sample that was negative for all HCV markers; 81 samples were considered to be in the pre-seroconversion phase, and 26 were collected after seroconversion. All samples were tested with HCV Ag-Ab ULTRA assay and the two MP-NAT procedures that are routinely used in France (pools of 8 for TMA and pools of 24 donations for Roche molecular system).

From the 44 samples collected in the window period that were MP-NAT positive, 31 (70.5 %) were also positive with Monolisa HCV Ag-Ab. All samples collected after seroconversions were detected with the HCV Ag-Ab assay. The HCV Ag-Ab assay was able to detect HCV infection an average of 26.8 days earlier than the most sensitive anti-HCV assay. The mean delay in the detection of HCV infection was 5.1 days between MP-NAT and Monolisa HCV Ag-Ab ULTRA assay.

In a second study carried out by the same team (Laperche et al, 2005) [23], 191 samples collected from 23 hemodialysed patients who developed anti-HCV Ab (seroconversion) during the follow-up were tested. Monolisa HCV Ag-Ab Ultra assay was able to detect 40.8 % (29/71) of HCV RNA positive/anti-HCV negative samples collected in the window period. The mean delay between positive results by Monolisa HCV Ag-Ab ULTRA assay and the first HCV Ab assay was 30.1 days.

In the third study (Ansaldi et al, 2006) [22], sensitivity was assessed by testing 93 PCR-positive and anti-HCV negative sera from well documented seroconversion panels. 91.4 % were found to be positive with Monolisa HCV Ag-Ab Ultra assay. The reduction in the diagnostic window period observed was an average of 24 days.

The fourth study (Lambert et al, 2005) [20] was also carried out on commercial seroconversion panels. The serologic profile for one representative panel is shown in Figure 3. The first bleed date was non viremic. Anti-HCV was detected at day 86 and HCV RNA and HCV Ag were detected at day 13. For this panel, Monolisa HCV Ag-Ab ULTRA assay was able to detect HCV infection 73 days before anti-HCV Ab assay and at the same time as HCV NAT in single units and HCV Ag assay. Among 10 seroconversion panels, beginning with HCV RNA-positive/anti-HCV Ab negative samples, the HCV Ag-Ab assay detected exposure to HCV an average of 33 days earlier than anti-HCV Ab assays. Among a total of 145 HCV RNA-positive/anti-HCV Ab negative samples tested, Monolisa HCV Ag-Ab Ultra assay was able to detect 126 (87 %) specimens.

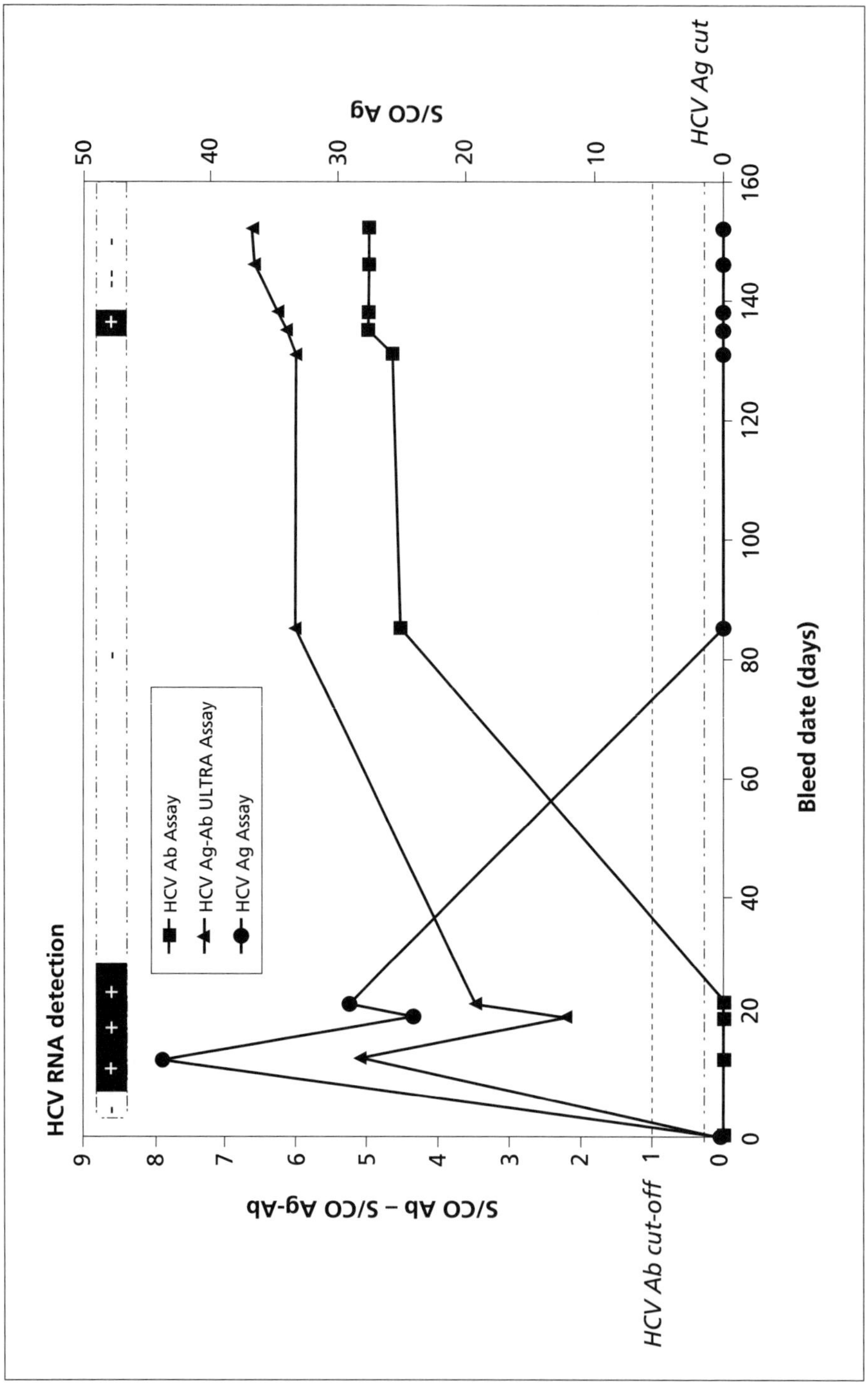

Fig. 3: HCV markers in seroconversion panel BBI PHV-917. Kinetics of the markers are represented with triangles for Monolisa HCV Ag-Ab ULTRA curve, with squares for Monolisa HCV Ab curve, and with circles for Ortho HCV Ag curve.

The aim of the last study (Schnuriger et al, 2005) [24] was to determine the potential clinical benefit of the new assay in the setting of acute HCV infection in HIV infected patients. 80 HCV seronegative (HCV neg-HIV pos) and 80 seropositive samples (HCV pos-HIV pos) from HIV positive patients were tested. Monolisa HCV Ag-Ab Ultra assay reduced the seronegative window period with an average of 49 days in this population. Use of such assays in the setting of high risk behavior individuals, particularly in HIV infected patients, would allow an earlier HCV diagnosis and rapid clinical management.

Conclusion

Monolisa HCV Ag-Ab ULTRA assay showed a specificity of 99.86 % (95 % IC: 99.78 %-99.91 %) among a total of 15,302 samples.

The different evaluations also confirmed a notable improvement in the detection of HCV infection in comparison to current HCV Ab assays. Depending on the evaluation, Monolisa HCV Ag-Ab ULTRA was able to detect 40 to 90 % of HCV RNA positive/anti-HCV negative samples collected during the window period.

The mean delay in detecting HCV infection between HCV RNA and HCV Ag-Ab ULTRA assay was approximately 5 days in these evaluations.

Considering a theoretical seronegative window period of 66 days, and knowing that this window period could be reduced by 37 days (average of all evaluations), the yield in reduction of the HCV transfusion transmitted residual risk using HCV Ag-Ab assay would be approximately 50 % (Fig. 4). In France, on the basis of the mathematical model developed by Shreiber et al [25], the HCV residual risk was recently estimated at 0.10 per million donations with MP-NAT and 0.64 per million donations without MP-NAT [15]. According to Laperche et al [21], the use of HCV Ag-Ab assay would lead to a reduction of the residual risk to 0.38 per million donations. Assuming that each of the 2.5 million allogenic units of blood collected annually in France is converted on average to 1.2 transfusable components, the Laperche study indicates that there would be 2 cases of transfusion-transmitted HCV infection per year without NAT, and that HCV Ag-Ab assay could prevent at least one of these cases [21].

Today, the question of NAT's cost-effectiveness is debated. Several models have demonstrated that HCV NAT is not cost-effective in any blood bank [26], even for developed countries already using this technology. These expenses could be better used for other health care priorities [27].

The classical way to calculate the cost benefit for any health care decision is to calculate the cost for "one quality-adjusted life per year saved". For blood banks this cost means the cost that blood banks use to implement the HCV NAT in terms of reagent and facilities and the benefit in terms of avoided contamination and, more precisely, of quality-adjusted life-year saved. It is a complex calculation with many variables due to the cost of reagent, the benefit of this treatment (or cost of HCV NAT implementation in this case), the morbidity of the disease, etc. The reference often cited as cut-off to make decisions for treatment or drug reimbursement in the USA is $ 50,000 [27]. The cost of HIV and HCV NAT calculated for US blood banks [26] was 100-fold more expensive (NAT would cost between $ 4.7-11.2 million per quality-adjusted life-year saved in the USA). In France, before implementation of HCV NAT in pooled samples in French blood banks, HCV NAT was not cost-effective [28], with a hypothesis of 5 cases per million donations of HCV infection averted with HCV NAT assay (in pooled samples of 50 units) and at a "neat cost per additional year of life saved" of 84.6 million Euros. After implementation of HCV NAT in France, the official rate of positive cases that are HCV NAT/Ab negative is 0.4 cases [9] per million donations, 10-fold less than the expected rate.

In that context, Monolisa HCV Ag-Ab ULTRA assay could be a reasonable solution for blood screening in developing countries for reasons such as low yield versus benefit and high cost-effectiveness ratio.

In conclusion, this new assay offers an advantage over existing antibody screening assays in that it detects HCV infection much earlier without the operational disadvantages of adding a supplemental test and requests only a switch from current the HCV Ab assay to this new HCV Ag-Ab combined assay. Monolisa HCV Ag-Ab ULTRA assay allows for a significant improvement in transfusion safety with a better cost-effectiveness, especially in comparison to HCV NAT.

References

1 WHO: World Health Report 2002. Annex table 2: deaths by cause, sex and mortality stratum in WHO regions, estimates for 2001. www.who.int/entity/whr2002.

2 Kuo G, Choo QL, Alter HJ, et al: An assay for circulating antibodies to a major etiologic virus of human non-A, non-B hepatitis. Science 1989; 244: 362-364.

3 Courouce AM, Pillonel J: Transfusion-transmitted viral infections. Retrovirus and Viral Hepatitis Working Groups of the French Society of Blood Transfusion. N Engl J Med 1996; 335: 1609-1610.

4 Barrera JM, Francis B, Ercilla G, et al: Improved detection of anti-HCV in post-transfusion hepatitis by a third-generation ELISA. Vox Sang 1995; 68: 15-18.

5 Busch MP: Closing the windows on viral transmission by blood transfusion, in Stramer SL (ed): Bethesda, MD, 2001, pp 33-54.

6 Pillonel J, Laperche S, Saura C, et al: Trends in residual risk of transfusion-transmitted viral infections in France between 1992 and 2000. Transfusion 2002; 42: 980-988.

7 Mine H, Emura H, Miyamoto M, et al: High throughput screening of 16 million serologically negative blood donors for hepatitis B virus, hepatitis C virus and human immunodeficiency virus type-1 by nucleic acid amplification testing with specific and sensitive multiplex reagent in Japan. J Virol Methods 2003; 112: 145-151.

8 Orton SL, Stramer SL, Dodd RY, Alter MJ: Risk factors for HCV infection among blood donors confirmed to be HCV RNA-positive, anti-HCV non-reactive. Transfusion 2004; 44: 275-281.

9 Velati C, Laperche S, Hossenlopp C, Rougier P: NAT screening in Europe. Vox Sang 2004; 87 (Sup3): P3-19: 26.

10 Chaivetta JA, Escobar M, Newman AM et al: Incidence and estimated rates of residual risk for HIV, hepatitis C, hepatitis B and human T-cell lymphotropic viruses in blood donors in Canada, 1999-2000. CMAJ 2003; 8: 767-773.

11 Busch MP, Kleinman SH: Nucleic acid amplification testing of blood donors for transfusion-transmitted infectious diseases. Transfusion 2000; 40: 143-159.

12 Operskalski EA, Mosley JW, Tobler LH, et al: HCV viral load in anti-HCV-reactive donors and infectivity for their recipients. Transfusion 2003; 43: 1433-1441.

13 Laperche S, Bouchardeau F, Maniez M, et al: Nucleic acid testing in blood donations reactive to hepatitis C virus antibody, but with an extremely low viral load. Vox Sang 2004; 86: 198.

14 Busch MP, Tobler LH, Gerlich WH, et al: Very low level viremia in HCV infectious unit missed by NAT. Transfusion 2003; 43: 1173-1174.

15 Pillonel J, Laperche S: Trends in risk of transfusion-transmitted viral infections (HIV, HCV, HBV) in France between 1992 and 2003 and impact of nucleic acid testing (NAT). Euro Surveill 2005; 10 (2).

16 Seme K, Poljaj M, Babic DZ, Mocilnik T et al: The role of core antigen in management of hepatitis C: a critical review. J Clin Microbiol 2005; 32: 92-101.

17 Raker CA, Tabor E, Okayama A, et al: HCV core antigen as an alternative to NAT to detect HCV viremia. Transfusion 2004; 44: 307-308.

18 Marshall DA, Kleinman SH, Wong JB, et al: Cost-effectiveness of nucleic acid test screening of volunteer blood donations for hepatitis B, hepatitis C and human immunodeficiency virus in the United States. Vox Sang 2004; 86: 28-40.

19 Jackson BR, Busch MP, Stramer SL, AuBuchon JP: The cost-effectiveness of NAT for HIV, HCV, and HBV in whole-blood donations. Transfusion 2003; 43: 721-729.

20 Lambert N, Vermet L, Bordier M, et al: Performance features of the new Bio-Rad HCV antigen and antibody assay: Monolisa HCV Ag-Ab Ultra. Vox Sang 2004; 87 (Sup 3: P4-22): 61-62.

21 Laperche S, Elghouzzi MH, Morel P, et al: Is an assay for simultaneous detection of hepatitis C virus core antigen and antibody a valuable alternative to nucleic acid testing? Transfusion 2005; 45: 1965-1972.

22 Ansaldi F, Bruzzone B, Testino G, et al: Combination hepatitis C virus antigen and antibody immunoassay as a new tool for early diagnosis of infection. J of Virol Hepatitis 2006; 13:5-10.

23 Laperche S, Le Marrec N, Girault A, et al: Simultaneous detection of Hepatitis C virus (HCV) core antigen and anti-HCV antibodies improve the early detection of HCV infection. J Clin Microbiol 2005; 43: 3877-3883.

24 Schnuriger A, Dominguez S, Valantin MA, et al: Early detection of hepatitis C seroconversion using a new combined antigen-antibody detection assay: potential use in high risk individuals. 8th Annual meeting of ESCV 27-30 April 2005.

25 Schreiber GB, Busch MP, Kleinman SH, Korelitz JJ: The risk of transfusion-transmitted viral infections. The Retrovirus Epidemiology Donor Study. N Engl J Med 1996; 334: 1685-1690.

26 Jackson BR, Busch MP, Stramer SL, AuBuchon JP: The cost-effectiveness of NAT for HIV, HCV, and HBV in whole-blood donations. Transfusion 2003; 43: 721-729.

27 Allain JP: Transfusion risks of yesterday and of today. Transfusion Clinique et Biologique 2003; 10:1-5.

28 Loubieres S, Rotily M, Durand-Zaleski I, Costagliola D: Including polymerase chain reaction in screening for hepatitis C virus RNA in blood donations is not cost-effective. Vox Sang 2001; 80: 199-204.

Dr. N. Lambert, Bio-Rad Laboratories, R & D Blood Virus Division, 3 bd R.-Poincaré, F-92430 Marnes-la-Coquette, France.
E-mail: nadine.lambert@bio-rad.com

Dax EM, Farrugia A, Vyas G (eds): Advances in Transfusion Safety – Volume IV.
Dev Biol (Basel). Basel, Karger, 2007, vol 127, pp 123-133.

Characterization of Scrapie-Infected and Normal Hamster Blood as an Experimental Model for TSE-Infected Human Blood

L. Gregori, R.G. Rohwer

Medical Research Service, Veterans Affairs Medical Center, Baltimore, Maryland, USA, and Department of Neurology, University of Maryland, Baltimore, Maryland, USA

Key words: Scrapie, prion, blood, leukoreduction, infectivity.

Abstract: Ideally, the distribution and separation properties of blood-associated infectivity in humans infected with transmissible spongiform encephalopathies (TSEs) would be investigated using endogenously infected human blood. However, technical limitations prevent these studies. We report here an extensive comparison of component separations of TSE-infected and normal hamster blood with normal human blood to evaluate its suitability as a model for TSE-infected human blood. Two leukotrap filtration systems were used to assess the similarities and differences in cell separation and distribution between human and hamster blood. Human-sized units of scrapie-infected hamster whole blood pools were produced, leukoreduced and processed following current standard blood bank procedures. Three centrifugation steps were performed, and all but one centrifugation resulted in cell separations both similar to those obtained with human blood and in compliance with the American Association of Blood Banks standards. Analysis of white blood cell removal by leukoreduction indicated that all filters performed within specification. The only deviation from human blood was for hamster platelets, which were not retained by the whole blood leukoreduction filter and partitioned together with red blood cells when blood was centrifuged to produce platelet rich plasma. This study indicates that hamster blood is a realistic substitute for human blood for investigations of the component distribution of TSE infectivity in blood.

Introduction

Transmissible spongiform encephalopathy (TSE) diseases are fatal central nervous system infections that can incubate asymptomatically in humans and animals for decades. TSE infectivity has been demonstrated in the blood of several animal species, both during symptomatic and pre-symptomatic stages of disease (Rohwer laboratory, ongoing studies) [1-5]. Three recent reports of transfusion transmission of variant Creuztfeldt-Jakob disease (vCJD) have confirmed that TSE-infected humans, like TSE-infected animals, contain TSE infectivity in their blood when still asymptomatic and that this infectivity is transmissible by blood transfusion [6-8].

All three of the transfusion transmissions that have been observed to date have been from non-leukoreduced red blood cell (RBC) concentrates [6-8]. The RBC fraction, while predominantly red blood cells, also contains contaminating white blood cells and plasma, and any one or all of these components could be sources of infectivity. An accurate knowledge of the component distribution of blood-associated TSE infectivity is essential for a reliable evaluation of the risks from blood products and indispensable to the implementation of effective risk reduction measures. Unfortunately, we currently lack a means of determining the component distribution of TSE infectivity in human blood. This is because there are as yet no ways of measuring the concentration of TSE infectivity in human blood and blood components. Moreover, developing and validating a means has been greatly complicated by the lack of TSE-infected human blood in quantities sufficient for component separations, titrations and assay development. A great deal of effort has been expended in trying to develop a bioassay animal with sufficient sensitivity to detect the low levels of TSE infectivity expected in human blood. As yet, none of the various transgenic variants of the human prion gene, nor a variety of inbred rodent strains, have demonstrated the required level of susceptibility to infection by human TSE strains [9-12]. When transmissions to rodents have occurred, they have had long incubation times, suggesting a weak host susceptibility, insufficient for transmission from low titer tissues such as blood.

The distribution of TSE infectivity in blood has been studied most effectively in hamsters, mice and sheep infected either experimentally or naturally. An advantage of these models is that the blood can be titered in the same species from which it was drawn, thus circumventing the species barrier that has prevented measurement on human blood. Sheep are the only practicable source of blood from naturally acquired infections. They also have the advantage of large blood volumes. However, few titrations have been attempted in sheep, and the complexity of multiple breeds and diverse genotypes presents a challenge to data interpretation. Furthermore, control, certified scrapie-free flocks are difficult to obtain and maintain in North America, especially if they carry scrapie-susceptible genotypes. The mouse model offers the advantages of well characterized antibodies for blood cell isolation and identification, and a growing inventory of transgenics deficient in various blood constituents as well as mouse adapted TSE strains originating from all naturally infected species. However, the small blood volume of the mouse and the relatively long incubation time of many mouse TSE models are significant drawbacks. In contrast, the golden Syrian hamster is large enough to produce useful volumes of blood, yet small enough to be held in the large numbers required for precise measurement of the concentrations of TSE infectivity in blood and blood components. Our laboratory has developed and characterized the golden Syrian hamster infected with the 263K strain of scrapie to study TSE infectivity in blood. Other advantages of the 263K hamster model are the high brain titer, relatively short incubation time (approximately 60 days following intracerebral inoculation of high titer inocula), a very predictable and reproducible clinical course, and an easily recognized progression of clinical milestones. Unlike sheep and human blood, hamster blood from different individuals can be mixed without hemocompatibility issues.

We have also developed a highly sensitive and precise means of assaying the low levels of TSE infectivity in hamster blood, which we call limiting dilution titration [13]. Using this method, we have consistently obtained titers of 10 infectious doses (ID)/ml for large pools of whole blood collected from hamsters in symptomatic disease [1,13,14]. (One infectious dose is by definition the minimal unit of infectivity capable of starting an infection.) In contrast to blood pools, the concentration of TSE infectivity in blood from individual scrapie-infected animals has varied from 4-24 ID/ml. To make sure that our studies represent average behavior and that we are not misled by idiosyncratic outliers, we have conducted most of our experiments on blood pools collected from twenty or more animals. We have also developed the ability to collect human-sized unit-quantities of rodent blood (500 ml or more) during only a few hours, which has made it possible to conduct studies for which scale-down processing was not an option, such as leukoreduction [13].

The relevance of the hamster model to human blood infection depends, importantly, on the similarity of the separation properties of hamster and human blood. We report here an extensive analysis of the distribution and separation properties of hamster blood cells following standard protocols for component separations and using identical equipment to that currently in use in North American blood banks. These results are compared with the expectations for human blood as specified by the American Association of Blood Banks (AABB) [15].

Materials and Methods

Blood production

Four-hundred weanling golden Syrian hamsters (Harlan, Madison, WI) were inoculated intracerebrally with 50 μl each of brain homogenate containing approximately 250 infectious dose$_{50}$ (ID$_{50}$) of hamster-adapted 263K scrapie. This inoculum was prepared by dilution of a previously titered stock of 10 % scrapie-infected hamster-brain homogenate prepared by exhaustive ultrasonication in phosphate buffered saline (PBS), pH 7.2. The dilution buffer was PBS supplemented with 0.1 % fetal calf serum (HyClone, Logan, UT), and 1 x penicillin/streptomycin (GIBCO, Carlsbad, CA). Two separate human-size blood pools were collected at 111 and 115 days post-inoculation when the animals were at the clinical phase of the disease just before losing the ability to rear. Human-sized units of normal hamster blood for pilot studies were produced from approximately 100 animals of 4 months of age.

Bleeding procedure

Animals were anesthetized under CO_2 until unresponsive, and the heart was exposed in a careful dissection that prevented contamination of the heart by other tissue. The pericardium was removed by rolling onto a sterile dry swab. Blood (3.5 ml) was drawn from the right ventricle into a 5 ml syringe equipped with a 22G needle (Becton-Dickinson, Franklin Lake, NJ) that had been preloaded with 0.5 ml of CP2D anticoagulant (Pall Corp. Port Washington, NY). Great care was taken not to touch any tissue other than the heart and to touch the heart only with the needle. After each collection, the blood was mixed with the anticoagulant for several minutes on a slowly oscillating table at room temperature before being pooled into the blood bag. Only bleeds containing the appropriate blood volume with no visible clots were pooled. Human-sized units of 500 ml or more of blood were produced from approximately 130 to 150 animals of 5-6 months of age. For the study with the Leukotrap WB system, the blood was collected over a 7 hour period. For the study with the Leukotrap RC-PL system, the blood was collected in 4 hours. Both collections were within the time limit (8 hours) for blood processing specified by the AABB.

All measurements were gravimetric and were converted to volumes using the experimentally obtained density of hamster whole blood, 1.04 g/ml, and red blood cell concentrate, 1.07 g/ml. We used 1.00 g/ml as the density of all other fractions.

Leukotrap RC-PL system

Results with the Leukotrap WB system have been published elsewhere [13]. A human-sized unit of hamster whole blood prepared from approximately 140 scrapie-infected animals was used to challenge the Leukotrap RC-PL system. An aliquot (35 ml) was removed and the remainder (464.3 g) was centrifuged at 2800 rpm (2270 x g) for 3 minutes 44 seconds using a Sorvall RC-3C centrifuge. The bag was carefully placed in a bag expressor and platelet rich plasma (PRP) was expressed out through an ATSLPL in-line filter. The filtration was stopped when red blood cells were visible in the filter but before they could enter the receiving bag. Leukoreduced PRP (84.1 g) was left to rest for 45 minutes at room temperature before an aliquot (17 ml) was removed and the remainder was centrifuged at 3600 rpm (3800 x g) for 7 minutes on a Sorvall RC-3C centrifuge. The platelet concentrate (PC) was separated by expressing platelet poor plasma (PPP) into an in-line satellite bag. The resuspended PC (15.6 g) was mixed under gentle agitation overnight at room temperature before an aliquot was removed for cell composition analysis. The red blood cell (RBC) component from the soft spin centrifugation was mixed with 100 ml AS-3 (cell preservative) contained in a satellite in-line bag, and a 35 ml aliquot (RBC + AS-3) was removed for cell composition analysis. The remainder (429.8 g) was leukoreduced by passage through an RCM1 in-line filter by gravity (60 inches of height) to produce leukoreduced RBC (405.6 g).

Cell count

The distribution of cells in each component of the normal and infected blood was measured with a HemaVet five part differential cell counter (CDC Technologies, Oxford, CT) custom calibrated for counting hamster blood cells. The residual white blood cell concentrations in the leukoreduced samples were below the limit of detection of this instrument (200 cells/µl). Manual count of white blood cells was conducted on a Neubauer hemocytometer after lysing the red blood cells and staining of the white blood cells with crystal violet. At least three separate determinations were averaged for each measurement. Flow cytometric quantitation of white blood cells was conducted by the Canadian Blood Service on samples that had been treated with a white blood cell preservative, Leukofix (Pall Corp. Port Washington, NY) and stained with propidium iodide to detect nucleated cells [16].

Results

In pilot studies with full, human-sized units of normal hamster blood, we confirmed the feasibility of collecting human-sized units of blood within the time constraints for processing set by the AABB [15]. Two in-line leukoreduction systems produced by Pall Corp. were tested: Leukotrap WB and Leukotrap RC-PL. The details of the Leukotrap WB system study with titration of the whole blood pre- and post-leukoreduction have been reported elsewhere [13].

The Leukotrap RC-PL system (Fig. 1) was first investigated with normal hamster blood. Under the standard conditions used for the separation of human blood, the first centrifugation (soft spin) produced less total plasma, between 18-25 %, from hamster than from human blood (lower limit 33 %), and the platelet recovery was also lower for hamster blood. Decreasing the centrifugation speed to 1900 x g or 2000 x g for 5 minutes did not significantly change the volume of PRP recovered or the platelet recovery. Increasing the centrifugation speed to higher than the standard value increased the volume of PRP collected but dramatically reduced the platelet content in the PRP fraction, as most of the platelets co-sedimented with the red blood cells. At the end of several tests, we concluded that under the standard conditions the volume of hamster plasma produced represented an adequate volume to test the filtration and comprised the best compromise between platelet recovery in platelet rich plasma and plasma separation from RBC.

The Leukotrap RC-PL system was challenged with a human-sized unit of scrapie-infected hamster blood. During the process, an aliquot of each fraction was removed and its cell profile analyzed. We also collected and analyzed aliquots of leukoreduced PRP (LR-PRP) and pre-leukoreduction RBC (with AS-3). These are intermediate fractions that are usually not collected. Table 1 shows the distribution of the major blood cell types for each fraction assayed. The white blood cell count in samples collected post leukoreduction are summarized in Table 2 and described below. The total number of white cells in the hamster whole blood pool was 2.2 x 10^9, and, as anticipated based on human blood, after the first centrifugation the majority of hamster

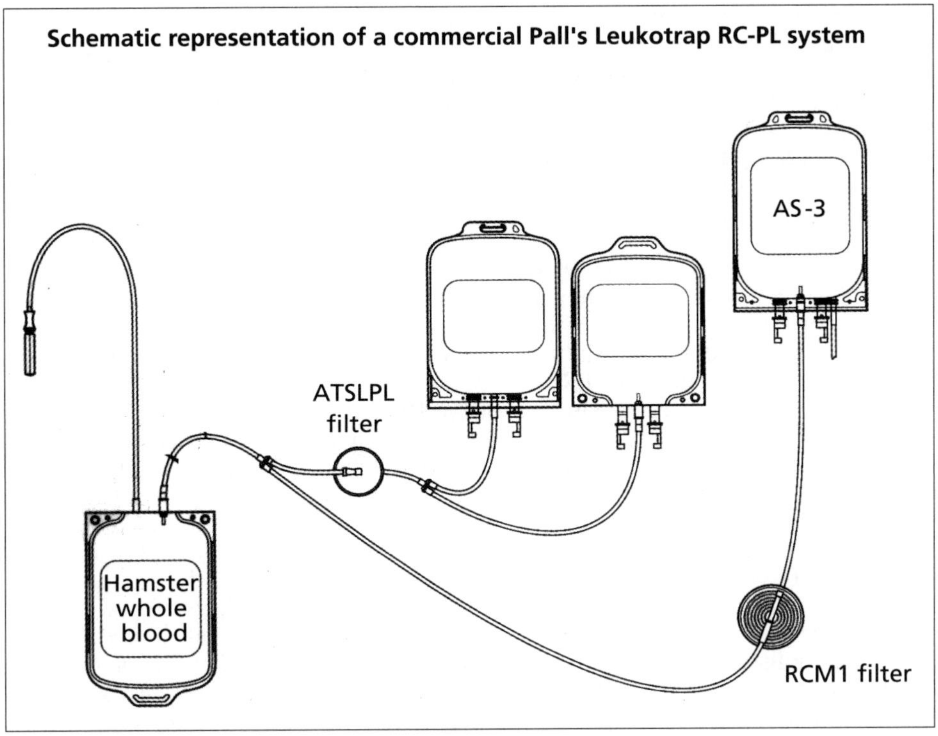

Fig. 1 : A human-size unit of hamster infected blood was placed in the blood collection bag and processed according to the specification of the PL-RC leukoreduction system. The ATSLPL and RCM1 filter are the platelets and red blood cells leukoreduction filters, respectively. At the end of the process, the following leukoreduced fractions were recovered: platelets poor plasma, platelets concentrate and red blood cells.

Table 1 : Cell recovery from the Leukotrap RC-PL system.

	Volume (ml)	Total WBC	% rec	log_{10} reduction	Total RBC	% rec	Total PLT	% rec
Whole blood	446.4	2.2×10^9	100	–	3.8×10^{12}	100	1.4×10^{11}	100
LR-PRP	84.1	3.4×10^5	0.015	- 2.8**	0	–	2.1×10^{10}	15
RBC + AS-3	401.7	2.0×10^9	91	–	3.7×10^{12}	97	1.4×10^{11}	100
LR-RBC + AS-3	379.0	2.2×10^6	0.1	- 2.9	3.2×10^{12}	84	7.7×10^{10}	55
LR-PRP*	67.5	2.7×10^5	100	–	–	–	1.5×10^{10}	100
PPP	51.3	1.6×10^5	59	–	0	0	2.3×10^9	15
PC	15.3	7.8×10^4	29	- 4.4	3.0×10^9	0	1.2×10^{10}	75

LR = leukoreduced; WBC = white blood cells; rec = recovery; AS-3 = red blood cells preservative.

* Only 67.5 ml LR-PRP were centrifuged to generate PPP and PC fractions.

** log_{10} of white blood cells reduction for the platelet filter was calculated as the WBC ratio log_{10} (LR-PRP/PRP) where the concentration of WBC in PRP was determined as the difference between the total WBC in whole blood and RBC.

white blood cells (91 %) partitioned in the RBC fraction (2 x 10^9 cells). The PRP fraction produced by the centrifugation was directly leukoreduced with the ATSLPL filter, and 84.1 ml of leukoreduced PRP (LR-PRP) were collected. Since an aliquot of pre-leukoreduction PRP could not be removed without significantly altering the configuration of the filtration system, it was not possible to directly establish the leukoreduction performance of the ATSLPL filter. However, by difference between the total white blood cells in whole blood (2.2 x 10^9) and the cells recovered in the RBC fraction (2.0 x 10^9) we could estimate that the ATSLPL filter was challenged with approximately 2 x 10^8 white blood cells. Following leukoreduction, the total white blood cell contamination in the LR-PRP fraction was 3.4 x 10^5, corresponding to 2.8 $\log_{10}$ reduction (Table 1) and indicating that the ATSLPL filter performed close to specification with hamster white blood cells. As mentioned above, the soft spin centrifugation of hamster blood exhibited differences from the human blood separation, with less recovered volume of PRP and poorer platelet recovery in the hamster LR-PRP fraction (15 %). Leukoreduction of the RBC fraction reduced the total white blood cells from 2.0 x 10^9 to 2.2 x 10^6, corresponding to 2.9 $\log_{10}$ of leukoreduction. The contamination of the RBC fraction with white blood cells was below the allowed limit (< 5 x 10^6 cells/RBC unit) and the total red blood cell recovery was close to the AABB limit (> 85%) [15,17]. Thus, both leukoreduction filters performed at or close to specification with hamster blood fractions and removed close to 3 $\log_{10}$ of white blood cells. The LR-PRP fraction was further processed to produce PPP and PC fractions. Only a portion (67.5 ml) of the total LR-PRP volume was centrifuged because approximately 17 ml of LR-PRP were kept for cell composition analysis and for possible future infectivity assays. Following centrifugation of LR-PRP, the total platelet count recovered in the PC unit for hamster blood (1.2 x 10^{10} cells/unit) was lower than that seen with human blood (> 5.5 x 10^{10} cells/unit). This recovery corresponded to 75 % of the platelets in the LR-PRP fraction and 11 % of the total platelets in whole hamster blood, assuming that the PC was prepared from the entire volume of LR-PRP (84.1 ml). The white blood cell contamination in the PC fraction (7.8 x 10^4 cells/unit) was well below the maximum allowed (< 8.3 x 10^5 cells/unit).

Table 2 shows the actual values for the manual and the flow cytometric determinations of white blood cells for each fraction assayed. To verify that both cell counting methods were consistent with the HemaVet results, whole blood was also analyzed (Table 2). The value obtained manually (4650 cells/µl) closely matched the value for the same sample determined with the HemaVet (4928 cells/µl). The two quantitation methods showed different white blood cell values for a few fractions. This difference was probably due to the low reliability of the manual count, for which only a few cells per measurement could be found. In general, the values from the two methods were in good agreement and within the acceptable experimental errors. The average value between the two methods was used to calculate the white blood cell concentration for all post-leukoreduction fractions in Table 1.

A direct comparison of the major cell types and other parameters in normal and infected hamster and human blood is reported in Table 3. The values for hamster blood were obtained from three replicate measurements of blood pools of approximately 100 normal animals and approximately 140 infected animals. The values for normal hamster blood determined with the HemaVet matched those reported for this animal species [18]. Values for total white blood cell count were very close for normal and infected hamster blood. However, in the blood of infected animals, there was an increase in the monocyte count compared with normal hamster blood and a significant increase in the relative percentage of neutrophils as compared with lym-

Table 2: White blood cells count in various fractions produced with the Leukotrap RC-PL system.

	Manual count (cell/μl)	**Flow cytometry (cell/μl)**	**Average (cell/μl)**
Whole Blood	5100	4200	4650
PRP	6.9	1.4	4.1
PPP	5.0	1.5	3.2
PC	4.4	5.8	5.1
LR-RBC	2.2	9.7	5.9

Table 3: Distribution of cellular types and other parameters in normal and infected hamster blood compared to normal human blood.

	Hamster*		**Human [19]**
Parameters	**Normal**	**Infected**	**Normal**
WBC (10^3/μl)	5.5 ± 1.0	4.9 ± 0.4	3.7-9.5
Neutrophils (%)	17.3 ± 3.6	51.7 ± 2.8	46-64
Lymphocytes (%)	78.8 ± 6.7	43.5 ± 1.9	27- 34
Monocytes (%)	1.9 ± 1.4	3.7 ± 1.6	5-6
RBC (10^6/μl)	8.4 ± 0.3	8.5 ± 0.2	4.3-5.7
MCV (fl)	49.1 ± 1.0	48.2 ± 0.8	82-98
HB (g/dl)	13.3 ± 0.1	13.4 ± 0.3	13.3-16.7
HCT	41.3 ± 1.0	41.2 ± 0.8	39-50
Platelets 10^3/μl	400 ± 85	308 ± 32	143-332
MPV	4.2 ± 0.4	4.1 ± 0.2	7-10

MCV = mean corpuscular volume; HB = hemoglobin; HCT = hematocrit; MPV = mean platelet volume.
* The values were determined from large pools of normal (approximately 100 animals) and infected (approximately 140 animals) hamster blood using the HemaVet blood cell counter.

phocytes (the two most abundant white blood cell types). These differences were not attributable to the difference in age of the normal hamsters (4 months) compared to that of the infected hamsters (5-6 months), as the cell distribution of normal hamster blood did not dramatically change with age (data not shown). Comparison between normal human and hamster blood did not reveal any unexpected features [19]. The more noticeable differences were the increased ratio of neutrophils to lymphocytes and the two-fold greater concentration of red blood cells in the hamster. However, the hematocrit (HCT) for the two species was approximately the same since the hamster red blood cells are about half the size of human red blood cells, as indicated by the mean corpuscular volume (MCV) values. Furthermore, in the hamster the mean platelet volume (MPV) was also lower than in human blood.

Discussion

In this study we compared component separations of hamster blood and human blood to evaluate the suitability of using TSE-infected hamster blood as a substitute for human blood in evaluating commercial leukoreduction filters to remove TSE infectivity from blood and blood components. To accomplish this, we measured the actual level of white blood cell reduction in each component and the recovery of each component compared to AABB standards for human blood.

We investigated the separation of hamster blood components using two commercial in-line leukoreduction systems: the Leukotrap WB and the Leukotrap RC-PL. An extensive exploration of the centrifugation parameters used for the component separations in both processes showed that the Leukotrap WB filtration and subsequent separation of hamster blood into red blood cells and plasma could be conducted in good compliance with AABB specifications while following the standard protocol for human blood [13,17]. The only exception was in the platelet distribution: human platelets are removed by the WBF2 leukoreduction filter [20], while most hamster platelets passed the filter and 71 % were recovered in the RBC concentrate component [13].

The RC-PL system performed very close, but not completely, to specifications. The soft spin centrifugation of whole hamster blood to produce PRP and RBC could not be adjusted to produce exactly the same separation obtained for human blood. After this centrifugation, the recovery of platelets in the PC fraction was below the AABB standard for human blood and the PPP volume was also reduced compared to the human specification. As a consequence, the ATSLPL filter was challenged with a lower platelet concentration than it would have been with human blood, while the RCM1 filter was exposed to a higher concentration of platelets. However, the distribution of white blood cells and the performance of the leukofilters with respect to removal of white blood cells were not affected by this deviation. We calculated that the ATSLPL filter removed approximately 2.8 $\log_{10}$ of white blood cells, while the RCM1 filter showed a reduction of 2.9 $\log_{10}$ in white blood cells. More importantly, both of the final leukoreduced components, RBC and PC, contained white blood cells below the limit set by the AABB. Thus, since one of the principal objectives of the study was to test the filters' ability to remove hamster white blood cells, we can conclude that both filters were challenged with realistic concentrations of white blood cells and performed adequately.

Hamster platelets appear to behave differently from human platelets. Unlike the human counterpart, hamster platelets were not removed by the WBF2 leukoreduction filter [13] and could not be separated from red blood cells under soft spin conditions. Moreover, under these conditions, not only was the platelet recovery in PRP low, but the volume of PRP was also below that usually obtained with human blood, suggesting that factors in addition to platelet size and density may have contributed to the deviation. In a detailed analysis of the various parameters of normal human blood compared to hamster blood, we observed that the median red blood cell and platelet volumes in hamster blood were smaller (approximately half) than those in human blood, while the red blood cell total count was higher for the hamster (approximately twofold). It seems likely that the lower PRP volume recovered was due to slow sedimentation of the smaller, but more numerous, red blood cells present in hamster blood compared to human blood. To improve the congruence of the separation of hamster and human blood, different centrifugation conditions seemed to be required for the hamster. Despite many attempts, none of the modifications in centrifugation that we tested resulted in a separation in which the majority of the platelets remained in the plasma supernatant separate from the red blood cell pellet. Despite these differences in platelet and red blood cell properties, overall the hamster blood behaved remarkably similar to human blood, and the white blood cell fraction separated within the specifications for human blood.

The comparative analysis between infected and normal hamster blood indicated an increase in neutrophil and monocyte concentrations in the blood of clinically infected animals. This difference is probably the result of the disease state of the animals at the time of blood collection. A more detailed flow cytometric analysis to identify the specific cells involved in the infectious process was frustrated by a lack of cell-specific antibodies for selective quantitation of hamster blood cells.

Human platelets and lymphocytes display readily detected levels of PrP^c, the normal form of the prion protein, on their cell surfaces and human platelets have been shown to contain most of the cell-associated PrP in blood [21,22]. In contrast, Holada and Vostal failed to detect PrP^c on any hamster peripheral blood cells [23] using a panel of different anti-PrP antibodies. This difference would be critical if PrP^c was a reliable indicator of TSE infectivity. In fact, the normal form of the prion protein is widely distributed in many organs and cell types that show little if any evidence of infection even during the symptomatic stages of the disease. It is only the abnormal, infection-specific isoform(s) of the prion protein, PrP^{TSE}, not PrP^c, that is correlated with the presence of infectivity. For human blood, infectivity has been shown only in RBC concentrate [6-8], a fraction that, even without leukoreduction, contains only a small proportion of the whole blood platelets. In our own study, purified platelets from infected hamster blood were not found to be infectious when inoculated into healthy animals [14]. Nevertheless, unless or until a means is found to quantitate the distribution of TSE infectivity in endogenously infected human blood, it will not be possible to rule out the presence of at least some infectivity in human platelets.

In a centrifugal separation of TSE- infected hamster whole blood, approximately 45 % of the endogenous infectivity was recovered in the buffy coat, approximately 30 % in the plasma layer and the remainder in the red blood cell concentrate [Rohwer lab, unpublished]. The results of two studies on the distribution of TSE infectivity in mouse blood were consistent with this result [1,5]. This distribution was also confirmed in our whole blood leukoreduction study, where 42 % of the initial TSE infectivity was removed by the leukoreduction filter [13]. Approximately one half of the endogenous TSE infectivity in whole blood is associated with the white cells. At least in the hamster, there is no intrinsic association of blood infectivity with platelets [see above and 14], and a similar ongoing study in our laboratory is suggesting that there is no intrinsic association of TSE blood infectivity with purified red blood cells either. As a consequence, the other half of endogenous infectivity is probably localized in plasma. Other studies from our laboratory indicate that the association of infectivity with white blood cells may be superficial and unstable, as it is easily released into the plasma fraction [Gregori and Rohwer, work in progress]. Based on these data, it seems likely that the transfusion transmissions of human vCJD infectivity by non-leukoreduced RBCs were caused by residual plasma and white blood cells.

In the studies presented here, hamster blood behaved very similarly to human blood during component separations. Small physical differences in the size and possibly the densities of hamster versus human platelets and red blood cells present some limitations. However, neither platelets nor red blood cells are intrinsically infected or appear to be involved in replication and/or transport of TSE infectivity in hamster blood. This suggests that neither cell type is responsible for the transmission of TSE infectivity in human infected blood. The very large differences in total blood volume and, consequently, total infectivity present in the blood compartment may also impact the pathogenetic significance of TSE infected blood to rodents compared to larger animals. In conclusion, the 263K scrapie-infected hamster is a useful and relevant animal model for investigations of many critical aspects of TSE infection by human blood.

Acknowledgements

We are grateful to the BL3 animal facility staff for excellent animal care and to Health Canada for providing the expertise in blood separation and the flow cytometry analysis of the samples produced from hamster blood. We also thank Dr. Ellen Elliott for the helpful review of this manuscript.

This work was supported by Health Canada and by NHLBI grant R01 HL 63930 and N01-NS-0-2327 to RGR.

References

1 Brown P, Rohwer RG, Dunston BC, MacAuley C, Gajdusek DC, Drohan WN: The distribution of infectivity in blood components and plasma derivatives in experimental models of transmissible spongiform encephalopathy. Transfusion 1998; 38: 810-816.

2 Houston F, Foster JD, Chong A, Hunter N, Bostock CJ: Transmission of BSE by blood transfusion in sheep. Lancet 2000; 356: 999-1000.

3 Hunter N, Foster J, Chong A, McCutcheon S, Parnham D, Eaton S, MacKenzie C, Houston F: Transmission of prion diseases by blood transfusion. J Gen Virol 2002; 83: 2897-2905.

4 Taylor DM, Fernie K, Reichl HE, Somerville RA: Infectivity in the blood of mice with a BSE-derived agent. J Hosp Infect 2000; 46: 78-79.

5 Cervenakova L, Yakovleva O, McKenzie C, Kolchinsky S, McShane L, Drohan WN, Brown P: Similar levels of infectivity in the blood of mice infected with human-derived vCJD and GSS strains of transmissible spongiform encephalopathy. Transfusion 2003; 43: 1687-1694.

6 Llewelyn CA, Hewitt PE, Knight RS, Amar K, Cousens S, Mackenzie J, Will RG: Possible transmission of variant Creutzfeldt-Jakob disease by blood transfusion. Lancet 2004; 363: 417-421.

7 Peden AH, Head MW, Ritchie DL, Bell JE, Ironside JW: Preclinical vCJD after blood transfusion in a PRNP codon 129 heterozygous patient. Lancet 2004; 364: 527-529. A new case of variant CJD associated with blood transfusion.

8 http://www.cjd.ed.ac.uk/TMER/TMER.htm

9 Nonno R, Bari MA, Cardone F, Vaccari G, Fazzi P, Dell'omo G, Cartoni C, Galeno R, Sbriccoli M, Lipp HP, Bruce M, Pocchiari M, Agrimi U: Efficient transmission and characterization of Creutzfeldt-Jakob disease strains in bank voles. PLoS Pathog. 2006; 2: e12: Epub 2006 Feb 24.

10 Scott MR, Peretz D, Nguyen HO, Dearmond SJ, Prusiner SB: Transmission barriers for bovine, ovine, and human prions in transgenic mice. J Virol 2005; 79: 5259-5271.

11 Weissmann C, Flechsig E: PrP knock-out and PrP transgenic mice in prion research. Br Med Bull 2003; 66: 43-60.

12 Taguchi Y, Mohri S, Ironside JW, Muramoto T, Kitamoto T: Humanized knock-in mice expressing chimeric prion protein showed varied susceptibility to different human prions. Am J Pathol 2003; 163: 2585-2593.

13 Gregori L, McCombie N, Palmer D, Birch P, Sowemimo-Coker SO, Giulivi A, Rohwer RG: Effectiveness of leucoreduction for removal of infectivity of transmissible spongiform encephalopathies from blood. Lancet 2004; 364: 529-531.

14 Holada K, Vostal JG, Theisen PW, MacAuley C, Gregori L, Rohwer RG: Scrapie infectivity in hamster blood is not associated with platelets. J Virol 2002; 76: 4649-4650.

15 Standards for Blood Banks and Transfusion Services, 22nd ed. Arlington, VA American Association of Blood Banks, 2003.

16 Vachula M, Simpson SJ, Martinson JA, Aono FM, Hutchcraft AM, Balma DL, Van Epps DE: A flow cytometric method for counting very low levels of white cells in blood and blood components. Transfusion 1993; 3: 262-267.

17 Textbook of Blood Banking and Transfusion Medicine 2nd ed. Sally V. Rudmann, 2005.

18 Laboratory Hamsters, in Van Hoosier GL, McPherson CV (eds): American College of Laboratory Animal Medicine Series, 1987.

19 A beginner's guide to blood cells, Bain BJ (ed): Publisher Blackwell Science Ltd, 1996.

20 Data sheet: Pall Corporation, Leukotrap® WB Filtration System at http://www.pall.com

21 Barclay GR, Houston EF, Halliday SI, Farquhar CF, Turner ML: Comparative analysis of normal prion protein expression on human, rodent, and ruminant blood cells by using a panel of prion antibodies. Transfusion 2002; 42: 517-526.

22 MacGregor I, Hope J, Barnard G, Kirby L, Drummond O, Pepper D, Hornsey V, Barclay R, Bessos H, Turner M, Prowse C: Application of a time-resolved fluoroimmunoassay for the analysis of normal prion protein in human blood and its components. Vox Sang 1999; 77: 88-96.

23 Holada K, Vostal JG: Different levels of prion protein (PrPc) expression on hamster, mouse and human blood cells. Br J Haematol 2000; 110: 472-480.

Dr. R.G. Rohwer, VA Maryland Health Care System, Medical Research Service 151, 10 North Greene Street, Baltimore, MD 21201-1524, USA.
E-mail: rrohwer@umaryland.edu

Dax EM, Farrugia A, Vyas G (eds): Advances in Transfusion Safety – Volume IV.
Dev Biol (Basel). Basel, Karger, 2007, vol 127, p 135.

SESSION IV

Regulation as a Driver for Blood Safety

Chairs: *J. Epstein and D. Maher*

Dax EM, Farrugia A, Vyas G (eds): Advances in Transfusion Safety – Volume IV.
Dev Biol (Basel). Basel, Karger, 2007, vol 127, pp 137-146.

Iron and Blood Donation – An Under-Recognised Safety Issue

A. Farrugia

Office of Devices, Blood and Tissues, Therapeutic Goods Administration, Woden, ACT, Australia

Key words: Iron, haemoglobin, donor health.

Abstract: A growing body of evidence suggests that iron status is frequently affected by blood donation. Iron deficiency may be assessed through iron storage depletion measured by serum ferritin. These measurements indicate a high incidence of iron deficiency in repeat donors. This is not ameliorated through increasing pre-donation haemoglobin cut-offs. Depletion of tissue – rather then storage – iron, may be assessed by measurement of the serum transferrin receptor; such measurements in repeat donors indicate tissue iron depletion, but to a much lesser extent than storage iron depletion. A fuller understanding on how repeat donation affects donor health will allow better haematological criteria for donor selection to be developed. Blood agencies and standard-setting authorities need to accord the issue of donor iron and donation status as high a priority as that of any blood safety issue involving patient safety, if the safety and supply of the blood system is to be maintained.

INTRODUCTION

While the issue of the appropriate level of haemoglobin pre-donation has been long-standing in blood banking, it has been exacerbated in recent years by the increasing pressure on the blood supply. This is especially so in the established blood systems of the developed world, where a combination of an aging population and a shrinking donor base has resulted in chronic shortages of donations. The measures directed at increasing product safety through the deferral of groups judged on the basis of epidemiological criteria to be at higher risk for transmitting infections (e.g., variant Creutzfeldt-Jakob disease) have unfortunately led to the loss of the most committed and safest part of the blood donor population. Given that low haemoglobin is still the major cause of donor deferral in many blood systems [1], it is understandable that decision makers in blood management still subject this issue to scrutiny and debate [2].

Measurement of haemoglobin prior to donation serves to assure that the donor is not anaemic. This consideration is obscured by an inadequate recognition of current definitions of anaemia – see below – but does also provide a general measure of donor health. In addition, it serves to ensure that a minimal dose of haemoglobin is delivered to the recipient in the final red cell product. Both of these considerations are underpinned by standards such as those of the American Association of Blood Banks and the Council of Europe. In most instances, the standards fail to recognise current perspectives on these issues, which have a bearing on pre-donation haemoglobin. It is beyond the scope of this review to comment on the optimal "dose" of haemoglobin in a red cell product; such a commentary would be more appropriate in the context of the optimal haemoglobin level post-transfusion, which has been assessed as being restrictive rather than liberal in at least one study [3].

What is the "Normal" Haemoglobin?

The different pre-donation haemoglobin levels used in blood systems are shown in Table 1. Blood systems have adopted different levels for reasons which are not entirely clear. The World Health Organisation (WHO) defines males who are below 13 g/dl and females who are below 12 g/dl as anaemic [4]. This definition is deplored by one source [5], ignoring as it does significant racial differences in normal haemoglobin values [6]. A recent review shows that the WHO definition would misclassify considerable numbers of individuals as "normal" when haemoglobin ranges based on extensive data bases would suggest that levels below 13.7 g/dl in white American males in the years when they are eligible to donate blood would have only an approximately 5 % chance of being a normal value. Meanwhile, the corresponding value for women of all ages would be 12.2 g/dl [7]. Issues of technological precision, standardization and small sample numbers necessarily influenced the 1968 WHO recommendation.

Such technological issues are of great importance in blood systems management. The influences of technological methods and sample type on haemoglobin level measurements in blood collection have been described [8-10]. While it is desirable to avoid subjecting donors to an extra venipuncture in procuring a pre-donation sample, capillary blood from the ear lobe overestimates haemoglobin and a finger-prick sample is satisfactory. The widely used gravimetric test using copper

Table 1 : Pre-donation haemoglobin levels.

Agency	**Hb – males (mg/dl)**	**Hb – females (mg/dl)**
WHO	13	12
Council of Europe	135	125
United Kingdom Blood Transfusion Service	130	120
New Zealand Ministry of Health	135	125
American Association of Blood Banks	125 – no sex difference	
Food and Drug Administration	125 – no sex difference	
Health Canada	125 – no sex difference	
Australian Red Cross Blood Service Pre 2004	125	115

sulphate was judged by Boulton et al [8] to be a satisfactory screening test as long as failures to achieve the pre-donation thresholds were confirmed using a venous sample assessed on a portable analyser. Radtke et al [10] still find an overestimation when using finger-prick relative to venous blood on these instruments, emphasizing the need for non-invasive methods to assess pre-donation haemoglobin status [11].

Iron and Blood Donation

Donation of a unit of blood results in the loss of 200 – 250mg of iron in the form of haemoglobin. Menstruating women have a higher estimated daily iron requirement than men (7 – 20 mg vs 5 – 10 mg), as well as lower iron stores (300 mg vs 1,000mg). Even in the absence of iron deficiency anaemia, a sensorimotor disorder [12], cognitive impairment [13] and other effects on learning capacity [14] ensue from iron deficiency. Conversely, iron depletion through blood donation has been associated with a decreased incidence of adverse cardiovascular events [15,16] and vascular function is improved in repeat blood donors with low iron stores compared with low-frequency blood donors [17]. This suggests that iron's role as a pro-oxidant/pro-atherosclerotic factor may offer benefit at some level of iron depletion.

The effect of iron depletion on the various haematological parameters has been described [18,19]. Progressive iron depletion leads to iron deficient erythropoeisis (IDE) followed by iron deficiency anaemia (IDA) as a relatively late consequence of iron depletion (Fig. 1). These studies have led to the recognition of the depletion of *storage* iron, followed by the depletion of *tissue* iron, as a result of iron depletion. They have also established the serum ferritin measurement [20] as the parameter of choice in assessing iron stores, and the serum soluble transferrin receptor's (STR) numbers to reflect the functional cellular need for iron [21].

The Iron Status of Blood Donors

Many studies show that iron stores, as assessed through serum ferritin measurement, decline with repeat blood donation [22]. Iron deficiency is generally defined by a serum ferritin measurement of ≤ 12 µg/l, but this measurement is insufficient to determine the clinical significance and full haematological status of iron-depleted donors. For example, studies on different populations of repeat donors show differences in the level of anaemia in donors with relatively similar donation histories and ferritin levels, emphasizing the contributory roles of environmental factors, particularly diet [23,24]. The problem is exacerbated for women, and the demonstrated progression to iron deficiency anaemia in some donor populations is of concern (Fig. 2). Ferritin is elevated in the anaemia of chronic disease and inflammation, limiting its use in assessing donors for iron deficiency even if a pre-donation test were possible.

As discussed above, the growing understanding of the role of STR in assessing the status of functional tissue iron has led to this parameter being proposed as a laboratory indicator of donor eligibility with regard to iron status. Boulton et al [25] applied the "STR-Ferritin" ratio concept developed by Punnonen et al [26], to show that above a certain value this index in repeat blood donors was associated with significant decreases in red cell volume (MCV), presumably indicating a microcytosis (iron-depletion induced). Although Boulton et al's study expressed

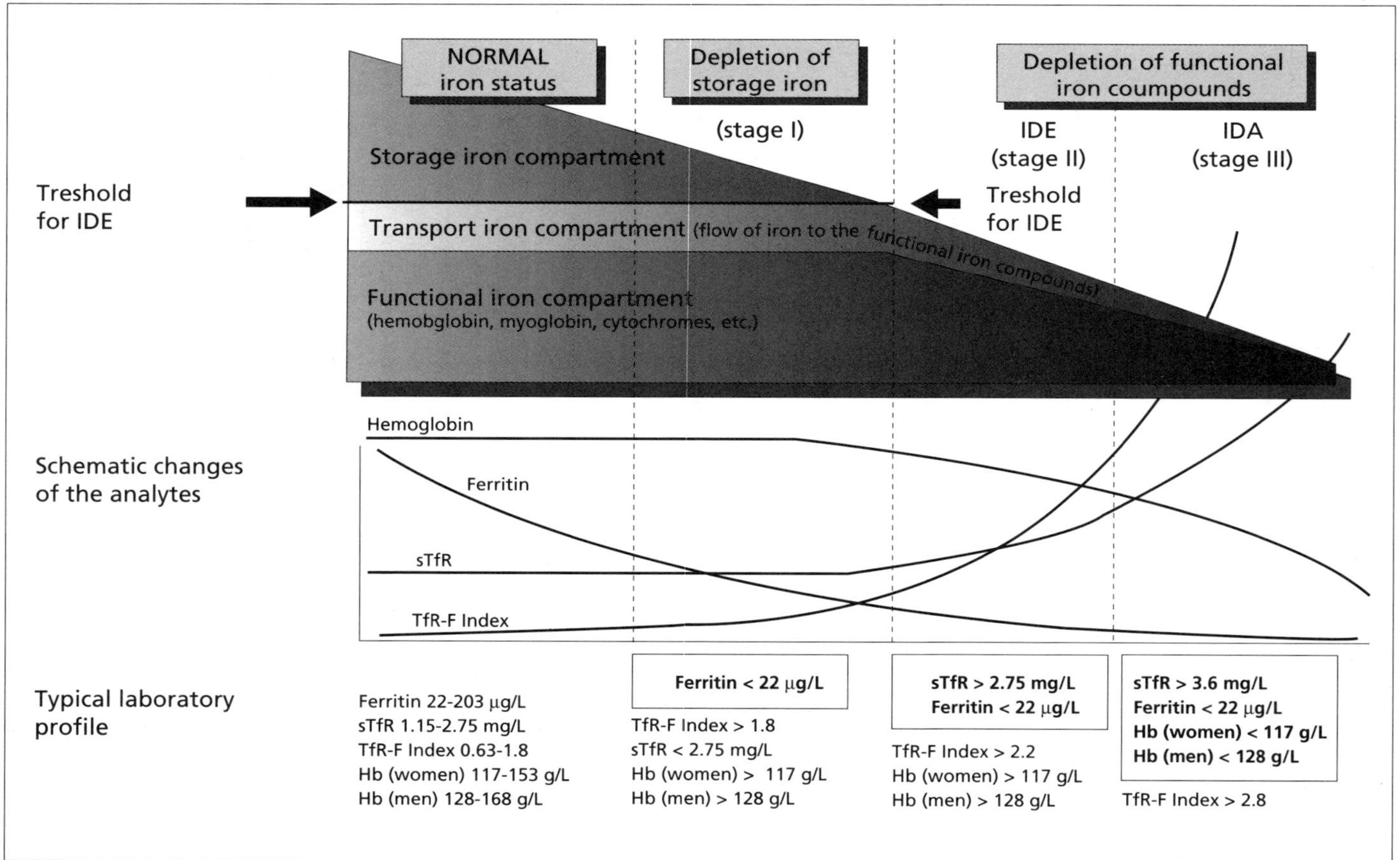

Fig. 1: Phases of advancing iron deficiency. The gradual diminution of the different iron compartments and the concomitant changes seen in the laboratory analytes are presented schematically in relation to the separate stages of advancing ID [19].

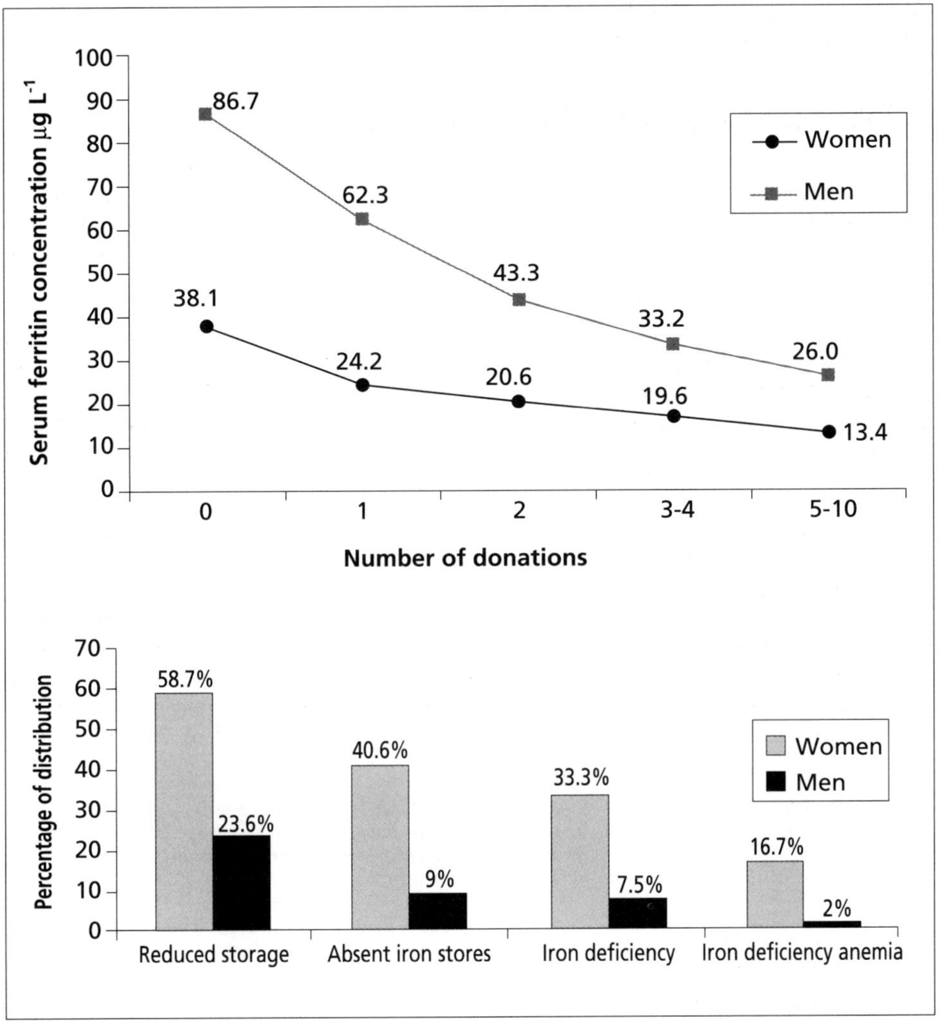

Fig. 2: Haematological status of blood donors at the Yazd Blood Transfusion Center, Iran, 2003 [24].

reservations about the use of the index, principally because of the wide normal range in serum STR, a more recent Norwegian study [27] questions the use of ferritin as an indicator of iron status in an otherwise healthy donor population. This study shows that only a minority of donors with low haemoglobin and/or low iron stores (as assessed by ferritin) have STR levels above a "normal" range. This suggests that STR can be used as a more specific indicator of functional iron deficiency than ferritin, allowing substantial numbers of donors who would be otherwise deferred as "iron-deficient" to donate on the presumption that depletion of storage iron is non-detrimental. In this context, Flesland et al's [27] comment that "The clinical importance of low iron stores without concurrent iron deficiency is not known" is well taken. Either way, STR measurements are expensive and the absence of an international standard for STR impedes the introduction of these assays in the mainstream blood banking practice.

Whither on Donor Haemoglobin?

The issue of what pre-donation haemoglobin level is best remains. Many of the studies cited in this Chapter show that many donors deferred for low haemoglobin levels have satisfactory storage iron status. Conversely, donors who pass any of the currently accepted criteria cannot be guaranteed to have such a status. In a large study carried out at the request of the Therapeutic Goods Administration[1] (TGA), the Australian Red Cross Blood Service (ARCBS) found that a significant proportion of donors were (storage) iron deficient irrespective of the haemoglobin level chosen as the cut-off (Table 2). The TGA's efforts were directed towards increasing the ARCBS' pre-donation haemoglobin levels to those recommended by the Council of Europe. The levels held for many years at 125 and 115 mg/dl for males and females, respectively [28], were judged to be unsatisfactory and were associated with high levels of (storage) iron deficiency in a preliminary study [29]. These data, generated in 2004, contrast with data for the general Australian population generated in 1998. For the general Australian population in 1998, using similar criteria, the level of iron deficiency in males was negligible, while in females it was 5-7 %. These studies indicate that the putative problem of iron deficiency in blood donors cannot be addressed through lowering the pre-donation haemoglobin thresholds. It will, at least in the Australian context, lead to donor losses without significantly ameliorating the storage iron profile of the donor population. Recognition of the iron storage issue and improved donor management can be attained through donor selection algorithms as exemplified by the ARCBS' approach (Fig. 3). The lack of

Table 2: Australian blood donors – iron storage status of donors with different pre-donation haemoglobin levels. A population of 3022 donors – 1535 males and 1487 females – from all the States and Territories of the Australian federation was studied. Iron deficiency was defined as a serum ferritin < 12ug/L. Council of Europe thresholds are shown for comparison.

	Total donor population iron deficient (%)
ARCBS Hb threshold from 1/1/04	
Males – 128g/L	6.2
Females – 118g/L	22.0
ARCBS Hb threshold from 1/1/05	
Males – 130g/L	6.0
Females – 120g/L	20.6
Council of Europe Hb threshold	
Males – 135g/L	5.3
Females – 125g/L	18.9

[1] At the time of writing this chapter, the Therapeutic Goods Administration is the regulator of the Australian therapeutics sector, including the blood industry.

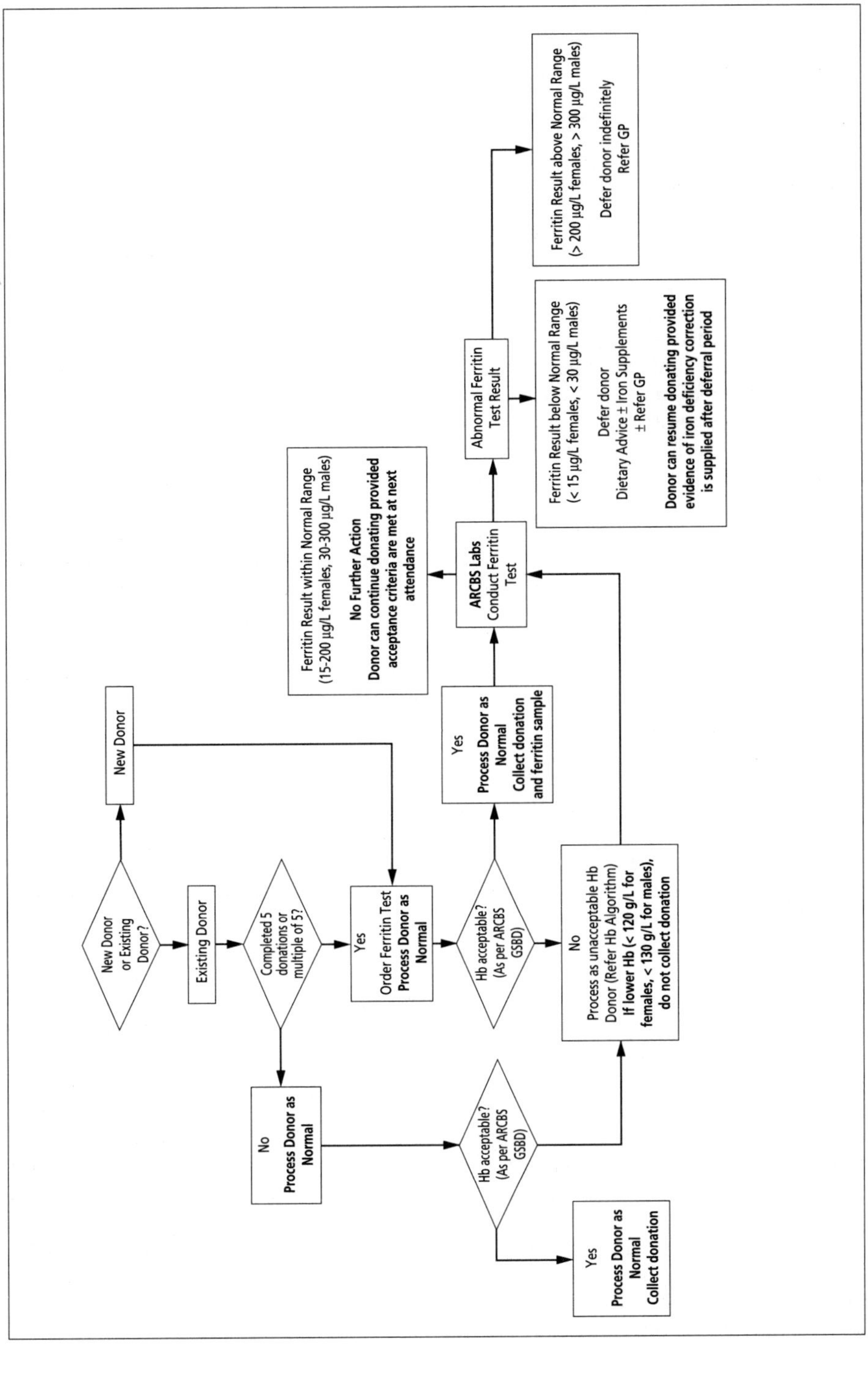

Fig. 3: Proposed algorithm for managing donors with iron deficiency. Australian Red Cross Blood Service 2004.

an STR assay, the difficulty of accessing a venous pre-donation sample for iron-related indices and the overall cost are all impediments to the improved understanding, retention and care of donor haemtalogical status.

Conclusions

Over the past 25 years, transfusion medicine has been shaped by the drive to ensure optimal outcomes for patients through increasingly sophisticated and costly product safety measures. These have included substantially complex donor selection procedures, which have made the donation process onerous and intrusive. While the issue of donor haematological status has continued to be assessed, it is this author's view that this has been as much as from the traditional paradigm of ensuring supply as from a basic concern for donor health.

It is therefore appropriate that the potential harm for donors is more strongly reflected in the various standard setting environments, and the following extract from the current Council of Europe Guide is timely:

> *"It is recognised that blood donation may result in iron deficiency in repeat blood donors. This problem may arise without being evident through pre-donation haemoglobin measurement. This may be especially important in women in the child-bearing years. Blood collection agencies should include appropriate measures to minimise this problem, and to protect donor health.*
> *Such measures may include the use of tests to assess iron status, the provision of materials for donor education particularly in regard to the importance of an iron rich diet, the tailoring of donation frequency based on iron status and if appropriate the supplementation of dietary iron through appropriate prophylactic medication.*
> *At the same time, agencies should recognise that many donors currently deferred because of low haemoglobin are in a satisfactory state of health and, once their iron status is confirmed as satisfactory, they may be re-entered into donation programs. Therefore, managing the problem of iron-deficiency contributes to the maintenance of donor health and the sufficiency of the blood supply."* [30]

It is clear that this issue requires more research. The differentiation between the depletion of storage and functional iron needs to be supported by clinical studies. If verified, the findings will lead to a substantial improvement in donor management. Similarly, the clinical significance of iron depletion requires clarification, given the emerging evidence of its benefit in certain cardiovascular states. Supporting donor iron status through appropriate supplementation needs to be assessed through appropriate trials. Assays for parameters such as ferritin and STR are needed, and non-invasive ways of assessing these would improve donor care. More work is needed to determine the influence of factors such as diet on the haematological status of blood donors; clearly, situations for otherwise healthy donors are not applicable in other environments. All these measures demand resources. The blood industry and their regulatory authorities need to work together to influence policy makers in making these resources available.

References

1 Blanco C et al: Maintaining iron balance in women blood donors of childbearing age: summary of a workshop. Transfusion 2002; 42: 798-805.

2 Newman BH: Adjusting our management of female blood donors: the key to an adequate blood supply. Transfusion 2004; 44: 591-596.

3 Herbert PC et al: A multicentre randomized controlled clinical trial of transfusion requirements in critical care. NEJM 1999; 340: 409-417.

4 Blanc B, Finch CA, Hallberg L, et al: Nutritional Anaemias. Report of a WHO Scientific Group. WHO Tech Rep Ser 1968; 405: 1-40.

5 Cook JD, Flowers CH, Skikne BS: The quantitative assessment of body iron. Blood 2003; 101: 3359-3364.

6 Johnson-Spear MA, Yip R: Hemoglobin difference between black and white women with comparable iron status: justification for race-specific anemia criteria [see comments]. Am J Clin Nutr 1994; 60: 117-121.

7 Beutler E, Waalen J: The definition of anemia: What is the lower limit of normal of the blood hemoglobin concentration? Blood 2005 [epub ahead of print].

8 Boulton FE et al: Improved strategy for screening prospective blood donors for anaemia. Transf Med 1994; 4: 221-225.

9 Wood E et al: Accuracy of predonation Hct sampling affects donor safety, eligibility, and deferral rates. Transfusion 2001; 41: 353-359.

10 Radtke et al: Hemoglobin screening in prospective blood donors: Comparison of different blood samples and different quantitative methods. Transfusion and Apheresis Science 2005; 33: 31 – 35.

11 Lotfi R et al: A noninvasive strategy for screening prospective blood donors for anemia. Transfusion 2005; 45: 1585-1592.

12 Silber MH, Richardson JW: Multiple blood donations associated with iron deficiency in patients with restless legs syndrome. Mayo Clin Proc 2003; 78: 52-54.

13 Bruner AB et al: Randomised study of cognitive effects of iron supplementation in non-anaemic iron-deficient adolescent girls. Lancet 1996; 348: 992-996.

14 Ramakrishnan U: Functional consequences of nutritional anemias, in Ramakrishnan U (ed): Nutritional Anemias. Boca Raton, FL, CRC Press, 2002, pp 43-68.

15 Salonen JT et al: Donation of blood is associated with reduced risk of myocardial infarction. The Kuopio Ishaemic Heart Disease Risk Factor Study. Am J Epidemiol 1998; 148: 445-451.

16 Meyers DG et al: A historical cohort study of the effect of lowering body iron through blood donation on incident cardiac events. Transfusion 2002; 42: 1135-1139.

17 Zheng H et al: Iron stores and vascular function in voluntary blood donors. Arterioscler Thromb Vasc Biol 2005; 25: 1577-1583.

18 Skine et al: Serum transferrin receptor: A quantitative measure of tissue iron deficiency. Blood 1990; 75: 1870-1876.

19 Suominen et al: Serum transferring receptor and transferrin receptor-ferritin index identify healthy subjects with subclinical iron defects. Blood 1998; 92: 2934-2939.

20 Cook JD et al: Serum ferritin as a measure of iron stores in normal subjects. American Journal of Clinical Nutrition 1974; 27: 681-687.

21 Beguin Y: Soluble transferrin receptor for the evaluation of erythropoiesis and iron status. Clinica Chimica Acta 2003; 129: 9-22.

22 Finch C et al: Effect of blood donation on iron stores as evaluated by serum ferritin Blood 1977; 50: 441-447.

23 Punnonen K, Rajamäki A: Evaluation of iron status of Finnish blood donors using serum transferrin receptor. Transfusion Medicine 1999; 9: 131-134.

24 Javadzadeh Shahshahani H et al: A study of the prevalence of iron deficiency and its related factors in blood donors of Yazd, Iran, 2003. Transfusion Medicine 2005; 15: 287 – 293.

25 Boulton F, Collis D, Inskip H, et al: A study of the iron and HFE status of blood donors, including a group who failed the initial screen for anaemia. Brit J Haematol, 2000; 8: 434-439.

26 Punnonen K, Irjala K, Rajamaki A: Serum transferring receptor, ferritin and TfR-F Index in identification of latent iron deficiency. Eur J Haematol 1998; 60: 135-137.

27 Flesland O et al: Transferrin receptor in serum. A new tool in the diagnosis and prevention of iron deficiency in blood donors Transfusion and Apheresis Science 2004; 31: 11-16.

28 Raftos J et al: Iron stores assessed in blood donors by hematoflourometry. Transfusion 1983; 23: 226-228.

29 Doherty K: Polymorphisms in the HFE gene protect against iron deficiency associated with blood donation. Proceedings of the 34th Annual Scientific Meeting of the Australasian Society for Blood Transfusion, 2000, p 103.

30 Council of Europe publications. Guide to the preparation, quality assurance and use of blood components. 11th edition 2006.

Prof. A. Farrugia, Office of Devices, Blood and Tissues, Therapeutic Goods Administration, PO Box 100, Woden, ACT, Australia 2606.
E-mail: albert.farrugia@health.gov.au

Dax EM, Farrugia A, Vyas G (eds): Advances in Transfusion Safety – Volume IV.
Dev Biol (Basel). Basel, Karger, 2007, vol 127, pp 147-152.

The European Blood Directive – Its Role in Blood Safety

R. Seitz

Division of Haematology/Transfusion Medicine, Paul-Ehrlich-Institut, Langen, Germany

Key words: European Communities (EC), legislation, blood safety.

Abstract: New EC legislation ensures a high level of quality and safety of blood and blood components, whatever the intended purpose, throughout the community. Though the initial intention was to strengthen regulatory oversight in the field of blood transfusion services, the Directive 2002/98/EC also has strong implications for the collection and testing of plasma for fractionation. Within the legal framework, as set out by Directive 2002/98/EC, mandatory minimal requirements are laid down by the Commission in further " daughter " Directives, with the assistance of a committee. While allowing some flexibility to the member states to find their specific solutions and regulatory mechanisms in transposition of the Directive, the new legislation advances the approximation of the provisions, thus strengthening the blood supply in the EC. This is an important step towards the ultimate goal to further improve the quality and safety of blood and blood components and to contribute to the confidence of the patients in a safe blood supply in the EC.

INTRODUCTION

The European Communities (EC), i.e. the European Union (EU), currently with 25 member states (Table 1), and three countries belonging to the European Economic Area (EEA), do not so far have the character of a nation, as for example the United States of America. The EU is a complex political structure held together on the basis of a Treaty [1], which is continuously updated and confers important competences to the EU institutions, i.e. the Council, the European Commission, and the European Parliament. Thus, the EC has the power to enact legislation either when harmonisation of existing provisions is essential, or when problems cannot be solved by laws of the member states but only on the community level. Such legal documents can be "Regulations", which are immediately binding in the whole EC, or "Directives", which have to be transposed into national laws within a certain period.

Another supranational institution is the Council of Europe, which is a European "UN-like" organisation with more than 40 member states. An important part of the Council of Europe is the European Directorate for the Quality of Medicines (EDQM), which includes the European Pharmacopoeia. There are also several observer states

Table 1: Member states of the EC.

	Member states
EU until 1st May 2005	Austria, Belgium, Denmark, Finland, France, Germany, Greece, Ireland, Italy, Luxembourg, Portugal, Spain, Sweden, The Netherlands, United Kingdom
Countries joining EU on 1st May 2005	Cyprus, Czech Republic, Estonia, Hungary, Latvia, Lithuania, Malta, Poland, Slovakia, Slovenia
EEA	Iceland, Liechtenstein, Norway

beyond Europe including Australia, Canada, and recently, U.S.A. The Council of Europe also publishes recommendations in the field of blood transfusion.

Until recently, national systems of blood services have developed and grown independently within the EC, with considerable diversity of organisation, funding, regulatory oversight, and responsibilities. This has not necessarily lead to differences in quality of the services, since comprehensive and well-respected guidelines have been available. Probably the most influential guidance document in Europe is the Council of Europe Guide [2]. However, it has the character of a recommendation and does not have the power of a mandatory legal document.

This situation was addressed by new EC legislation. As necessary for all legislative initiatives of the EC, the basis is the Treaty. It states in Article 152 (ex Article 129), paragraph 4: "The Council, acting in accordance with the procedure referred to in Article 251 and after consulting the Economic and Social Committee and the Committee of the Regions, shall contribute to the achievement of the objectives referred to in this Article through adopting… measures setting high standards of quality and safety of organs and substances of human origin, blood and blood derivatives; these measures shall not prevent any Member State from maintaining or introducing more stringent protective measures…".

Scope and Objectives of DIRECTIVE 2002/98/EC

As outlined above, until recently there has been a considerable diversity of blood services in the EC member states. The goal of Directive 2002/98/EC [3] is the approximation of provisions in this field. To this end, the Directive lays down standards of quality and safety of human blood and blood components in order to ensure a high level of human health protection. In the explanatory recitals the following is stated: "It is essential that whatever the intended purpose, Community provisions should ensure that blood and its components are of comparable quality and safety throughout the blood transfusion chain in all Member States, bearing in mind the freedom of movement of citizens within Community territory." This sentence contains two very important aspects. First, the focus is on the free movement of citizens (i.e. potential patients) in the EC, but not on free movement of the blood components. This is in line with the wording in the Treaty cited above: "these measures shall not prevent any member state from maintaining or introducing more stringent protective measures…". Second, Article 2 of Directive 2002/98/EC states that it "shall apply to the collection and testing of human blood and blood components, whatever their intended purpose, and to their processing, storage, and distribution when intended for transfusion". This created a new link between the industrial plasma derivatives, which had been regulated since 1989 by the pharmaceutical legislation, and the blood components for transfusion.

This new situation was a cause for some dispute. In the transfusion sector, the declared policy of international organisations such as the WHO and the Council of Europe is to rely on "voluntary and unpaid blood donations". Member states wished to incorporate this as a mandatory requirement in the Directive. However, this might have created considerable problems with the supply of stable plasma products, since much of the plasma collected within the EC and imported from outside Europe (U.S.A.) comes from reimbursed or paid plasmapheresis donors. An extensive debate about this issue included ethical aspects and the question of whether reimbursement might (still) be a factor possibly compromising the safety of stable plasma products. The scientific committee of the European Medicines Agency (EMEA), made the following statements [4]: "...The safety of plasma derived medicinal products is optimised by the stepwise application, in the course of collection, manufacture, and batch release testing, of a number of complimentary measures, which are under regulatory control. Both non-remunerated and remunerated donors contribute to the supply with safe plasma-derived products... The question of whether or not non-remuneration is important for the safety of blood and blood components for transfusion is a separate issue outside the scope of this document". Anyway, there have been no documented transmissions of relevant viruses (HIV, HBV, or HCV) by industrial plasma products in the past ten years.

At the end, the Directive was adopted with the following wording. Article 20, 1: "Member States shall take the necessary measures to encourage voluntary and unpaid blood donations with a view to ensuring that blood and blood components are in so far as possible provided from such donations". And Article 4, 2: "This Directive shall not prevent a Member State from maintaining or introducing in its territory more stringent protective measures which comply with the provisions of the Treaty. In particular, a Member State may introduce requirements for voluntary and unpaid donations, which include the prohibition or restriction of imports of blood and blood components, to ensure a high level of health protection...". This means that the EC as such would not ban plasma from reimbursed donors, but each member state would have the opportunity to do so.

An important definition used in the Directive should be mentioned: "'blood establishment' shall mean any structure or body that is responsible for any aspect of the collection and testing of human blood or blood components, whatever their intended purpose, and their processing, storage, and distribution when intended for transfusion. This does not include hospital blood banks; 'hospital blood bank' shall mean a hospital unit which stores and distributes and may perform compatibility tests on blood and blood components exclusively for use within hospital facilities, including hospital based transfusion activities".

Provisions

As outlined above, an EC Directive is a legal text which is not immediately applicable but has to be transposed into the national legislation of member states by a stated date, which was in this case not later than 8 February 2005. The blood

Directive provides a legal frame, which outlines the goal to reach an equivalently high standard all over the EC, but gives the member states some flexibility. An example of this is the wording that blood establishments need "designation, authorisation, accreditation or licensing by the competent authority".

The Directive contains a number of chapters, addressing the following items:

- Designation of competent authorities.
  In several member states, there used to be fairly autonomous national systems without stringent regulatory oversight. Now, every member state has to designate a competent authority or authorities.

- Designation, authorisation, accreditation or licensing of blood establishments by authority.
  The goal is clearly to achieve a sufficient level of reliability and accountability to ensure compliance of blood establishments within the requirements as set out in the Directive. However, the member states have the choice of which regulatory mechanism would best achieve this goal on their territory.

- Inspection by authority and control measures.
  This is for several member states a new element, particularly for those which did not yet have a competent authority in place. This does not mean that in those countries the blood sector was without control, since there have been systems of self-inspection and audits in operation. However, the Directive makes it clear now that such inspection and control measures shall be carried out by officials representing the competent authority who must be empowered to inspect all facilities, take appropriate samples and examine relevant documents. It is a considerable challenge to build up in every member state a staff for this purpose with the necessary manpower and skills.

- Responsible person, personnel.
  The Directive requires the designation of a responsible person in charge of ensuring proper collection and testing of every blood unit, providing information to the competent authority and implementing the relevant regulatory requirements. In some member states, this person has to be a licensed physician, preferably with board certification in transfusion medicine. The Directive, however, requires as minimal standard that "he/she shall possess a diploma, certificate or other evidence of formal qualifications in the field of medical or biological sciences awarded on completion of a university course of study or a course recognised as equivalent by the Member State concerned", as well as practical post-graduate experience in relevant areas for at least two years, in one or more authorised blood establishments. Certain tasks may be delegated to other persons who shall be qualified by training and experience to perform such tasks and be provided with timely, relevant and regularly updated training.

- Quality system for blood establishments.
  The wording used in the Directive is: "Member States shall take all necessary measures to ensure that each blood establishment establishes and maintains a quality system for blood establishments based on the principles of good practice." In several countries, a system strictly according to good manufacturing practice (GMP) rules is clearly required. However, again, the Directive allows, to some extent, flexibility, using in the recital (17) the expression: "taking into account the principles of good manufacturing practice".

- Documentation, record keeping.
  All relevant data have to be documented and records have to be kept for at least 15 years. All data of potential relevance for traceability, possibly necessary look-back procedures, have to be kept for at least 30 years. The latter very stringent requirement was apparently adopted with a view to infections with excessively long incubation periods such as variant Creutzfeldt-Jakob Disease.
- Haemovigilance.
  The Directive puts considerable weight on the provisions to ensure traceability. This means that blood and blood components collected, tested, processed, stored, released and/or distributed on the territory of the member states can be traced from donor to recipient and vice versa. This includes, explicitly, blood and blood components imported from developing countries. All serious adverse events (including accidents and errors) related to the collection, testing, processing, storage and distribution of blood and blood components, which may have an influence on their quality and safety, as well as any serious adverse reactions observed during or after transfusion, which may be attributed to the quality and the safety of blood and blood components, have to be notified to the competent authority.
- Quality and safety of blood and blood components.
  The Directive stipulates essential elements, such as exchange of information with and examination of donors to ensure their eligibility, testing of donations, storage conditions, and quality controls.

Technical Requirements

In essence, the Blood Directive outlines the fundamental principles, and to which areas standards shall apply, but it does not fix technical requirements in all detail. It installs, however, a mechanism producing mandatory technical requirements by giving the EU Commission a mandate to adopt further Directives which list in Annexes the minimal standards required in the EC. The Commission is assisted in this task by an expert committee with representatives of all member states. The first of these "daughter" Directives, Directive 2004/33/EC [5], provides detailed provisions regarding the following areas: information to prospective donors; information required from donors; eligibility of donors; storage, transport and distribution conditions for blood and blood components; quality and safety requirements for blood and blood components (specifications and required quality testing); autologous donations; and validation.

Transposition, Example Germany

As outlined above, the Blood Directive allows the member states to implement or maintain more stringent measures. Thus, Germany can continue its long-standing regulatory system, which is continuously refined and updated. An important milestone was the Transfusion Act [6], which came into force in 1998. Technical details are stipulated in guidelines [7] issued by the German Medical Association together with the Paul-Ehrlich-Institut. One element above the minimal standards fixed by the Directive is, e.g., that a licensed physician is required as the responsible person in every blood establishment. Furthermore, a manufacturing license is needed for blood establishments, requiring a functioning quality system and GMP, reinforced by regular official inspections by the regional ("Länder") authorities. Like any medicinal products, blood components for transfusion also need a marketing authorisation on the basis of a dossier defining methods of manufacture and quality controls, verified by inspections by experts of the Paul-Ehrlich-Institut.

References

1 Consolidated version of the treaty establishing the european community. Available in the internet under: http://europa.eu.int/eur-lex/en/treaties/dat/C_2002325EN.003301.html.

2 Guide to the preparation, use and quality assurance of blood components, Recommendation No. R (95) 15, yearly updated, Council of Europe.

3 Directive 2002/98/ec of the European parliament and of the council of 27 January 2003 setting standards of quality and safety for the collection, testing, processing, storage and distribution of human blood and blood components and amending Directive 2001/83/EC.

4 CPMP Position Statement EMEA/CPMP/BWP/1818/02.

5 Commission Directive 2004/33/EC of 22 March 2004, implementing Directive 2002/98/EC of the European Parliament and of the Council as regards certain technical requirements for blood and blood components.

6 Gesetz zur Regelung des Transfusionswesens, Bundesgesetzblatt (German Federal Law Gazette) I 1998, 1752. Last update on 10 February 2005.

7 Richtlinien zur Gewinnung von Blut und Blutbestandteilen und zur Anwendung von Blutprodukten (Hämotherapie). Available in the internet under: http://www.bundesaerztekammer.de/30/Richtlinien/Richtidx/Blutprodukte2005Nov/Haemo2005.pdf.

Useful Internet Addresses

- Paul-Ehrlich-Institut
  http://www.pei.de
- European Commission
  http://ec.europa.eu/index.htm
- European Medicines Agency (EMEA)
  http://www.emea.europa.eu
- European Directorate for the Quality of Medicines (EDQM)
  http://www.pheur.org/site/page_628.php
- German Medical Association
  http://www.bundesaerztekammer.de/05/90Englisch/index.html

Prof. Dr. R. Seitz, Division of Haematology/Transfusion Medicine, Paul-Ehrlich-Institut, Langen, Germany
E-mail: seira@pei.de

Dax EM, Farrugia A, Vyas G (eds): Advances in Transfusion Safety – Volume IV.
Dev Biol (Basel). Basel, Karger, 2007, vol 127, pp 153-158.

Supply and Safety Through One Agency – The Singapore Experience

D. Teo, P.S. Lim

Health Sciences Authority, Singapore

Key words: Blood safety; regulation of blood; Health Sciences Authority; Health regulation in Singapore; blood products.

INTRODUCTION

Singapore Healthcare System

Singapore is an island city-state with a total land area of 697.1 sq km. The Singapore population of about 4.2 million is relatively young, comprising three major ethnic racial groups – Chinese, Malays, and Indians. The state of health in Singapore is good by international standards, with an average life expectancy of 78.9 years and an infant mortality rate of 2.2 per 1,000 live births. Currently, the leading causes of morbidity and mortality are major non-communicable diseases such as cancer, stroke and cardiovascular disease.

The healthcare system in Singapore is delivered through a network of public and private healthcare facilities under the central development and planning coordination of the Ministry of Health (MOH). The public healthcare system includes 7 public hospitals, 6 national specialist centres, and 17 outpatient polyclinics; private healthcare is provided by 16 private hospitals and numerous private GP clinics.

In addition to the formulation of policies and health services development work, the MOH is also responsible for regulating health standards.

The Health Sciences Authority

The Health Sciences Authority (HSA) was formed as a statutory board under the MOH in April 2001. It was a merger of three government departments – the Singapore Blood Transfusion Service, the National Pharmaceutical Administration, and the Institute for Science and Forensic Medicine. Because of this merger, seven Professional Centres now reside under one roof. This effectively brought the national blood service (now called the Centre for Transfusion Medicine or CTM) within the same agency as the national regulatory body for medicinal products (now called the Centre for Drug Administration or CDA).

BLOOD SUPPLY IN SINGAPORE

The CTM fulfills 95 % of the blood needs in Singapore and provides blood and blood components to all public and private hospitals in the country. The remaining 5 % is provided by the National University Hospital Blood Centre, which collects blood for about 50 % of its own hospital needs. In 2004, 78,308 whole blood donations and 8,238 apheresis donations were collected by the CTM and processed into 192,137 blood components, which were distributed to the hospitals for use. The range of blood products provided include red cells, fresh frozen plasma, platelets (whole blood derived and apheresis), cryoprecipitate, fibrin glue, washed red cells, leucoreduced blood products, and irradiated blood products. Additionally, between 8,000-10,000 kg of plasma are shipped to the CSL Bioplasma facilities in Melbourne each year for processing to albumin, intravenous immunoglobulin, Factor VIII and Factor IX concentrates under contract fractionation agreement.

Singapore maintains a policy of self sufficiency in fresh blood and blood products, and blood is rarely imported into the country except in instances of rare blood types when the national service is unable to provide the needed units. There is no policy of self sufficiency for plasma derivative products, and so the supply includes a mix of derivatives produced by CTM through contract fractionation and commercial plasma derivatives.

REGULATION OF BLOOD SUPPLY

The supply and safety of the blood supply is ensured through a team approach involving various members of the Health Team, in particular:

Ministry of Health

New policies and changes in policies that have significant impact on blood safety and quality require endorsement by the Director of Medical Services, MOH. In addition, two MOH Divisions oversee various aspects of CTM's operations and services. They are:

- *Health Regulation Division* (HRD) – which looks into the regulation of processes and premises. All premises providing services related to the collection, processing, testing and distribution of fresh blood and blood products are regulated under the *Private Hospital and Medical Clinics Act.* Specifically, blood collection activities, which involve donor selection and whole blood and apheresis donation require licensing as a Medical Clinic, and the processing and testing activities require licensing as a Clinical Laboratory. Licensing of the facility is required biennially, and involves inspection of the premises and audit of its processes and quality systems by teams comprising inspectors from the MOH and external independent assessors.
- *Communicable Disease Division* – All data pertaining to blood safety, including data on infectious disease markers in the donor population, are regularly submitted to the MOH for review. All cases of HIV infections in blood donors must be notified to the MOH under the *Infectious Diseases Act.*

Professional bodies

All practising doctors must be registered by the Singapore Medical Council and all practising nurses by the Singapore Nursing Board. These professional boards ensure that professional standards of practice and competence are met; the Singapore Medical Council additionally requires all registered doctors to maintain a minimum level of continuing education through the compulsory enforcement of a system of Continuing Medical Education (CME) points. This ensures that all professional personnel dealing with blood and blood products have the proper qualifications and remain current in their knowledge of blood-related or transfusion medicine issues.

Expert committees

Expert panels constituted from national medical and technical experts, such as the AIDS Task Force and the Advisory Committee for Hepatitis & Related Disorders, also provide advice to the MOH and CTM on matters relating to HIV and Hepatitis, respectively. The role of other expert committees will be discussed further in the presentation.

Health Sciences Authority

The two main professional centres overseeing blood safety in HSA are the Centre for Drug Administration (CDA) and the CTM. The rest of the paper will now focus on their respective roles in ensuring an adequate and safe blood supply for Singaporeans.

Centre for Drug Administration, CDA

Blood products are regulated as biological products by the CDA under the *Medicines Act*[1], which was introduced in 1987. Under this Act, all medicinal products must be registered and licensed so that desired standards of safety, efficacy and quality are met. CDA is the health product regulatory authority, which plays a similar role as the Australian Therapeutic Goods Administration (TGA), US Food and Drug Administration (FDA) or the UK Medicines and Healthcare Products Regulatory Agency (MHRA).

All plasma derived products are also registered and licensed by the CDA. These include plasma derivatives produced by CTM through contract fractionation. All applications for product registration undergo stringent screening that includes the pre-licensing product evaluation process and post-licensing monitoring. Product evaluation is carried out by CDA scientific evaluators and a panel of independent external evaluators and assessed against specific pre-set criteria. The evaluations are further scrutinised by the Biologicals Expert Panel and the Medicines Advisory Committee before the decision is made to register the product.

Currently, local fresh blood products are not required to undergo product registration. However, all blood products intended for import into Singapore must obtain approval by the CDA to ensure that the products meet quality and safety standards.

---

1 Biologicals, under the Medicines Act, refer to products derived from living sources that are intended for use in the prevention, treatment or cure of diseases to humans. They include: blood products, allergenic extracts, vaccines, proteins and peptides, monoclonal antibodies, somatic cell or tissue products, gene therapy products, xenotransplantation products, and stem cell products.

Centre for Transfusion Medicine, CTM

CTM is the national blood bank and centre of excellence for transfusion medicine in Singapore. CTM has in place stringent internal control procedures to ensure blood supply for the nation is safe. The procedures include:

- use of blood donor selection and screening criteria based on standards and guidelines developed by international blood bank organisations, e.g. Council of Europe, AABB, World Health Organisation;
- blood collection, processing, testing and release procedures that follow standards and guidelines developed by international blood bank organisations, e.g. Council of Europe, AABB, World Health Organisation;
- screening for infectious agents – including Hepatitis B by HBsAg and HBV-NAT, Hepatitis C by anti-HCV and HCV-NAT, HIV-1 & 2 by anti-HIV-1/2 and HIV-NAT, and syphilis by TPHA;
- implementation of a comprehensive quality system in all processes and procedures; and
- legislative support – false blood donor declaration during the pre-donation screen by blood donors is liable to prosecution under the Infectious Diseases Act.

Supply and Safety Through One Agency

As both CDA and CTM are Centres under the umbrella of HSA, concerns may be raised on potential conflicts of interests. This, however, is managed through the following mechanisms:

Clearly defined mission, accountabilities

HSA's mission, as a government statutory board, is to excel in applying science to support healthcare services and regulation, serve the administration of justice and enhance safety in our community. Within these broad goals, there is a clear delineation of roles and responsibilities of each professional centre within HSA, with the Director of each Centre holding sole responsibility for the professional standards of performance within his/her Centre. In the case of blood safety, the mission of the CTM is clearly defined as the provision of a safe and adequate national supply of blood and blood products. Its accountability is to not only HSA but to MOH and to the Singapore public. A continued strong emphasis on professional integrity as a core value within the organisation contributes to ensuring that organisational interests do not supercede the responsibility to provide an adequate and safe national blood supply.

Clear and transparent deliverables

Specific quantifiable deliverables are set to measure its performance, including such set targets as the number of units collected and processed, infectious disease testing quality control indicators, and red cell and platelet unit outdates. To ensure that supply is appropriate to clinical needs, indicators are set to measure elective operations postponed due to lack of blood and unmet requests for blood products.

A national haemovigilance programme has also been in place since 2003 to monitor blood transfusion safety, and this includes transfusion transmitted infections.

As a form of good corporate governance practice, the performance indicators and data on deliverables are provided on quarterly and annual bases to both the HSA Senior Management and its Board of Directors, as well as to the MOH. Results of the haemovigilance programme are provided on a half-yearly and yearly basis to all Hospital Transfusion Committees and Medical Boards for information.

The use of clear and quantifiable indicators and deliverables enables the performance of the CTM in fulfilling its blood supply responsibilities to be presented in a way that can be easily understood by its stakeholders and the public. Data regarding blood donor infectious disease markers and post-transfusion infections is regularly collated by the MOH as part of infectious disease statistics routinely published. Transparency increases the public's confidence that their blood supply is safe.

Checks and balances within each regulatory process

Within each regulatory process, checks and balances are also introduced to ensure independent evaluation. The process of product registration within the CDA includes peer review post-evaluation of each product, which may include evaluation by external evaluators and, later in the process, further deliberation on product safety by two independent expert panels. External evaluators for CTM products are carefully selected to ensure no conflict of interest, and, where necessary, overseas evaluators may be used.

Similarly, whilst the MOH regulates processes, premises and personnel involved in blood safety, its various responsible divisions are advised by panels of independent external expert advisors, which include private sector experts.

Regulation of products, processes and premises depend on compliance with preset standards and specifications that are based on international standards. The use of specifications and clear requirements allow for objective assessment and evaluation of the adequacy of the product or process.

External evaluation

CTM also sought accreditation by internationally recognised bodies such as the AABB to ensure that CTM continues to maintain standards of best practices in its quality systems. The appointment of CTM as a WHO Collaborating Centre for Transfusion Medicine is an additional driver to ensuring that it maintains high standards of quality and safety.

Relationship with other organizations

The role of other organisations in ensuring supply and safety cannot be underestimated. In 2001, the CTM entered into a Memorandum of Understanding with the Singapore Red Cross (SRC), to delegate the national blood donor recruitment programme to the SRC. Under this agreement, the SRC assumed the role of recruiting blood donors and organising blood donation drives, while the CTM focused on the "regulated" functions of donor selection, blood collection, processing, testing and distribution. The Singapore Red Cross adheres to the principles of the International Confederation of Red Cross & Red Crescent, which further ensures that it adheres to international best practices in ensuring safe blood.

Hospitals, through their Hospital Transfusion Committees and through the regular dialogues and meetings with key MOH officials, keep watch on the policies and performance of CTM to assure adequate supplies of safe blood to support their clinical programmes.

What Else Can Be Done

Further measures can be considered to strengthen the robustness of the regulatory process for blood. Within the HSA, recommendations will be made to constitute an independent Blood Advisory Committee that will advise on key decisions and policies relating to blood supply quality and safety. This is similar to the Medicines Advisory Committee, which advises on medicinal products. An additional platform under consideration is the introduction of a schedule of meetings of the Hospital Transfusion Committee Chairpersons, which will provide a formal route of feedback from hospitals on issues pertaining to blood supply.

Conclusion

HSA is a statutory board under the Ministry of Health. The blood supply in Singapore is provided nationally by the Centre for Transfusion Medicine, which is one of seven professional centres in the Health Sciences Authority. The activities of the CTM are regulated in part by the Centre for Drug Administration of the HSA, and in part by various professional divisions within the Ministry of Health. HSA has therefore put in place various internal control procedures to ensure no compromise to blood supply and safety.

This model has worked well for Singapore in ensuring adequacy and safety of blood supply while optimizing operational efficiency by sharing of resources across the nation and various agencies, in particular within HSA. The key success factors for this model include clarity of mission and transparency of deliverables coupled with an openess to external (including international) scrutiny and supportive partners.

Dr. D. Teo, Health Sciences Authority, 11 Outram Road, Singapore 169078, Singapore.
E-mail: Diana_Teo@hsa.gov.sg

Dax EM, Farrugia A, Vyas G (eds): Advances in Transfusion Safety – Volume IV.
Dev Biol (Basel). Basel, Karger, 2007, vol 127, p 159.

SESSION V

Transfusion and Blood Safety in the Asia-Pacific

Chairs: *Lin Che-kit and P. Flanagan*

Dax EM, Farrugia A, Vyas G (eds): Advances in Transfusion Safety – Volume IV.
Dev Biol (Basel). Basel, Karger, 2007, vol 127, pp 161-168.

The New Japanese Blood Law: Its Impact on Blood Safety and Usage

K. Tadokoro

Blood Service Headquarters, Japanese Red Cross, Tokyo, Japan

Key words: Blood Law, hemovigilance, look-back, appropriate use, stable supply.

Abstract: The New Blood Law and the amendments of the Pharmaceutical Affairs Law were enforced in 2003 for the purpose of securing a stable supply of blood based on domestic voluntary donations and promoting the appropriate use. The safety of blood has been increased dramatically by various safety measures. Adverse reactions/infections reports and nationwide look back studies showed the remaining risk of screening test-negtive, ID-NAT-positive blood transfusion: HBV 1: 130 x 10^3, HCV 1:22 million, HIV 1:11 million. Eight items of safety measures were announced by JRC in 2003 and are being achieved. Implementation of further safety measures requires public understanding and support. Supply of blood has been decreasing owing to the guidelines for appropriate use of blood, the mandated informed consent for transfusion and the enforcement of the Laws. However, additional safety measures and the rapid progress into highly aging society necessitate an expansion of the donor pool, especially among young generations. Public understanding and close collaboration among stakeholders are necessary to achieve what the new laws ask.

The History of the Blood Program

The Japanese Red Cross (JRC) blood bank was opened in Tokyo in 1952, following public and commercial blood banks. Paid donations sharply increased in the late 1950's with the prosperity of commercial banks. "Yellow blood" from anemic, frequent and paid donors that caused the high incidence of post-transfusion hepatitis (PTH) became a social problem. In 1964, a Government Cabinet decision was made to establish a system to secure an adequate supply of stored blood by voluntary donations through the cooperation between government, local authorities and JRC blood centers. With public understanding and cooperation, voluntary non-remunerated donations increased gradually. Commercial blood banks for blood transfusion were closed in 1972, and those for plasma derivatives in 1992. The incidence of PTH, 50.6 % at the period of paid donation, decreased gradually with the transition to the voluntary donation and the introduction of apheresis and 400 mL donation in addition to 200mL donation. The improvement of screening tests also reduced PTH dramatically. No PTH case was found in the prospective study after the implementation of the 2nd generation anti-HCV screening test in 1991.

However, HIV infections through imported unheated coagulation factors in the 1980's and the subsequent lawsuits provoked social concern about the safety of blood and blood products and the management of a blood program. Discussion of a new legal framework of the blood program started in 1996.

The Law on Securing a Stable Supply of Safe Blood

The Law on Securing a Stable Supply of Safe Blood (The New Blood Law) was enforced in July 2003 after several years' discussions. This law provides the following basic principles for guiding the management of the blood program and defines the responsibility of stakeholders involved in the blood program.

- **Basic principles**
  1. To enhance the safety of blood products.
  2. To secure the stable supply of blood products through the domestic non-paid blood donations.
  3. To promote the appropriate use of blood products.
  4. To ensure fairness and improve transparency in managing the blood program.
- **Responsibilities of stakeholders involved in the blood program**
  1. The national government.
     - (i) To plan and implement basic and comprehensive measures for securing stable supply of safe blood.
     - (ii) To provide Japanese citizens with education and enlightenment to enhance their understanding of and cooperation with blood donation.
     - (iii) To plan measures for promoting the appropriate use of blood products.
  2. The local authorities (prefectural and municipal governments).
     - (i) To deepen local residents' understanding of blood donation.
     - (ii) To take measures to assist blood collecting services in receiving blood.
  3. Blood collecting services (JRC blood services).
     - (i) To promote and receive blood donations.
     - (ii) To cooperate with manufacturers in improving the safety of blood and securing a stable supply.
     - (iii) To protect donors.
  4. Blood manufacturers/sales contractors (Marketing license holders: JRC blood services).
     - (i) To secure stable supply of safe blood products.
     - (ii) To improve technology.
     - (iii) To collect and provide information to improve the safety.
  5. Medical Professionals.
     - (i) To use blood products appropriately.
     - (ii) To collect and provide information to improve the safety.

The Pharmaceutical Affairs Law was also amended in July 2002 and fully enforced in April 2005. Through these amendments, blood products, including blood for transfusion, plasma derivatives and the functionally equivalent recombinant products, are defined as special bio-products, which have more risk of infection than other bio-products and are to be controlled by the additional regulations. For example, market license holders of these products must use a label to indicate a special bio-product and keep the records for 30 years. They are also obliged to report information regularly to the Ministry of Health, Labor and Welfare (MHLW) on relating infections and perform look back studies.

Adverse Reactions and Infections Reporting System (Hemovigilance) in Japan

JRC established a nationwide adverse reactions and infections reporting system to monitor the safety of blood and blood products in 1992. Although this system is based on voluntary reports from physicians, JRC blood service is mandated to report them to the MHLW if the case is severe, fatal or unknown. The number of reports has been increasing year by year along with growing public interest in the safety of transfusion medicine. This nationwide system revealed rare cases of transfusion-transmitted (TT) infections. Causal relation to transfusion is judged based on individual donation (ID)-nucleic acid amplification testing (NAT) of repository donor specimens that have been stored since 1996 to be stored for 11 years. Mini-pool NAT screening for HBV, HCV and HIV was implemented in October 1999.

Although about 20 cases of TT HBV infection were reported annually before NAT screening, the number of TT HBV infection cases decreased to 6-7 annually after NAT. No case of TT HCV infection has been found for 4 years after NAT, though 5 to 7 cases were reported annually before. While 3 cases of TT HIV infection were reported before NAT, only one case has been found in the 4 years after NAT (Figs. 1 and 2).

Results of Look-Back Studies and the Remaining Risk of Viral Infection

While national guidelines for look-back studies had been discussed for years in the Central Panel for Pharmaceutical Affairs without conclusion, look-back was conducted by JRCBS mainly for previous donations from NAT screening positive-converting donors based on ID-NAT results. In the face of enforcement of the laws, triggered by finding a case of HBV transmission from an ID-NAT negative donation, MHLW issued a directive to look back at the previous donations within one year before the donor converted positive in a serological test or a mini-pool NAT for HBV, HCV, HIV and syphilis.

From April 1999 to October 2004, approximately 28 thousand donors turned positive for the above marker(s) and the repository specimens of the previous donations were subjected to ID-NAT.

The result: Among 19,071 previous donations from HBV marker positive-converting donors, 239 donations were found to be screening test negative but ID-NAT positive for HBV (Table 1). Out of 239 HBV ID-NAT positive donations, 90 were

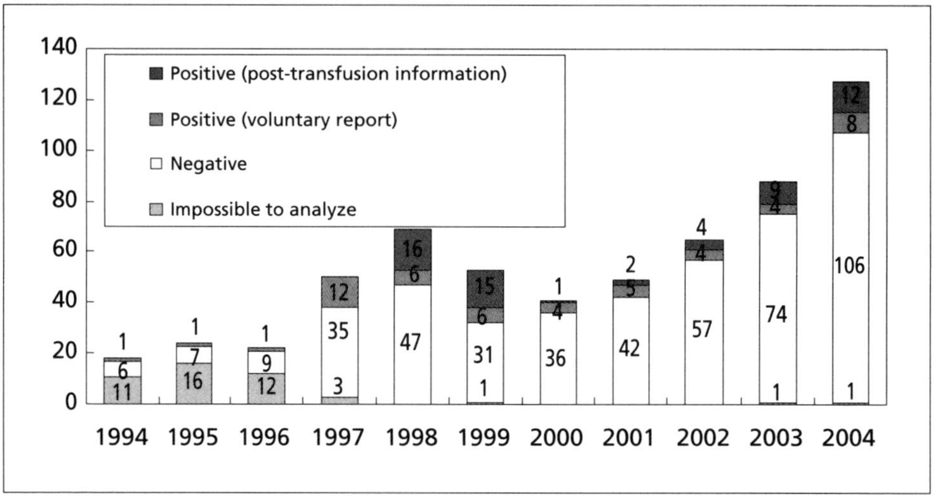

Fig. 1: Reported cases suspected of a transfusion-transmitted HBV infection and the results of individual donation-NAT of the relevant donor specimens.

* The causal relation to transfusion was estimated based on the individual donation-NAT results of the implicated donor repository specimens and the homology of the gene sequence.

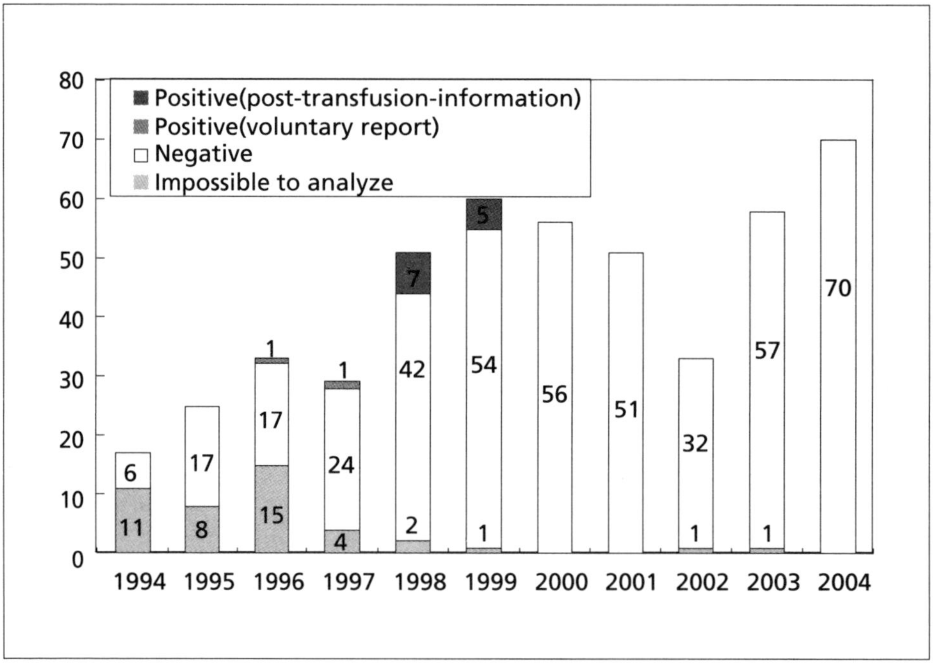

Fig. 2: Reported cases suspected of transfusion-transmitted HCV infection and the results of individual donation-NAT of the relevant donor specimens.

Table 1: The results of look-back study for HBV (April 1999-October 2004).

		Total	**Anti-HBc negative**	**Anti-HBc positive**
Previous donations subjected to ID-NAT			19,071	
ID-NAT	Positive (%)	239[3] (1.25)	90	149
Clinical outcome	(–)→(+)[1]	10	9	1
	NT→(+)[2]	7	3	4
	Unchanged	58		
	Died	93		
	Not tested, unknown	15		

1 The recipient converted positive for a HBV marker(s) after transfusion.

2 Not tested before transfusion, but positive for a HBV marker(s) after transfusion.

3 From the 239 donations, 298 blood components were supplied to medical institutions.

negative for anti-HBc, indicating that the donors were in the window period and 149 were anti-HBc weak positive below the screening test cut off level, indicating that the donors were chronic carriers or in the late phase of infection. Among these ID-NAT positives, 142 donations with ID-NAT positive for HBV were found for 4 years from February 2000 to January 2004 when the 50-sample mini-pool NAT screening was conducted. The projected number of screening negative but HBV ID-NAT positive donations was 36 per year. The information including the ID-NAT result was given to relevant medical institutions. Among the recipients of these components, 183 cases were reported from medical facilities. Among 75 reports, informative for the estimation of the infectivity of these components, 10 patients converted positive after transfusion. Among these 10 patients, 9 were transfused with anti-HBc negative blood and one with anti-HBc weekly positive blood. Seven patients were positive for HBV, with no information available for pre-transfusion samples. Among these 7, 3 received anti-HBc negative blood and 4 anti-HBc weekly positive ones. These results suggest that the infectivity of the HBV window period donations is 28.1 ~ 37.5% (9/32~12/32) and that from carriers or those in the late phase of infection is 2.3 ~ 11.6% (1/43~5/43) [1]. Fifty-eight patients remained negative. Calculating from the annual projected number of ID-NAT only positive donations, the rate of window period donations to donations from a carrier or those in the late phase of HBV infection and the respective infectivity, it was estimated that at least 6 to 10 cases of HBV infection would be found annually by look-back study.

When we add 6 or 7 cases of HBV infection reported annually from medical institutions, it was estimated that annually 42 or 43 donations (1 : 130,000) would be screening test negative but ID-NAT positive for HBV, and 13 to 17 cases (1 : 340,000 to 1 : 450,000) of HBV infection would occur annually.

In the four years with the 50 sample mini-pool NAT, two screening test negative but HIV ID-NAT positive donations were found. One was plasma for plasma derivatives and retrieved during the inventory hold. However, fresh frozen plasma (FFP) from the other transfused to one patient caused HIV infection. The remaining risk of HIV-RNA positive donation is one every two years or 1 : 11,000,000. In this period, one screening negative but HCV ID-NAT positive donation was found. The remaining risk of HCV-RNA positive donation is 1 : 22,000,000. However, no information on the recipient was obtained because the recipient died from the original disease before look-back.

JRC's Planned Safety Measures

Along with the nationwide look-back studies, JRC announced the planned safety measures in July 2003 :

1. Implementation of personal identification of donors at the reception.
2. Preparation of JRC's own guidelines for look back studies.
3. Inventory hold of FFP for 6 months.
4. Further enhancement of NAT screening precision : down-sizing of sample pools from 50 to 20 and evaluation of next generation systems.
5. TTI surveys for all transfused patients in selected medical institutions.
6. Epidemiological study on hepatitis E virus.
7. Implementation of pre-storage leukocytes reduction
8. Evaluation of technology for pathogen-inactivation for blood for transfusion.

Donor identification was implemented in October 2004. JRC's own guidelines for look-back studies were prepared, authorized by MHLW and put into practice in August 2004. FFP has been supplied after the inventory hold for 6 months since July 2005. The pool size of NAT screening was reduced from 50 to 20 in August 2004 and the next generation NAT systems are being evaluated, focusing on the reduction of HBV infection.

Pre-storage leukocytes reduction was implemented for platelet concentrate (PC) in August 2004 and is being prepared to implement for FFP in 2005 and for red cells in 2006.

Other measures are now under way. In addition, the incidence of bacterial contamination of PC is being reevaluated using automated bacterial screening kits, although reported cases of bacterial contamination are very rare (one confirmed case so far) for PC probably due to the short expiration period of 3 days.

An implementation of further safety measures that would cost a huge amount of money and affect the quality of blood needs public understanding and support.

Appropriate Usage and Supply of Blood

Usage and supply of blood, especially of PC, had been increasing mainly due to the introduction of advanced medical technologies and the expansion of a senior population in need of transfusion. Approximately 16 to 18 million units of blood were used annually in about 14 thousand medical institutions in recent years.

MHLW issued guidelines for the appropriate use of blood and those for the practice of transfusion medicine in 1986 and 1989, respectively. The latter recommended that medical institutions establish an internal committee for transfusion medicine to decide on the policies for the appropriate use and proper management of blood. Informed consent for transfusion became mandatory, so that transfusion was covered by the public health insurance in 1997, which forced physicians to learn more about blood and transfusion and raised awareness about the safety and appropriate usage of blood. The indication of FFP usage was restricted to the replacement of coagulation factors in the revised guidelines for an appropriate use of blood in 1999.

Owing to these measures and the two laws, annual supply units decreased. Annual consumption of RC/WB and FFP per 1,000 population was 3.6L and 2.6 L, respectively, and the FFP/(RC + WB) ratio was 0.72 in 2000 [2]. The supply of RCC/WB, PC, and FFP in 2004 was 99 % (5.76 million units, one unit = 200 mL), 98 % (7.82 million units), and 64 % (3.04 million units), respectively, compared to each in 1999 (Fig. 3).

An internal committee for transfusion medicine was established in 94 % of medical institutions, and the appropriate use was discussed in 86 % of those with over 300 beds, but 71 % and 65 %, respectively, of those with less than 300 beds [3].

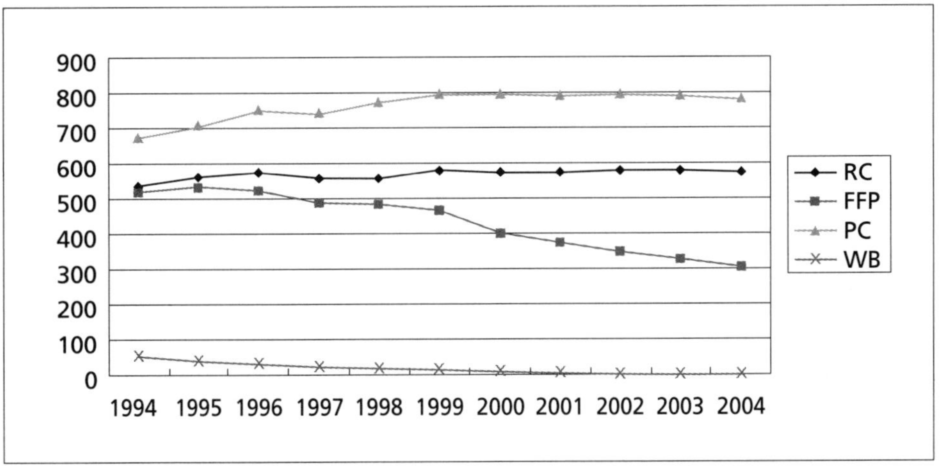

Fig. 3: Annual supply of blood. Annual supplied units (x 10^4) are indicated. One unit is 200 mL.

The Expansion of The Donor Pool and Appropriate Usage to Secure Stable Supply of Safe Blood

In spite of the current decreasing trend of the blood supply, expansion of the donor pool is essential in order to secure a stable supply of safe blood.

More stringent selection of eligible healthy donors is required to enhance the safety of blood. The rate of donors deferred by the donor interview is increasing yearly, from 7.6 in 1996 to 8.7 in 2003. It was anticipated that 3.6 % of potential donors would be lost by the introduction of policy to prevent transfusion-transmitted vCJD by deferring donors who stayed in England for more than one day in spring 2005, though the shortage of blood is avoided by the cooperation in the donor recruitment campaign among JRCBS, government, local authorities and media.

On the other hand, Japan is rushing into a highly aging society that will need more transfusion. The number and rate of young donors below 30 years of age are decreasing. An expansion of the donor pool, especially among young generations, is indispensable.

Public understanding and close collaboration among stakeholders are necessary to achieve what the New Blood Law asks.

References

1 Satake M, Taira R, Yugi H, Tadokoro K: Lookback study for transfusion-related HBV infection in Japan, Tansfusion 2005; 45: suppl abstract S25.

2 Takano M: Report on the average consumption of blood products in Japan, MHLW Special Research Program, 2004.

3 Takahashi K: Report the establishment of transfusion management system controlling safety management and appropriate use in concert with the New Blood law. Research Program on Regulatory Science for Medicine and Medical Devices. 2005.

Dr. K. Tadokoro, Blood Service Headquarters, Japanese Red Cross, 1-3, Shibadaimon 1-chome, Minato-ku, Tokyo, 105-8521 Japan.
E-mail: k-tadokoro@bs.jrc.or.jp

Dax EM, Farrugia A, Vyas G (eds): Advances in Transfusion Safety – Volume IV.
Dev Biol (Basel). Basel, Karger, 2007, vol 127, pp 169-173.

Domestic and Imported Products – The Malaysian Experience in Assuring Safe and Sufficient Plasma Products

Y. Ayob

National Blood Centre, Kuala Lumpur, Malaysia

Introduction

A country's socioeconomic status is often a determinant of the level of available healthcare services, which can be clearly reflected in the development of blood transfusion services and the standard of care accorded to patients requiring blood and blood products. In many developing countries, public health issues such as sanitation, infectious diseases, family planning and the management of acute conditions often take priority over care for lifelong diseases and/or rare diseases like congenital bleeding disorders. In developed countries where the standards of healthcare are high, blood and blood products are safer and more readily available, while patients in developing countries have little or no access to these products or to proper care. An analysis of FVIII consumption relative to economic status demonstrates this point [1]. The use of recombinant products in the treatment of haemophilia in the developed world has further widened the gap between the two types of economies.

Currently, the safety of plasma derived products depends on the reduction of viral load in the source plasma and the inactivation or elimination of infectious agents that may escape employed screening tests. In order to reduce viral load in the source plasma, other strategies are adopted such as donor selection, appropriate screening tests and inventory hold of donated units before processing.

Managing Blood and Blood Products in Malaysia

Malaysia, a developing country of 25 million people, has a well coordinated blood transfusion service that is funded by the government's Ministry of Health Strategies to ensure safe blood supply, with emphases on safe donors, quality management systems and appropriate use of blood. Currently, the service is undergoing a process of reorganization with consolidation of services such as processing and testing in order to further improve efficiency and quality of service and products. A policy of self sufficiency that has been adopted since the early 1980s has helped to increase blood collection (Fig. 1). At a rate of 20 per 1000 population self sufficiency in fresh blood components would be attained. However, the demand for factor concentrate cannot be met by the national blood program, and as a result, commercial blood products have to be imported. The supply is supplemented by a contract fractionation program providing factor concentrates, albumin and intravenous immunoglobulin.

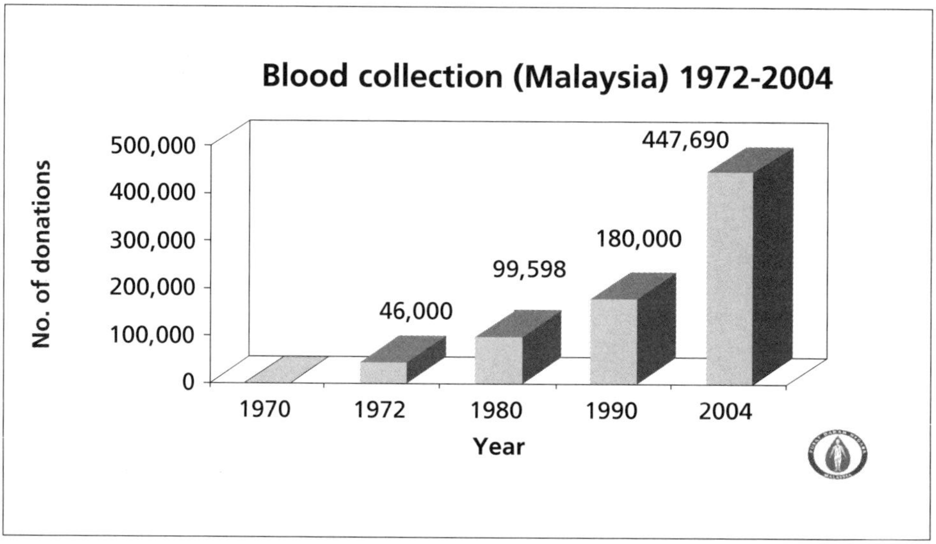

Fig. 1: A 10 fold increase in collection over 3 decades.

Contract Fractionation

With the advocacy of blood component therapy came an excess of available plasma. After the emergence of HIV/AIDS, Malaysia's Ministry of Health allocated a relatively large budget toward an HIV/AIDS prevention program. Through this program, all haemophiliacs were treated with commercial factor concentrate instead of cryoprecipitate or fresh frozen plasma, further adding to a plasma surplus.

Plasma that was not transfused was then sent off for contract fractionation, a program that began in 1990. The first products were received in 1991. Over the last 15 years, the amount of plasma sent for fractionation has progressively increased (Fig. 2). Manufactured products include factor VIII and IX concentrates, intravenous immunoglobulin and albumin. Yields have also improved (Fig. 3) so that by 2003, the Ministry of Health no longer needed to purchase any immunoglobulin for intravenous use. The amount of factor IX concentrate has reached 95 % to 100 % of requirements. However, the demand for factor VIII could not be met by the fractionation program even 15 years after its institution because the number of haemophiliacs has steadily increased over these years (Fig. 4) with the expansion and improvement in diagnostic services as well as access to comprehensive care.

Furthermore, because plasma from many centres has yet to be inspected by the fractionator to evaluate whether they (as the sources of plasma) meet the standard set by the regulators of the country where the fractionation plant is situated, all excess plasma can be sent for contract fractionation.

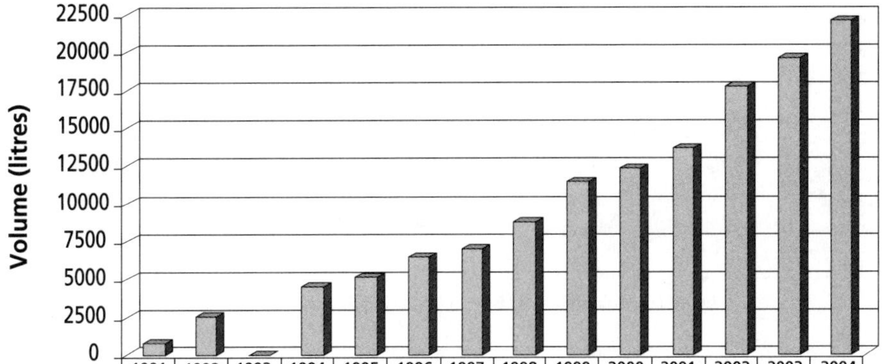

	1991	1992	1993	1994	1995	1996	1997	1998	1999	2000	2001	2002	2003	2004
Volume	840	2553	0	4556	5121	6474	7030	8751	11443	12350	13700	17768	19625	22091

Year

Fig. 2: Plasma volume of contract fractionation (1991-2004) – Malaysia.

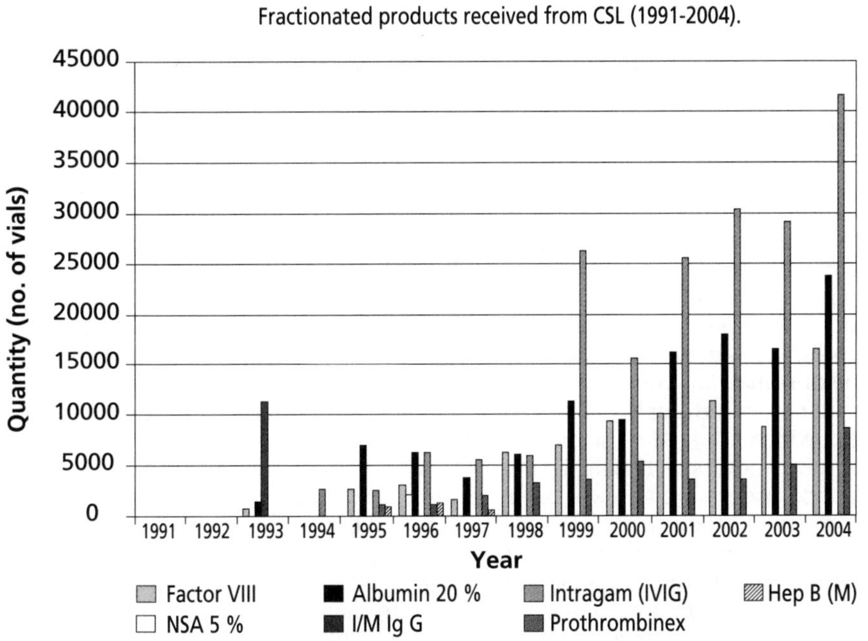

Fig. 3: Products obtained from contract fractionation (1991-2004) – Malaysia.

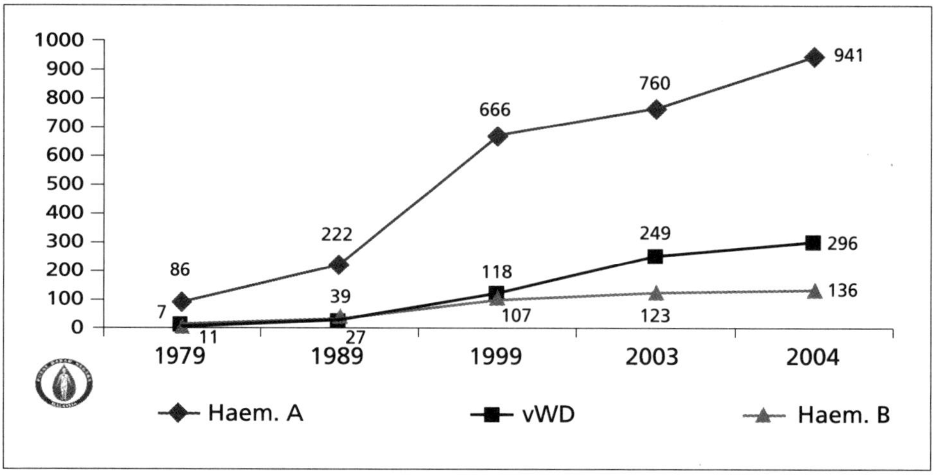

Fig. 4: Haemophilia A & B, von Willebrands disease in Malaysia.

Commercial Plasma Derived Products

To help haemophiliacs achieve their full potential and to prevent transfusion transmitted infection, the Malaysian government continues to fund the purchase of commercial factor VIII and factor IX concentrate from two sources. One product is acquired through bulk purchase by central tender, while the other is through a pharmaceutical company that has been chosen by the government through a process of privatization of its pharmaceutical services. The National Haemophilia Centre determines the specification of these products and evaluates them before purchase, which maintains the quality of the products throughout the country and keeps the cost down.

The importation of plasma products is regulated by the Drug Control Authority (DCA). In recent years the DCA has become more aware of the importance of safety of the source plasma. Currently all plasma derived products have to be registered by the DCA before they can be imported. Apart from documentation, the registration requires the submission of the Plasma Master File, which includes the details of the plasma origin including selection criteria for donors, epidemiology data for viral makers and emphases on safety and quality of blood bags, storage and their conformity with established international quality standards. This has prevented the registration of somewhat dubious products, a problem in the past, when the responsibility to ensure safe and quality factor concentrate rested solely on the National Blood Centre, which is also the Haemophilia Referral Centre. A situation in which the end-users were more strict than the regulators had created an awkward environment where end-users were accused of favouring certain manufacturers.

The 3 tier system, where 3 products are used to treat haemophiliacs, i.e. product from contract fractionation and 2 commercial products, has ensured sustainability of supply. Fluctuation of global production due to temporary closure of fractionation plants and reversion to plasma derived products when the supply of recombinant factor was interrupted were managed better than if dependency on one product was adopted.

Currently, factor concentrate consumption is approximately 16,000 international units (IU) of factor per patient. This is still below the required minimum level of 20,000 IU [2]. None of the suppliers of recombinant factor VIII concentrate are seeking registration. Eighty eight percent of the world supply of recombinant products goes to Europe and America. Even if factor concentrate is registered in Malaysia, the cost may still be prohibitive. However, recombinant factor VIIa is registered and available for use, though also limited by cost. The supply is limited to haemophiliacs with inhibitors. Special permission is required for use in other situations.

Conclusion

Developing countries are faced with limited resources in ensuring that safe, quality plasma products are in adequate supply. With inadequate blood transfusion services, the management of transfusion-dependent patients is often compromised. Where some resources are available, patients may be able to be managed using commercial products. However, there is often no regulation for registration and importation of these products. As a result, products that cannot be registered in developed countries end up in developing countries, a problem whose magnitude is unknown. Only anecdotal reports are exposed in the mass media, and often, the number of patients affected is not reported nor what happens to those involved. Malaysia is somewhat lucky because the government has made blood safety a priority of the Ministry of Health and is committed to national healthcare.

References

1 Stonebraker JS, Amand RE, Nagle J: A country-by-country comparison of FVIII concentrate consumption and economic capacity for the global haemophilia community. Haemophilia 2004; 9: 245-250.

2 Beal RW: Transfusion science and practice in developing countries: 'a high frequency of empty shelves'. Transfusion 1993; 33: 276-278.

3 Robert P: Access to Therapy: Data. Presented to the Plasma Forum of the Plasma Protein Therapeutics Association, Washington, June 2003.

Dr. Y. Ayob, National Blood Centre, Jalan Tun Razak, 50400 Kuala Lumpur, Malaysia.
E-mail: yasminpd@tm.net.my

Dax EM, Farrugia A, Vyas G (eds): Advances in Transfusion Safety – Volume IV.
Dev Biol (Basel). Basel, Karger, 2007, vol 127, pp 175-181.

Blood Safety – A Focus on Plasma Derivatives in Mainland China

Y.M. Zhu

Shanghai Blood Center, Shanghai, China

Key words: Plasma derivatives, safety, apheresis, quality assurance.

Abstract: Plasma derivative production in Mainland China can be encapsulated by two figures: 50 years of history and 5000 tons of annually processed source plasma. Demands for albumin, immunoglobulinin and main clotting factors can barely be met, despite a relatively low average usage among China's population of 1.3 billion. The tragedy of contamination among plasma donors in Henan province in the early 1990's has left shadows on the safety of the plasma derivative industry. However, during the last ten years the Chinese government has made great strides forward. The regulation of the entire operation has been strengthened, from law and standard setting and upholding to stricter licensing regulations for plasma centers and fractionators. Public concerns in blood safety are gradually being relieved, and confidence is returning. Nevertheless, the plasma donors and hemophilia patients infected a decade ago by infected blood or plasma products represent a set of severe social and medical problems that the government and society must still deal with.

History Retrospect

Plasma derivative production in mainland China began in the late 1950's. Freeze-dried plasma and fresh frozen plasma were used when products were not available. All six state-owned biological institutes and many blood centers began plasma protein production as the demand increased for these newly developed and marketed products. The production techniques were relatively simple (chemical or salt precipitation, for example), and the number of producers reached 60 in the 1980's.

Plasma fractionation was supervised entirely by the Ministry of Health (MOH) before the establishment of the State Drug Administration (SDA) in 1998. It was renamed the State Food and Drug Administration (SFDA) in 2003. In the late 1980's the MOH ordered that lab-scale production using traditional production methods stop, allowing only modified Cohn's Method (or Low-Temperature Alcohol Precipitation) based production be used. The number of producers subsequently diminished: only 17 were certified by the MOH as of 1995. When the SDA took over the administrative responsibility in 1998, it required that all fractionation facilities be inspected and licensed against cGMP standards. Thirty-three GMP licenses were issued to different fractionators by the end of 2004.

Despite the fact that the whole blood collected in blood centers is separated into components and that nationwide component transfusion is over 50 %, fresh frozen plasma is still widely used in hospitals today. This leaves very little plasma for fractionation. The vast majority of source plasma for production is collected in plasma centers using the apheresis method. The ever-increasing demands for plasma products have led to the evolution of a large number of fractionators and, consequently, a larger number of plasma collection centers. There were over 400 plasma centers in early 1990. The supervision and discipline of the centers was not strictly applied in some areas. The price for this mistake was very high. Because red cells from different donors of the same blood group were mixed and reinfused during manual apheresis procedures, a single window-phase HIV or other infectious diseases carrier could infect the entire group of apheresis donors [1-5]. In December 1996 the State Council issued a strict Executive Order (#208) to adopt automation for plasma apheresis in all plasma centers. Since January 1998, manual apheresis has been completely prohibited.

A series of other orders and regulations have been issued by health authorities. Plasma centers failing to obey these regulations have been closed. By 2004 the number of plasma centers again diminished to 153. A plasma fractionator may now receive source plasma from several designated plasma centers. At the same time, a plasma center can only admit donors from within the geographic boundary of its county and supply plasma to one fractionator defined by the MOH [6,7]. The MOH also requires that a plasma center shall have at least 10 auto-apheresis devices and a minimal annual collection of 10,000 liters of plasma. The MOH has published Standard Operating Procedure sample (SOP) as a guideline for plasma centers. Many of the current requirements for source plasma are adapted from, or similar to, those used in the developed world. They cover all aspects including accreditation and licensing, donor recruitment and management, and quality assurance control and documentation, etc.

As revealed officially by the MOH, by the end of 2004, confirmed HIV positive cases numbered 106,900 in Mainland China, and 23,955 had already developed AIDS. The total number of living HIV positive cases is estimated at 840,000, so that confirmed cases account for 12.7 % of the total number. This rate was only 7.4 % in 2003 [8]. Researchers have shown that, similar to other areas, drug abuse and sexual contact are the main routes of transmission. However, there still remains the unique and horribly effective path of transfusion transmission. Contamination between plasma donors in some plasma centers in Henan province in the early 1990's was the main route of transmission in that province. Unqualified personnel and poor management and supervision were claimed as the main causes. One unconfirmed research report estimated that the HIV positive rate among paid plasma donors in Henan is 9-44 %, with a total number of 1.2 million [9]. A more reliable finding was announced by the local authority on September 10, 2004 [10]. A door to door investigation that lasted for two months reported that there were 280,476 inhabitants who had made at least one paid plasma donation in the 1990's. Of those surveyed, 260,025 were tested for HIV antibody, the rest of whom were out of town when the survey was being conducted. Those who tested HIV antibody positive numbered 25,036, at a rate of 9.6 %. In the same survey, 11,815 were confirmed to have developed AIDS, including 2000 patients newly found in this survey. The HIV positive rate in the Henan population was estimated at 0.035 %. While the contamination between plasma donors is now under control, handling the consequences of this accident remains a major challenge.

CURRENT SITUATION

As of 2004, 33 fractionators were licensed by the FDA, and about 24 were in production. It is estimated that 5,000,000 liters of source plasma were processed in 2004, all using the Cohn method. The average turnover is 210 tons per facility, ranging from 70 to over 500 tons. Final products are sold directly to hospitals and pharmacies, or via exclusive distributors. Approximately 150 tons of albumin is used for the whole country: 90 % from local providers, and the rest is imported. Since the mid 1990's, the Chinese drug authority has banned import of plasma products, with albumin being the only exception.

16 plasma products are listed in the new edition of Chinese Pharmacopoeia 2005 (Table 1). Albumin prepared from Human Placenta has been removed from the list. Other products, such as FiberSelanat and Antithrombin-III, are produced in some companies, but the demands are rather limited.

Table 1: Plasma products listed in Chinese Pharmacopoeia 2005.

Categories	Plasma products
Albumin	Albumin Albumin, freeze-dried
Immunoglobulin	Immunoglobulin Immunoglobulin, IV Immunoglobulin, freezed-dried Immunoglobulin (pH4), IV Immunoglobulin (pH4), IV, freeze-dried
Specific immunoglobulin	Hepatitis B immunoglobulin Hepatitis B immunoglobulin, freeze-dried Rabies immunoglobulin Rabies immunoglobulin, freeze-dried Tetanus immunoglobulin Tetanus immunoglobulin, freeze-dried
Clotting factors	Coagulation factor VIII Fibrinogen Prothrombin complex

Under the State Council are the direct government agents that set up policies for source plasma and plasma derivatives. The division of Blood Product Management in the MOH closely regulates source plasma collection. Its responsibilities include establishing standards of operation and SOPs for plasma centers issuing permits for establishing a plasma center within designated provinces, organizing annual and random nation-wide audits of compliance of plasma centers evaluating the applications from fractionators for source plasma and allocating the approved amount to designated plasma centers. They also maintain a database for actual usage of source plasma. In cooperation with the MOH, the provincial health department (PHD) and local county health bureau (CHB) regulate the plasma centers in their regions. Their responsibilities include but are not limited to licensing and local auditing. SFDA, on the other hand, focuses on regulating fractionators, product distribution and pharmacovigilance. The guideline issued by SFDA is Good Manufacture Practices (GMP), and SFDA requires each of the fractionators to comply with GMP. SFDA has an annual and random auditing system and only issues drug production permits to those fractionators who comply absolutely with current GMP. A division of SFDA, National Institute for Control of Pharmaceutical and Biological Products (NICPBP) is the exclusive executing agent for GMP validation and for all required tests for plasma derivatives. SFDA requires that all batches of albumin from all companies be tested by NICPBP and the quality documented in SFDA before marketing is permitted. The Chinese Society of Blood Transfusion (CSBT) and its Biological Product Committee advise MOH and SFDA in setting national standards.

Safety and Quality Assurance

There are five layers of legislation and regulation bodies: the National People's Congress (NPC), the State Council (SC) or Provincial People's Congress (PPC), the MOH/SFDA or Provincial Government, National Standard Committees (NSC) and the local health authorities. All have issued laws or statues regulating plasma derivative production (Table 2).

Plasma centers are authorized for collecting source plasma but cannot collect whole blood or components for transfusion. One plasma center can only supply plasma to one fractionatior according to its geographic designation, which is controlled by the MOH. The MOH has defined a series of procedures and papers to ensure plasma centers meet all requirements (Table 3).

Table 2: Some laws, statutes, regulations and standards issued by Chinese government for the safety and quality of plasma products.
Abbreviations are defined in the text.

Category of legislation	Legislator	Examples
Laws	NPC	Blood Donation Law (Oct. 1998)
	NPC	Drug Administration Law (Dec. 2001)
	NPC	Infectious Disease Prevention Law (Dec. 2004)
Statutes	SC	Blood Derivatives (Dec.1996)
	SC	AIDS Prevention Plan (2001-2005)
Regulations	MOH	Blood Transfusion Services (Oct. 1998)
	MOH	Operational Techniques Standards for BTS's (Oct. 1998)
	SFDA	Batch Release of Biological Products (Jan. 2003)
Standards	NSC	Operational Standards for Blood Collection and Distribution
	NSC	Criteria of Plasma Apheresis Stations
Administration measures	MOH	Clinical Transfusion of Blood Measures

Table 3: Some documents required for plasma centers to ensure that plasma centers meet all legal requirements.

Type of document	by	Renewal	Audit
SOP	MOH	Progressive	/
Registration	PHD	Annual	Annual
Permit	CHB	Annual	Annual

Donor recruiting and management is the core business of a plasma center and, therefore, will occupy a major portion of this short review. There is a detailed document issued by MOH for reference [11]. However, a brief outline of the key elements will highlight the beauty of Chinese source plasma. The MOH classifies a geographic district of a county as a plasmapheresis region where only one plasma center can be set up. Tables 4 and 5 list the requirements for identifications and medical conditions for a qualified donor. Laboratory tests that are required are listed in Table 6.

Table 4: Identification and history review that must be met for a donor to qualify to donate plasma.

Item	Approved by
Local residency	Identification card issued by government
Physical examination	Authorized medical doctor's signature
Neg. for all required tests	Formal and authorized test reports
Donor register card	Plasma centers
Donor donation certificate	Plasma centers
Donor's files and records	Plasma centers
Medical history and records	Local hospitals

Table 5: Critical medical criteria that must be met if a donor is to qualify.

Age	M: 18-55, F: 18-50	
Body weight	M: > 50 kg, F > 45 kg	
Blood pressure	M: 12-20 kPa, F: 8-12 kPa	
Pulse	60-100 beats/min.	
Body temperature	Normal	
Skin	No tattoo or body piercing	
Chest X-ray	Normal	Checked annually
Sexual behavior	Not homosexual	
Surgeon scum	Case depending	Temporary or permanent deferral
Growth factor users	Permanent rejection	

Table 6: Laboratory test results are required to meet the criteria given for plasma donors.

Hemoglobin	**M ≥ 125g/L, F ≥ 115g/L**	
Serum protein	≥ 60g/L	Method depending
Blood types	A, B, O	1st time donor only
ALT	< 40u (Kinetic) < 25u (Reitmaim)	
Serum protein	Albumin ≥ 50 %	Annually
HBs Ag	Neg. (sen. ≤ 1ng/ml)	ELISA
Syphilis	Neg.	(RPR_TRUST_ELISA)
HIV-1/HIV-2 Ab	Neg.	ELISA
HCV Ab	Neg.	ELISA

All required laboratory tests are performed twice. Plasma is screened at plasma centers, and the reactive units are destroyed under the supervision of local CDC. Plasma units passing initial tests are shipped to fractionators and screened again in their laboratories using kits from different manufacturers. All screening kits are batch tested and released by the NICPBP before being put on the market. The possibility of NAT testing has been widely discussed and studied. Some of the fractionators have been performing NAT testing voluntarily. Normal holding periods practiced by most fractionators are now 60 days. SFDA requires that at least one step of viral inactivation is employed in the production process for any product. Since 2005, two steps of virus inactivation are required by Chinese Pharmacopoeia 2005.

Future Prospects

The Chinese plasma industry faces a number of challenges, which are generally similar to those topics of all of fractionators in the rest of the world. They include potential risks of emerging diseases, more sensitive screening methods, balance between supply and demand, recombinant products and substitutes. On the other hand, the Chinese concerns deserve reiteration.

- Plasma: The ever expanding market-demand for greater amounts of plasma and more kinds of product is evident in China. The young prefer to find new life in big towns and cities, leaving elders in villages where plasma centers are usually located. Thus, donor size is shrinking and aging.
- Fractionators: There are too many independent fractionators, leading to smaller scales of operation. thus weakening the capabilities of developing new products and adapting new standards. Some small companies are only able to produce albumin as their sole product and market it at a low price.
- Technology: The government has planned to introduce NAT testing and two steps of viral inactivation into plasma derivative production. It will still take some time to implement these initiatives.

- Legislation and standards: As mentioned above, some of the standards and regulations were formulated some years ago and no longer reflect new developments and needs.
- Pharmvigiliance: The nationally coordinated surveillance system on bioproducts and plasma products is being constructed by SFDA. Unqualified product call-back and early stage alarming are gradually being adopted.

The Chinese government has reiterated its commitment and taken on the entire responsibility for blood programs and the plasma industry to ensure adequate supply of the safest possible blood and plasma products to patients. The short supply of source plasma, decision to adapt new standards and new techniques, regular revision of laws and development of regulations and standards are all being considered and will contribute to an increasing safety of supply of plasma derivatives.

References

1 Hua Shan, et al: Blood banking in China. Lancet 2002; 360: 1770-1775.

2 Pomfret J: The high cost of selling blood as AIDS crisis looms in China. Foreign Service Section of Washington Post, Jan. 11, 2001.

3 HIV infection during selling blood in northwest. Oriental Daily (China), April 4, 2002.

4 HIV infection from plasma at Shanxi Province. Beijing Time, Oct. 16, 2001.

5 HIV infection-costs for selling plasma. West Commerce News, 2002.

6 MOH Instruction, Planning for source plasma, 40th File, 2002.

7 MOH Instruction, Notice for SOP for source plasma. 12th File, 2001.

8 MOH News Release, March 18, 2005.

9 Bates Gill and Jennifer Chang, HIV Crisis in China, Foreign Affairs, March/April, 2004.

10 MOH newspaper Jiangkang, September 13, 2004.

11 MOH documents, brochures for national training for source plasma centers. Chengdu, April, 2001.

Prof. Y.M. ZHU, Shanghai Blood Center, #1191 Hong Qiao Rd., Shanghai 200051, China.
E-mail: ymzhu@sbc.org.cn

Dax EM, Farrugia A, Vyas G (eds): Advances in Transfusion Safety – Volume IV.
Dev Biol (Basel). Basel, Karger, 2007, vol 127, pp 183-195.

Advances in Quality Assurance of Laboratory Testing for Transfusion Safety

E.M. Dax, S. Walker

National Serology Reference Laboratory, Australia and Australian Red Cross Blood Service Laboratories

Key words: Blood-borne virus tests, quality assurance programmes, accuracy, minimising wastage, regulation.

INTRODUCTION

Requirements for quality assurance of testing for blood-borne viruses and other laboratory processes are part of most international standards for the quality and safety of transfusions. Under the Code of Good Manufacturing Practice (cGMP) and other regulations or guidelines, all steps of transfusion processes are expected to be quality assured. For the laboratory processes employed to screen for possible infectivity of blood, the quality assurance requirements are sometimes defined more thoroughly. The Council of Europe Guidelines [1] has a complete section on laboratory testing and its quality assurance. The importance of quality assurance for the screening of donations for infectious markers is emphasized, and both general and specific approaches are suggested in these guidelines. The cGMP in Australia, Section 837, also requires that testing conducted for screening should be quality assured [2].

With the widening adoption of "zero-risk" policies for blood transfusion services, the laboratory components of blood safety have received a great deal of attention. The Precautionary Principle demands that testing for blood-borne pathogens is as complete as possible and that the testing is carried out without error. In the words of Resnik, "According to a version of the principle defended here, one should take reasonable measures to avoid threats that are serious and plausible" [3]. The reasonableness of a response to a threat depends on several factors, including benefit verses harm, realism, proportionality, and consistency. Screening of blood has become extensive and complex with the inclusion of nucleic acid test screening and tests or technologies to screen out emerging infections (e.g. West Nile fever or prion disease). The requirements for the quality of tests that identify donors who are virus/infection free have increased to previously unprecedented levels. At the same time, transfusion laboratories require that quality assurance ensuring that their performances are of the highest standard is in place. Quality assurance measures are those that check that the quality of tests and the testing process is adequate or meets targets. If tests are of poor or variable quality or they are not used properly, the performance cannot be adequate, no matter how rigorous quality and its assurance are.

Results of quality assurance measures ensure that tests and testing are operating to the standards required. As the sophistication of tests and testing has increased so has the demand for improved and more extensive quality assurance measures. However, the extensive resources needed to meet the requirements give rise to serious questions concerning quality programme advancement such as, "How much quality assurance is appropriate?", "Who should perform quality assurance?", "How can the effectiveness of quality assurance programmes be assessed?", "Which methods should be used?" and "Can quality assurance methods be improved upon?" In Australia the quality assurance for tests used in blood transfusion services is administered and supplied by the National Serology Reference Laboratory, Australia (NRL). Advances in quality programmes over the last few years have attempted to provide responses to these questions.

In developed countries all donations are screened for transfusion transmitted infections including HIV, hepatitis B and C, often HTLV and usually Syphilis. Other infections may be screened for in particular areas as reported in other Chapters of these Proceedings. In many developed countries screening for transfusion transmitted infections is accomplished by serological testing along with nucleic testing to guard against the possibility of missing a donation made during the serological window period. Quality assurance programmes need to accommodate methods and exercises for these advancements.

In Australia, core funding for the NRL comes from the Australian Government. Its international programmes are supported by the World Health Organisation, Centers for Disease Control and Prevention, Global AIDS Program and the Australian Agency for International Development (AusAID). The NRL is an independent body working under contract to the Australian Government, specifically on contract to the regulator, the Therapeutic Goods Administration. The system for assuring the quality of transfusion transmitted infection testing in Australia is depicted in Figure 1.

The importance of high sensitivity, high specificity performances with minimal batch-to-batch variation in screening tests has been recognised by transfusion services worldwide [4]. The demand for tests with these characteristics has been unprecedented over recent years. If tests perform poorly, false results will occur. False negative results obviously have disastrous consequences for transfusion services [5]. False positive results mean that donations are wasted, but also that donors have to be deferred and thus, the pool of donors may be depleted. If tests are not used appropriately there is also risk of incorrect results occurring. Laboratory tests from reputable manufacturers perform well, unless those using them are poorly trained or equipment is not operating properly. Better quality tests are identified through evaluation and performance monitoring, which is enforced through regulation. If poor quality tests are rejected in developed countries through regulatory processes, they sometimes appear in countries where regulatory systems do not exist or are weak. This means that testing in the blood services may be inferior, despite the best efforts of the staff of these transfusion services where only poor quality kits are made available or where kits are constantly changing.

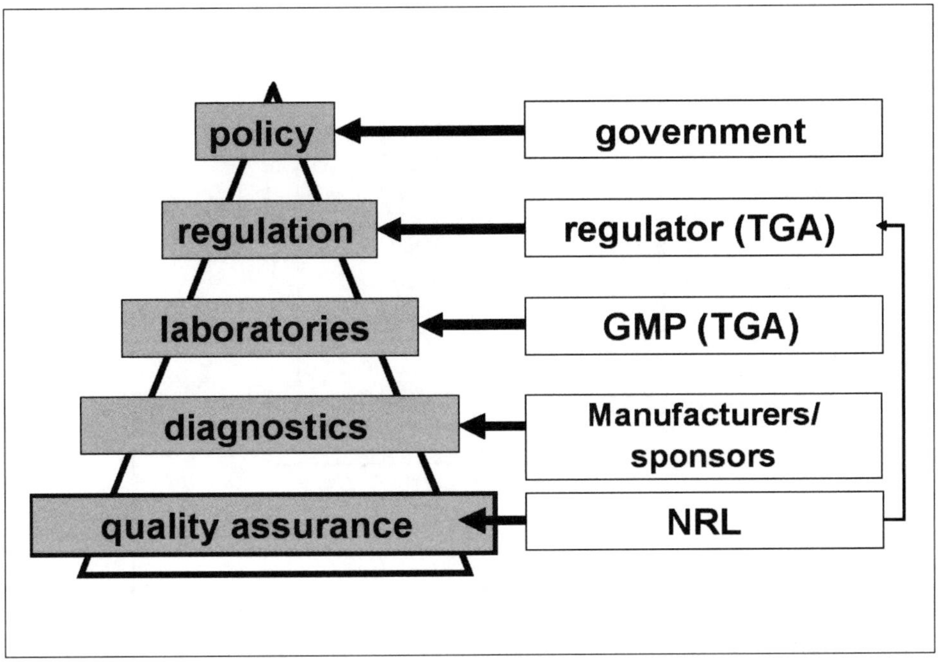

Fig. 1: The system for assuring the quality of testing for transfusion transmitted infections in Australia. TGA = Therapeutic Goods Administration, GMP = Good Manufacturing Process, NRL = National Serology Reference Laboratory, Australia which is the independent quality assuror for quality of tests used to screen for blood-borne virus. The government sets policy on transfusion safety which is carried out by the TGA. TGA regulates the quality and safety of kits as well as the quality and safety of the blood supply. It is responsible for audit of GMP in the services. NRL provides the checks and balance through its quality assurance programme and reports irregularities of significance to TGA.

Quality assurance is the overall mechanism that employs a set of methods to provide the checks and balances to assure the quality of tests and testing [6]. Often, suppliers of quality assurance offer only one of the various methods that are available. Further, the demands on quality assurors have increased as the complexity of blood screening has increased and the requirements for quality have accelerated. Advances in quality assurance include the ways that quality assurance is provided, the ability of the assurors to report on results quickly and the variety or combinations of methods available.

The Testing Process

No matter which test is being used to screen blood donations, the actual process involved in the testing is highly uniform [7]. Although the individual steps within the process may differ, the process remains as that depicted in Figure 2. All critical steps of the process must be quality assured. The most likely steps to yield false results if they are not followed, are the very ones that are most appropriately quality controlled. This means that well-constructed quality assurance schemes or programmes should be applied to all testing processes in all blood services.

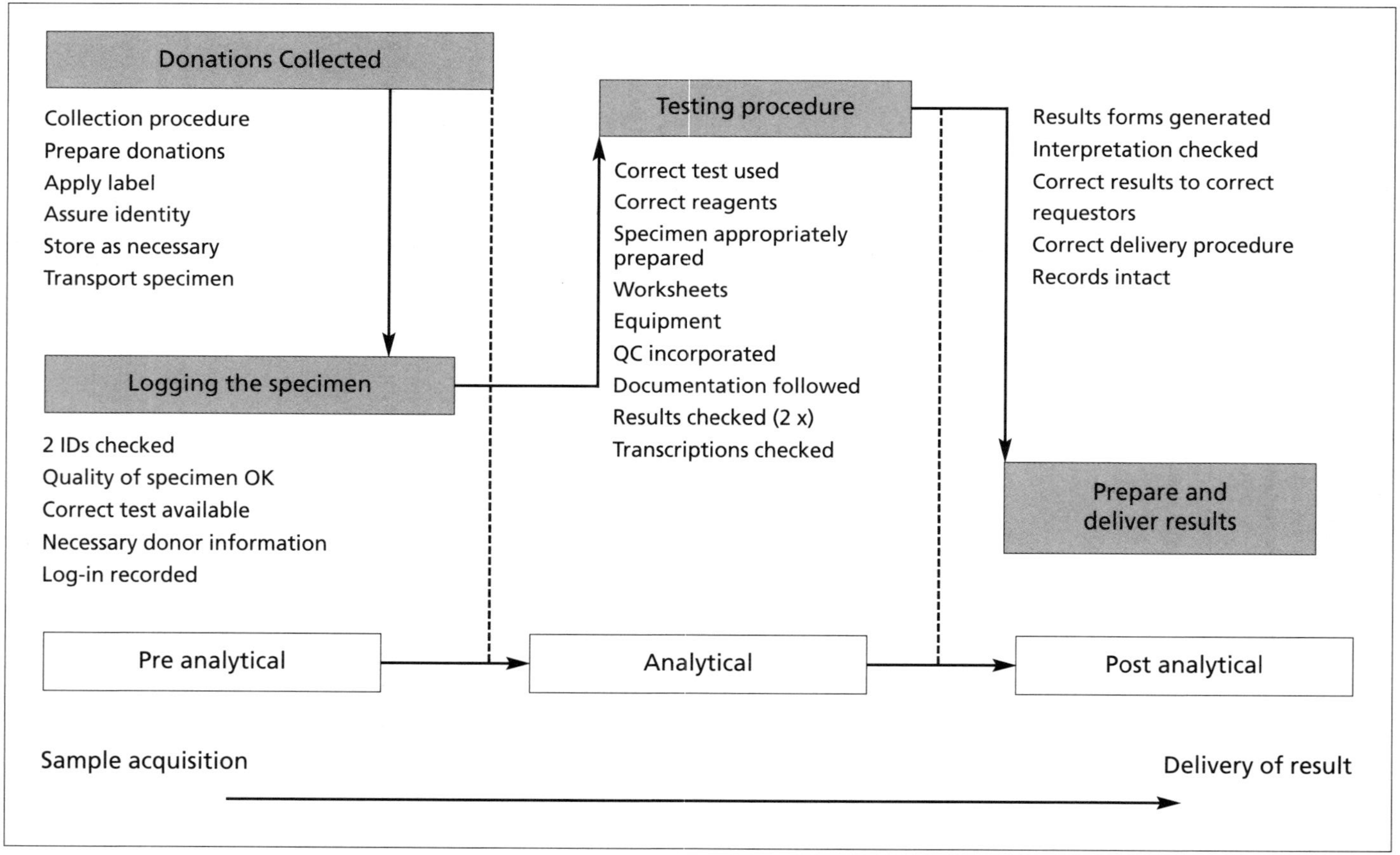

Fig. 2: The testing process is similar for testing all donations, no matter which test is used. Analysis of the process reveals the points at which quality assurance measures should be implemented i.e. where failures in the integrity of the process might occur. Some measure are quantitative such as monitoring quality controls in a statistical process control, while others are qualitative and are measures for checking that steps in the process have been carried out properly.

QUALITY ASSURANCE OF THE LABORATORY TESTING PROCESS

Laboratory-based personnel should all be trained to check every step of the processes in which they participate if quality goals are to be met. For example, in the testing process there should be procedures that check that sample is added to the testing well, procedures that assure that anything recorded manually is correct by having it checked by another person, a procedure that assures that the right result is ascribed to a particular sample, etc [7].

Quality assurance of testing processes is best carried out independently of the groups actually performing the testing. This does not exclude the laboratory's need for having a quality management system in place and assuring that the whole process is operating to the standards expected and with checks and balances in place. The external checks assure that the service is not its own "judge and jury". The quality services for the Australian Red Cross Blood Service laboratories include evaluation of test kits before they are registered for marketing, external quality assessment programmes to access periodically their entire testing processes, a quality control programme to monitor precision and accuracy and programmes that monitor the false reactor rates (specificity). These quality measures are independently administered. They are an adjunct to the laboratories' own quality management systems which supply quality measures such as internal audit, validation and routine examination of statistical process control etc. In more recent years, significant advancements in monitoring specificity and in conducting the NRL's quality control procedures have been made by quality assuring laboratories using an internet-based data collection and analysis system, designed and implemented by the NRL, called EDCNet.

Definitions of terminology for the quality assurance measures supplied by the NRL to the ARCBS are as follows:

- **Evaluation** is the full assessment of test kits' performances to ensure that the claimed manufacturing characteristics of the tests are met in national or other particular environments. Evaluation findings are only valid at the time of the evaluation and not for kits produced subsequently unless the performance is followed and assured with continuity.
- **Validation** is the assessment of a performance or claim of performance ensuring that the claim operates in a local (or laboratory) environment. Thus, a laboratory validation of a test kit should ensure that the test kit's performance is met in that particular laboratory.
- **Quality Assurance** is the overall assessment of a process that operates to provide the checks and balances that ensure that the process is operating as expected, and within statistical confines if the measure is quantitative.
- **Quality Assessment** is the procedure of checking that a process is operating to deliver the expected outcome. For laboratory quality assessment schemes (internal or external), panels or groups of samples akin to those tested in a laboratory are distributed periodically and the results are sent to the distributor for assessment and comparison with the results of like laboratories. This procedure assesses that a laboratory can deliver the correct results at a particular time. Because External Quality Assessment Schemes are administered intermittently, they cannot be an assessment mechanism for ongoing accuracy of kit performances, although poor kit performances may be detected.

- **Quality Control** is the procedure of determining the precision of a procedure by assessing whether the same result is achieved in a standard measure or index each time the procedure being controlled is performed. For quality controlling a test, a standard sample is assayed in each test run and the results are followed on a statistically managed chart to assure that the results are precise. If these results are compared with those of other laboratories using the same assay and same quality control sample, the accuracy can also be assessed by assuring that all laboratories are "hitting the same target value" [8].
- **Specificity Monitoring** is following the non-specific reactor rate (rate of false reactivity) over time as a measure of batch performance and/or indicator of test quality.

Assessment through Quality Assurance Procedures

Evaluation and monitoring

It is clear that quality procedures can assist in assuring the quality and improvement of laboratory procedures. Evaluations of test kits can prevent a test that does not meet transfusion service requirements from being used. Of particular concern to blood services is test specificity. If false reactor rates are too high, blood will be wasted unnecessarily, although in order to ensure adequate sensitivity, some false reactive tests have to be accepted. The reactor rates in the Australian Red Cross Blood Services (ARCBS) are monitored continually to ensure that test performances continue to meet evaluation specifications. The data are now collected electronically through EDCNet. Table 1 shows the reactor rates during 2005 for the

Table 1: The Australian Red Cross Blood Service (ARCBS) screens all donations for HIV, HCV, HBsAg and HTLV in the PRISM system (Abbott Diagnostics). The number of false reactive results is reported to the NRL electronically through an internet-based application. The reactor rates can be followed in real time. The reactor rates give a measure of the on-going specificity and hence, albeit indirectly, the tests' performances. They also provide a measure of blood wastage resulting from the rates of false reactivity which is indicated in the right hand column by the ratio of relative costs. The information shown was collected in 2005.

PRISM assay	Specimens	IR (IRR %)	RR (RRR %)	Donations discarded (per 100,000)	Ratio of relative costs
Anti-HCV	1,069,071	960 (0.08)	724 (0.05)	68	3.0
Anti-HIV	1,069,836	1,539 (0.14)	1,259 (0.11)	118	5.3
Anti-HTLV	1,069,328	487 (0.04)	329 (0.03)	31	1.4
HBsAg	1,073,794	495 (0.03)	240 (0.01)	22	1.0
Total	N/A	3,481	2,552	239	N/A

PRISM chemiluminescent immunoassays screening for the blood-borne viruses. The repeat reactor rate for the HIV assay was nearly four times that of the HTLV assay and more than twice that for the HCV assay. This means that the rate of discard of repeatable reactive donations is nearly four and over two times greater, respectively, albeit very low. Demonstration of these data ensures that batches of highest specificity are maintained in the ARCBS laboratories. Over time it has been shown that significant changes in the reactor rate herald batch or operator problems in the test or testing.

Quality control programmes

Quality controls used in every run of a testing procedure can monitor the precision of an assay's performance [8]. If the performances of laboratories using the same testing systems are compared, the accuracy of testing can be assessed. This is assured in the ARCBS by all laboratories using the same independent controls in their systems and working within the same limits, which are determined statistically over time. In Australia (and internationally in about 100 laboratories), the NRL distributes quality control samples. The same quality control sample is used in Australia so that both the precision and accuracy of the tests (notably the PRISM assays) can be monitored. In the international programme the same sample is also used so that national performances can be compared with international performances. The EDCNet system enables the laboratories to view their data through the internet-based system. The analysed data are displayed as soon as they are entered for individual laboratories and compared with the mean for all laboratories: thus, they can follow the precision and accuracy of their testing within real time. Because the appropriate information is collected from each Australian laboratory, the performances of instruments, assay batches (Fig. 3), reagents and operators can all be monitored. If discrepancies are found, the screening laboratory or laboratories is/are notified immediately.

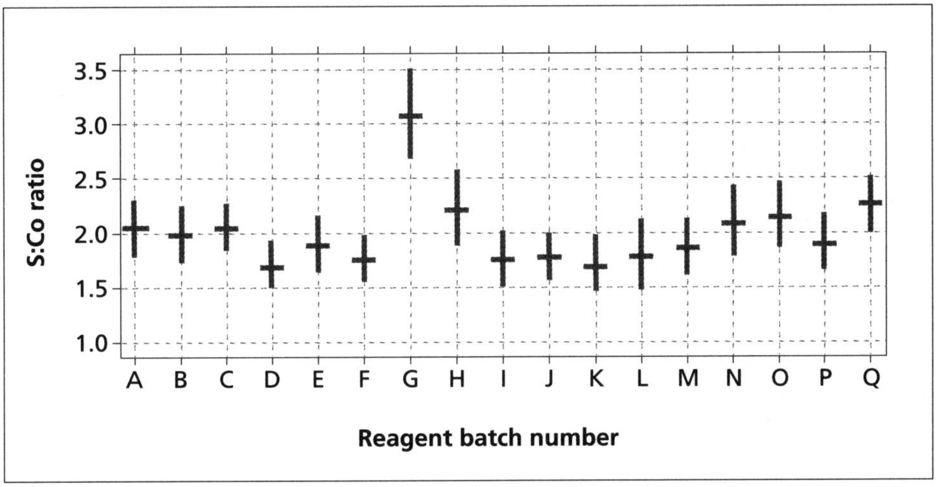

Fig. 3: A quality control sample (PeliSpy: Type 7) from VQC (the Netherlands) was tested in the PRISM anti-HTLV-I/II ChLIA (Abbott Diagnostics) in reagent batches designated A-Q. Ten laboratories reported 8,912 results. The mean ± 2SD of quality control sample results were for each anti-HTLV-I/II PRISM reagent lot. Reagent batch G produced results on average 60 % higher than the mean of all reagent lots.

External Quality Assessment Schemes (EQAS)

EQAS involves sending out panels of samples, each of known characteristics, to laboratories periodically (usually 2-4 times a year). The laboratories are instructed to treat the samples as though they were samples received for testing under usual circumstances. They are required to process the samples through their usual process. Therefore, EQAS assesses the entire process at a point in time. Very few errors occur in EQAS from the Australian Laboratories. However, when performances are compared internationally, there are more aberrations detected.

Although it is difficult to determine exactly the reasons for individual errors, most errors (~ 60 %) were due to technical and other difficulties. In HIV-related schemes, 20 % of the errors were due to laboratories testing negative samples on immunoblots. In HCV-related schemes, some of the errors were due to transcription and others were due to mixing up of samples. If the number of samples per panel in a scheme is larger than the few samples usually supplied in proficiency testing programmes, more complex errors can be defined. This is important in quality schemes for blood services where many have quality management systems in place and errors are often not systematic. Over years of administrating these schemes, the NRL has been able to identify specific problems by following errors defined in the schemes that appear to be random but have later been demonstrated as symptomatic of systematic problems.

Comparative studies on the quality of testing

The NRL, Australia, has in the last 2-3 years sent identical EQAS to laboratories in Australia and internationally. While this is hardly a controlled acquisition of information, it helps assess the state of laboratory services' testing for different purposes and using different methods. It also has helped in the comparison of performances of laboratories in highly regulated environments compared with those whose regulation is less well-established (Table 2). Another common source of error in non-regulated countries is rapid assays with inadequate sensitivity. For example, if low reactivity samples are presented in the assessment scheme, these deficiencies may be highlighted and established over time.

EQAS and QC for blood transfusion services

A search of the literature reveals that results of quality programmes are seldom published. In fact, if "quality assurance of blood transfusion testing" is entered into the PubMed search engine, no papers are revealed. While this does not mean that there is none [9-14], most reports are sent to individual laboratories participating in the quality programmes and few are accepted for reporting in the scientific literature. Others are embedded within programmes for many laboratory types such as the reports on the Model Performance Evaluation Program from the CDC, USA. This may be because of legal issues with any mistakes of blood transfusion services being revealed, thus accounting for this lack of information. At the same time, much is written about the necessity of quality assurance and the absolute necessity for blood services laboratories' belonging to quality programmes. A "Google" search for quality assurance programs & HIV testing yielded 1,350,000 results! Although not all those listed have been looked at, none was found that contained scientifically evaluated data from quality assurance programmes. There are functioning quality

Table 2: An EQAS panel consisting of 5 anti-HCV positive and 5 anti-HCV negative samples, was tested by laboratories in Australia (n = 102) and in the Southeast Asian and Western Pacific regions (n = 57). Aberrant testing result interpretations were those that did not agree with the reference laboratory status. The error rate was defined as the ratio between the total number of aberrant test result interpretations and the total number of reported test result interpretations and was expressed as a percentage. The overall error rate was lower in Australian laboratories than for laboratories in the Southeast Asian and Western Pacific regions, the majority (52.4 %) of aberrant test result interpretations reported by the laboratories in the Southeast Asian and Western Pacific regions were associated with rapid assays. Some rapid assays were unable to detect two positive samples that contained lower levels of anti-HCV (lower S/Co ratios were obtained for these samples in several other assays). Lack of sensitivity in the rapid assays may have been the cause of several of the aberrant test result interpretations. However, this is difficult to confirm as there was no source of comparison for the five rapid assays associated with aberrant test result interpretations for the two samples because each assay was used by only one laboratory.

Anti-HCV EQAS	**No. of laboratories reporting Aberrant Test Result Interpretations (%)**	**No. of Aberrant Test Result Interpretations/Total No. of Test Result Interpretations reported**	**Error rate (%)**	**Aberrant Test Result Interpretations for positive samples**		**Aberrant Test Result Interpretations for negative samples**	
				False negative rate %	Inconclusive/ indeterminate rate (%)	False positive rate (%)	Inconclusive/ indeterminate rate (%)
Australian	8 (8.0)	16/1353	1.2	0.9	0.4	0.4	0.7
International	11 (20.8)	21/815	2.6	2.3	1.8	0.8	0.0

programmes which have yielded important information. An example is that the quality assessment panels sent from Sanguin VQC were pivotal in establishing limits of detection and parity between laboratories in the establishment of nucleic acid testing [9-16].

Quality requirements and quality assurance

ARCBS laboratories are required to be licensed to the cGMP. Independent quality assurance is administered by the NRL. The original thesis for the present paper was to question whether the quality requirements for blood service laboratories, in general, were sufficient, appropriate, delivered as they should be, and whether they were as effective, or as useful as they might be. These are legitimate queries because the resources needed to meet the quality requirements when internal quality systems are operating often are considerable. Despite the extensive information acquired in NRL's quality assurance programmes along with searching the literature, it is difficult to offer definitive or proven evidence to answer these questions. There is no doubt that quality assurance results supply the evidence that shows whether processes and procedures are in control. The quality and correctness of the laboratories' results delivered through the quality programmes cannot be attributed directly to the quality assurance programmes alone, nor can correction of deduced causes of aberrations in laboratories' results or test kit operations be attributed to the programmes. The maintenance of quality outcomes is multi-factorial. Thus, it is impossible to assess through the information that is obtained in quality assurance programmes what the particular contributions of regulation, quality management, quality assurance, test kits' performances and so on, to maintaining the correctness of the process outcomes are. However, having established a multi-method quality programme that operates both nationally and internationally, the NRL is in a position to offer some insight.

Clearly, from our results, errors and aberrations in blood transfusion screening laboratories do occur (Table 2). Comparative results suggest that some tests operate better than others and these differences may be highlighted by quality assurance programmes and may be identified in any of the methods that NRL employs. Once the quality of test kits is established through evaluation and validation, following the performance of test kits by demonstrating their specificity may be a useful way to keep the reactor rates down. This method can also be used to demonstrate the ongoing quality of test kits and thus keep manufacturers delivering best quality product. This may be a way to assist in assuring efficiency in testing by maintaining test quality. Advances in this method are in the collection of the data through electronic means, facilitating the rapid reporting of collective results, the willingness of the groups involved to use the data appropriately and the ability to demonstrate batch variations in the test kits as they are being used.

So the questions on how to define the advancements in quality assurance remain. To support the arguments on how advancements have occurred in quality programmes, the questions posed at the beginning of the chapter should be addressed. On one hand, in developing countries it is known that laboratories, and often their performances, are inadequate. While this may be because resources, including trained staff, are lacking, it is also because quality management systems are lacking. No quality assurance programme can counter the errors or aberrations created by deficiencies in adequate resources or training. However, the NRL has been able to offer feedback education on the inadequacies identified by quality programmes that assist in improving laboratories and assisting them to better utilize the resources that they do have. In these cases, the answer to the question, "How much quality assurance is appropriate?" might be that extensive services are required for a considerable period of time. Where there are few mistakes, an extensive service may be considered inappropriate. In defense of a continuing and extensive quality programme, the NRL has found through its quality assurance programmes in Australia, staff or operators who required retraining, equipment that was malfunctioning, and has identified these malfunctions before they changed the outcomes of test performances, identified testing procedures that were inappropriate or incorrect, identified areas where testing strategies could be improved upon and so on. Compared with the cost of quality programmes, the savings to the blood service may be equivalent or cost-effective, especially if any claimed damages were factored into the calculations of cost-effectiveness. Thus, in advancing quality assurance, the programme administrators must take into account the stages of development of the participating laboratories, their resources and their need for education in quality matters.

Another question that arises with respect to advancing quality programmes is "Who [or what organisations] should perform quality assurance?" A tenet of quality assurance programmes is that they should be independently administered of the organisation requiring the quality assurance [16]. If they are not independent, the assuror is quality assuring its own processes and bias creeps in. Thus, numbers of regulators indicate that quality assessment (and possibly, by inference, assurance) must be "external". No evidence to support this contention is immediately obvious from the results in NRL's quality programmes. However, if evidence were collected independently, manufacturers and sponsors are more likely to respond to the evidence that a test were not operating as it should. Collective, independent evidence of poor performance is far more powerful than a single customer's complaints in getting responses from manufacturers. Comparison of performances between laboratories becomes vital to assuring the accuracy of performances. Quality assurance programmes can provide the source of comparison.

A continuing and difficult question to answer has been "How can the effectiveness of quality assurance programmes be advanced and assessed?" The more effective the quality programme is, the less likely there are to be aberrant results. While not evident in the programmes administered by the NRL to the ARCBS, other NRL programmes may provide evidence for this [17,18]. It is only possible to obtain definitive evidence in new programmes.

Finally, when considering advances in quality assurance, "Which methods should be used?" and "Whether quality assurance methods can be improved upon?" should be considered. Over the last few years the requirements for safety have increased. The sophistication of the tests themselves and the types of testing, including nucleic acid screening and new tests for new blood-borne viruses, have been introduced. While checks and balances within the kits themselves have been developed further, the complexities of the tests demand better quality assurance systems. The NRL has increased the efficiency of its methods, employing internet-based data collection with instant analysis of quality control material in response to the requirements. Regulators have also increased their requirements. For example, ISO 15189 requires that laboratories reporting results are able to quote the measurement of uncertainty. The TGA in Australia has proposed a new framework for regulating in vitro diagnostics that will include a requirement that the quality of all testing for blood-borne viruses be monitored to ensure satisfactory post-market performance. The NRL has responded by proposing that the most effective mechanism would be through quality control programmes. Development of EDCNet means that the data are collected and analysed immediately. The same data may be used to calculate the measurement of uncertainty [19]. Several companies have developed systems that are similar for their customers. Few have accompanied such systems in combination with other methods. Information to improve the quality of testing comes from all the types of quality assurance methods.

Advances in Quality Assurance Programmes

Quality assurance methods arose in the 1950s and many programmes still employ methods relatively unchanged from the early assessment methods. Many assurors are not ready with new quality assurance programmes at the time that new methods or technologies are introduced into the blood services, possibly because the funding of quality assurance is not necessarily planned into the introduction of new methods and technologies. Thus, one of the advancements that could be made in quality assurance is that the programmes be introduced at the time the new testing methods are introduced. This would provide a measure of the success of testing programmes and their efficiencies. Quality assurance programmes may be used as ideal methods for identifying where training is required, especially in newly established testing programmes. More quality assurance providers are offering feedback in their reports and approaching the provision of quality assurance with a view to providing education around the outcomes as needed. More advanced quality assurors can expect their staff to spend considerable time communicating with participating laboratories, responding to their queries and identifying areas for improvement and suggesting ways in which improvements may be achieved. To obtain an evidence-based grasp of laboratory quality the quality assuror is far better equipped to respond if the evidence is drawn from multiple quality methods administered in parallel rather than a single data collection method (e.g. EQAS only). Collection of the information through electronic means has shown that much of this information can be accumulated and analysed in real time. Future laboratories might expect their quality assurance to be immediate, and they could be informed immediately if aberrations occur.

Acknowledgements

The authors acknowledge the extensive work of the NRL staff and staff of the ARCBS laboratories in collecting the information necessary to produce the present commentary. Dr Darren Jardine, Dr Roderick Chapel and others at the NRL provided valuable comment and editing skills. Ms Helen Hasler provided efficient and effective manuscript management and coordination for the production of this paper.

References

1 Council of Europe Guide to the preparation, use and quality assurance of blood components 11th Edition 2005 Council of Europe Publishing.

2 Australian Code of Good Manufacturing Practice – Human blood and tissues 2000 http://www.tga.gov.au/docs/html/gmpbltic.htm.

3 Resnik DB: The precautionary principle and medical decision making. J Med Philos 2004; 29 (3): 281-299.

4 Busch MP, Watanabe KK, Smith JW, Hermansen SW, Thomson RA: False-negative testing errors in routine viral marker screening of blood donors. For the Retrovirus Epidemiology Donor Study. Transfusion 2000; 40 (5): 585-589.

5 Busch MP, Kleinman SH, Nemo GJ: Current and emerging infectious risks of blood transfusions. Jama 2005; 289 (8): 959-962.

6 Australian/New Zealand Standard Quality Management Systems – fundamentals and vocabulary AS/NZS ISO 9000:2000.

7 Constantine N, Saville RD, Dax EM: Retroviral Testing and Quality Assurance published by Malley Printers Ann Arbour MI (a not-for-profit publication).

8 Brooks ZC: Performance-driven quality control. 2001; AACC Press Washington DC, USA.

9 Davis C, Heath A, Best S, Hewlett I, Lelie N, Schuurman R, Holmes H: Calibration of HIV-1 working reagents for nucleic acid amplification techniques against the 1st international standard for HIV-1 RNA. J Virol Methods 2003; 107 (1): 37-44.

10 Holmes H, Davis C, Heath A, Hewlett I, Lelie N: An international collaborative study to establish the 1st international standard for HIV-1 RNA for use in nucleic acid-based techniques. J Virol Methods 2001; 92 (2): 141-150.

11 Saldanha J, Lelie N, Heath A: Establishment of the first international standard for nucleic acid amplification technology (NAT) assays for HCV RNA. WHO Collaborative Study Group. Vox Sang 1999; 76 (3): 149-158.

12 Koppelman MH, Assal A, Chudy M, Torres P, de Villaescusa RG, Reesink HW, Lelie PN, Cuypers HT: Multicenter performance evaluation of a transcription-mediated amplification assay for screening of human immunodeficiency virus-1 RNA, hepatitis C virus RNA, and hepatitis B virus DNA in blood donations. Transfusion 2005; 45 (8): 1258-1266.

13 Busch MP, Glynn SA, Wright DJ, Hirschkorn D, Laycock ME, McAuley J, Tu Y, Giachetti C, Gallarda J, Heitman J, Kleinman SH: National Heart, Lung, Blood Institute Nucleic Acid Test Study Group*. Relative sensitivities of licensed nucleic acid amplification tests for detection of viremia in early human immunodeficiency virus and hepatitis C virus infection. Transfusion 2005; 45 (12): 1853-1863.

14 Schirm J, van Loon AM, Valentine-Thon E, Klapper PE, Reid J, Cleator GM: External quality assessment program for qualitative and quantitative detection of hepatitis C virus RNA in diagnostic virology. J Clin Microbiol 2002; 40 (8): 2973-2980.

15 Valentine-Thon E: Quality control in nucleic acid testing – where do we stand? J Clin Virol 2002; 25 (3): S13-S21.

16 Lewis SM: Quality assurance programmes in the United Kingdom. Ann Ist Super Sanità 1995; 31 (1): 53-59.

17 Chappel RJ, Goris M, Palmer RF, Hartskeerl RA: Impact of proficiency testing on results of the microscopic agglutination test for diagnosis of leptospirosis. J Clin Microbiol 2004; 42: 5484-5488.

18 Sayer DC, Land S, Gizzarelli L, French M, Hales G, Emery S, Dax EM, Christiansen FT: A quality assessment program (QAP) for genotypic antiretroviral testing (GART) results in an improvement in the detection of drug resistance mutations. J Clin Micro 2003; 41: 227-236.

19 Dimech W, Francis B, Roberts G, Chappel R, Kox J: A proposed approach to estimating uncertainty of measurement in serological assays. Aust J Med Lab Sci 2005;26: 28-65.

Assoc. Prof. E.M. Dax, National Serology Reference Laboratory, Australia and Australian Red Cross Blood Service Laboratories, 4th Floor Healy Building, 41 Victoria Parade, Fitzroy 3065, Australia.
E-mail: liz@nrl.gov.au

Dax EM, Farrugia A, Vyas G (eds): Advances in Transfusion Safety – Volume IV.
Dev Biol (Basel). Basel, Karger, 2007, vol 127, pp 197-204.

Improved Safety of Clinical Blood Transfusion in Four Provinces of China 1997-2005

G. Whyte

International Education Development Unit, Faculty of Medicine, Nursing and Health Sciences, Monash University, Victoria, Australia

Professor Whyte was Director of the Australian Red Cross Blood Service in Victoria (1988-98) and Tasmania (1997-98)

Abstract: This paper outlines the activities of the Blood Component of the World Bank Health IX Program in China over the period 1997-2005. There has been a large and sustainable improvement in the safety of the systems that provide blood for transfusion in four provinces of China. This success is only one of the many great improvements that have occurred across the whole country.

CONTEXT

The Chinese Blood Banking System was described in 2002 [1]. It described the difficulty of recruiting volunteer donors in China and the reliance on paid and employer organised donations. Clinically, blood component use was low at 40 %, although increased from 20 % in 1996. Previously, all donors were tested twice for the viral indicators of infectiveness, once before donation to determine eligibility and again after donation of blood. Confirmatory tests for HIV are done at the provincial level by the provincial public health laboratories, which are also responsible for notifying and counselling donors.

The same article reported that intravenous drug usage was the leading risk factor for HIV, in addition to increasing numbers from sexual contact and mother to child transmission. There have also been reports of transmission to donors during the donation process by "underground for-profit plasma collection operations." Unlicensed centres had used non-sterile needles and pooled blood from donors of the same ABO group during plasma collection before red cells were returned to the donors, often without testing for HIV. The donors were often at high risk because they were drug users. For example, in Henan, a poor central province, HIV prevalence in the population as a whole was 2 per 1000 in 1997, while among blood donors it was

170 per 1000. By way of confirmation, in Hubei and Shandong, HIV prevalence in the population was 6 per 1000 in 1997, compared with a rate in whole blood donors of 26 per 1000 and apheresis donors of 259 per 1000.

Serious quality issues and procedural errors in testing of blood for transfusion were reported, aggravated by variable quality of testing kits.

Many of these factors had been identified in the mid 1990s and created the environment in which the World Bank developed a loan program with China to address the safety of blood transfusion as part of a larger program to address the transmission of HIV/AIDS and STDs in China.

Prevalence of HIV/AIDS in China

In 1985, the number of documented HIV/AIDS cases was 4 [2], rising to 1445 in 1994 [3]. However, UNAIDS estimated that there were truly about 400,000 cases across China in 2000 with a projected 10,000,000 cases in 2010 if no effective preventive action was taken [4]. We are therefore currently in a phase of rapid expansion of the spread of the disease in China.

The pattern of spread is different in China compared with Australia, as shown in Table 1. Australia has a typical Western pattern of spread, particularly through male to male sex, unlike China, where intravenous drug use is the dominant route. The high rate of "other" as a category in China reflects the quality of data available for analysis.

Table 1: Pattern of spread of HIV/AIDS in China and Australia.

Mode of transmission	China 1985-1994*	Victoria 1984-1993**
Sexual M/F	5.1	5.3
Sexual M/M	0	81.7
IDU	63.8	3.5
Blood	0	4.5
Other	31.1	1.3

* Am J Pub Health 1996; 86: 1116
** Med J Aust 1995; 163: 66

Health IX program

The Chinese national plan for HIV/AIDS prevention and control in 1998 gave little attention to blood transfusion as a major route of transmission of the disease, focussing on testing of blood [5]. However, by the next plan [6], a considerably expanded program had been put in place that covered voluntary donation and modernised laws and standards for collection and testing centres. The laws and standards covered test materials and protocols and required all staff involved in blood collection and transfusion to be trained and able to pass a professional examination; management systems to monitor quality were also installed.

In 2003, the Midterm review summarised the project as follows [7]: "The Health nine project HIV/AIDS/STD part is in the charge of Chinese government, loaned by WORLD BANK. Health nine project is a comprehensive prevention and control AIDS project, with the largest scale and investment up to now in China. It includes five components, such as policy development and organization construction, HIV/AIDS/STD intervention, HIV/AIDS/STD surveillance, blood management and central project. The project aims to strengthen the capacity to combat with HIV/AIDS/STD in China, as well as to provide experiences for the rest areas in the country. Four provinces (autonomous regions): Fujiang, Guangxi, Shangxi and Xinjiang, were selected as the project provinces. The whole project covers 35 prefectures, 57 counties, with the total population of 22.4 million. The Health project began in November of 1999."

The four provinces were chosen because they each had a high prevalence or risk of HIV/AIDS, but with different characteristics of the AIDS epidemic, and firm government commitment. For example, Fujian has many ports with extensive trading links by sea and therefore a risk of drug use and sexual transmission. Guangxi adjoins Vietnam and the truck routes, with the same risk factors and the additional risks to ethnic groups with different traditions. Shanxi has many coal mines with, therefore, many men working away from their families and at risk of sexual transmission. Xinjiang has long trade routes by truck along the old Silk Road, but also many large ethnic minorities with feelings of disenfranchisement from mainstream China and an increased susceptibility to risky behaviour.

The four components of the loan program were Policy development and institution building, HIV/AIDS/STD intervention, HIV/AIDS/STD surveillance and Blood Management. This paper is about the last component.

Components of the Blood Management program included civil works, equipment, vehicles, drugs, consumables, training, technical assistance and program support across 26 prefectures in the four provinces. The majority of funding (63.2 %) came from a low interest loan, and the remainder (36.8 %) was funded by the participating provinces. In 2003, the Chines government took a loan on future earnings to fund a large program to modernise all of China's blood transfusion systems (the National Debt Program). This new program was managed by the Ministry of Health and funded new facilities and equipment across the country's 27 provinces. It also provided training and quality systems across all provinces using the World Health Organisation manuals translated into Chinese.

Actions

Both programs have focussed on the following elements.

Volunteer unremunerated blood donations

The program has sought to develop a base of volunteer unremunerated blood donors from low risk populations. Most blood donors previously gave blood under some form of reduced option to refuse, for example as paid donors, as family donors or as donors organised through work groups. The program therefore sought to improve the regulatory and legislative framework to support voluntary unremunerated donation and to teach the public about the change. Donor recruitment was actively pursued and marketing techniques applied as appropriate for a customer service. This meant that time and place of collections were made more suitable for donors. The fixed sites were made more attractive, and staff were taught to be friendly. Mobile buses were purchased, often by local municipalities, to take the collection site to donors in universities, in markets, on busy streets and to workplaces. The number of repeat donors was made a key performance indicator, and the collection of larger donations (400ml rather than the traditional 200ml) was implemented.

Quality program

A comprehensive quality program was introduced that covered collection, testing, processing, storage and transport and across facilities, equipment, materiel, staff, standard operating procedures and information technology. Screening and testing equipment has been widely upgraded through both funding systems. Testing was initially upgraded and staff trained for the prefectural and city centres, but the increased safety of highly automated testing and the use of large machines with redundancy of critical processes and the improved safety from highly trained staff have led to a decision to centralise testing to provincial centres where possible. Similarly, local development of information technology systems has been discouraged and province-wide systems are being installed with a limited number of trusted suppliers. All staff members have been trained with WHO materials under the National Debt Program. Domestic testing kits are still overshadowed by imported kits, and this will continue until local kits are shown to have less batch to batch variation and perform as reliably as internationally sourced kits. All staff members have been required to sit a national examination about blood laws; a second failure results in redeployment of the staff member. Internal and external audits of standard operating procedures, review of records and development and recording of corrective actions are being promoted vigorously; the same progressive change in culture has been experienced when systems were changed in developed countries. A proposed national quality assurance scheme through four main centres has been moved back to the provincial centres with strengthened roles. Many centres have used ISO accreditation as a way to learn about quality systems.

Improved blood usage

Safe and efficient use of blood transfusion has been promoted vigorously through training sessions for hospital staff, by upgrading hospital blood banks and through the use of booklets promoting correct use of blood. All doctors are required to sit an exam about blood laws every two years as part of relicensure. However, the power differential between blood bank scientists and hospital clinicians continues to delay positive change, similar to what occurs in developed countries. Nevertheless, the use of blood components for transfusion rather than whole blood is an indicator of the effectiveness of education.

Outcomes

The proportion of blood transfused in project prefectures that is from voluntary unremunerated blood donors (VUBD) has increased over the life of the project, as shown in Table 2. The provision of mobile buses to service donors has been greatly appreciated and has facilitated the change to VUBD. A straw poll of donors indicated that they gave blood out of concern for their community. Many had heard of the blood bank through school. They had a good understanding of the transmission of HIV. Zaller et al have examined the attitudes of volunteer donors in one of the main sites, Urumqi in Xinjaing [8]. They found that fear of acquiring HIV from blood donation persisted and that motivating factors to donate blood included social pressure, desire to know results and altruism.

Table 2: Proportion of blood transfused that was collected from voluntary unremunerated blood donors in 26 prefectures of four provinces, 1997-2005.

% VUBD	1997	2003	2005
Fujian	10.7	86.3	93
Guangxi	7.7	84.2	81.8
Shanxi	9.0	100	100
Xinjiang	14.0	70.8	90.7

The total amount of blood collected from VUBD has generally increased over the last three years, with 2005 extrapolated from 6 months data. Some prefectures have shown a decline in collections, probably due to less demand due to less inappropriate usage. Table 3 shows these figures as collections per thousand population per year. Some of the provincial city collection rates are approaching developed world rates.

Table 3: Collections per thousand population per year in 26 prefectures of four Health IX project provinces, 1997-2005. (2005 figures extrapolated from 6 months data).

Collections /1000 pop'n	1997	2003	2005
Fujian	6.8	6.2	10.7
Guangxi	12.5	6.0	7.7
Shanxi	13.6	5.7	9.0
Xinjiang	7.9	9.6	14.0

Table 4 shows that the other targeted goal of an increased proportion of repeat donors has become more realized. Repeat donors have been previously tested and are loyal to the program, so they provide blood less likely to be in the window period for viral markers. They also require less recruitment, reducing costs and increasing the reliability of supply.

Larger donations of blood have been resisted, but with increasing size of donors with improving social conditions, more collections can be made as 400 ml compared with the previous 200 ml size. Larger donations mean that each individually transfused patient is exposed to fewer donors. The change is shown in Table 5.

Table 4: Repeat donors as a percentage of VUBD collections per year in 26 prefectures of four provinces 1997-2005.

% Repeat donors	1997	2003	2005
Fujian	0	16	36
Shanxi	0	–	45
Guangxi	0	32	38
Xinjiang	0	–	33

Table 5: Proportion of VUBD collections as 400 ml in 26 prefectures of four Health IX project provinces, 1997-2005.

% 400 ml donations	1997	2003	2005
Fujian	0	15	67
Shanxi	0	48	91
Guangxi	0	17	36
Xinjiang	0	34	41

Each donation is screened for antibody to human immunodeficiency virus (HIV), antibody to hepatitis C virus (HCV) and Hepatitis B virus antigen (HBV). Donors are also screened pre-donation for HBV because of the high prevalence of hepatitis B viremia in developing countries. Confirmatory tests for HIV are performed by the provincial Public Health Laboratory. All screening tests are in duplicate with one domestic and one imported test. HCV positivity is recorded for these purposes if 2 of 3 screens are reactive, although blood is not used if any screen is reactive. The brand of kit used in each institution depends on the purchasing authority in the province, which is becoming centralized. The results of screening tests are shown in Table 6.

It will be seen that the HIV prevalence in new donors is of concern in Xinjiang, where the situation is being closely monitored. On the other hand, the prevalence of HCV at about 5 per 1000 population is rather less than in developed countries. Finally, it is noted that pre-screening of donors for hepatitis B has reduced the load

Table 6: Virus markers per 1000 tests on first time VUBD from 26 prefectures of four project provinces, 2005.

2005	HIV pos screen	HIV pos confirmed	HCV pos	HBV pos	ALT
Guangxi	1.7	0.09	5.1	13.6	5.6
Shanxi	1.8	0	6.0	10.3	6.7
Fujian	4.0	0	5.2	14.7	13.7
Xinjiang	1.3	0.39	5.6	3.6	6.4

in new donors to about 15 per 1000. The implication is that the program to improve blood services has arrived in time for many patients requiring blood transfusion in China.

Finally, conversion of use of blood transfusion from whole blood to packed red cells reflects a growing awareness of appropriate blood transfusion. Although the use of components is often driven by the needs of the plasma industry, there is also a safety improvement. Whether the changes in China, shown in Table 7, are due to these factors or are reflecting perceived current practice in developed countries cannot be deduced. However, the changes are dramatic and are probably related to the wide distribution of the official publication on Guidelines for Clinical Blood Transfusion and the introduction of recommended cross match protocols for common surgical procedures.

Table 7: Use of red blood cell concentrates as a proportion of total blood transfused in 26 prefectures of four provinces 1997-2005.

Component use (%)	**1997**	**2003**	**2005**
Fujian	61	97	96
Shanxi	17	–	89
Guangxi	68	66	86
Xinjiang	50	–	93

An excellent example of the commitment of staff to achieving the very best blood transfusion service possible and the pride taken in a good job was demonstrated in Urumqi, provincial centre for Xinjiang. There are many other examples in the four provinces. However, in Xinjiang, many of the staff members of the regional blood service have purchased red and white uniforms and musical instruments and taught themselves to play well. On most Sundays, they give up part of their weekend to play as a band in parts of the city to recruit donors. That kind of dedication to the idea of a voluntary community based blood service is not often seen anywhere!

I am advised by the Ministry of Health that similar changes have been achieved across all provinces of China.

Acknowledgements

Grateful acknowledgements to Dr Yi Mei, Director of Blood Transfusion Services in the Ministry of Health in China, for leadership and for permission to publish this information. Grateful acknowledgements also to Mr Shiyong Wang of the World Bank in China for authorisation to use World Bank data gathered while I was a consultant with the Bank.

References

1 Hua Shan, Jing-Xing Wang, Fu-Rong Ren et al: Blood Banking in China. Lancet 2002; 360: 1770-1775.

2 Yu Esh, Qiyi Xie, Zhang K, Lu P, Chan LL: HIV infections and AIDS in China 1985 through 1994. Am J Pub Health 1996; 86: 1116.

3 De Kock KM, Weiss HA: The global epidemiology of HIV/AIDS. Trop Med & International Health 2000; 5: A3.

4 Portsmouth S, Stebbing J, Keyi X, Jinaping Z, Guohua P: HIV and AIDS in the People's Republic of China: a collaborative review. Int Jnl STD & AIDS 2003; 14: 757.

5 Dept of Disease Control Chinese national medium- and long term strategy for HIV/AIDS prevention and control (1998-2002). National Centre for STD & Leprosy Control, Ministry of Health, China, 2002.

6 Dept of Disease Control China's action plan for reducing and preventing the spread of HIV/AIDS (2001-2005). National Centre for STD and Leprosy Control, Ministry of Health, China, June 2001.

7 External mid-term review report World Bank Loan Health Nine Project: HIV/AIDS/STD prevention and control. Centre of AIDS prevention and control studies, School of Public Health, Beijing University. September 2003.

8 Zaller N, Nelson KE, Ness P, Wen G, Bai X, Shan H: Knowledge, attitude and practice survey regarding blood donation in a Northwestern Chinese city Transfusion Medicine 2005; 15: 277-286.

Dr. G. Whyte, International Education Development Unit, Faculty of Medicine, Nursing and Health Sciences, Monash University, Victoria 3800, Australia.
E-mail: gordon.whyte@med.monash.edu.au

Dax EM, Farrugia A, Vyas G (eds): Advances in Transfusion Safety – Volume IV.
Dev Biol (Basel). Basel, Karger, 2007, vol 127, p 205.

SESSION VI

Harmonising Practice and Product – The Role for Blood Safety

Chairs: *M. Busch and P. Strengers*

Dax EM, Farrugia A, Vyas G (eds): Advances in Transfusion Safety – Volume IV.
Dev Biol (Basel). Basel, Karger, 2007, vol 127, pp 207-214.

Modelling Outcomes of HCV in Recipients of Blood Products

G. Whyte

International Education Development Unit, Faculty of Medicine, Nursing and Health Sciences, Monash University, Victoria, Australia

Professor Whyte was Director of the Australian Red Cross Blood Service in Victoria (1988-98) and Tasmania (1997-98)

Key words: Hepatitis C, blood transfusion, natural history, blood products, modelling.

INTRODUCTION

Modelling of disease outcomes is helpful 1) at the individual level to advise infected patients about the likely outcome of their disease and 2) at the population level to model the effects of infection in a population and on hospitalisation rates and to develop cost benefit analyses. In the specific context of transfused patients, the disease models need to be adapted to transfusion rates of sub populations and take into account the mortality of transfused patients to give a realistic model. A recent example is the modelling exercise by Marshall et al [1], which concluded that "the cost effectiveness of adding PCR is outside the typical range for most healthcare interventions, but not for established blood safety measures." Since the introduction of PCR testing of all blood donations, the risk of hepatitis C virus (HCV) infection by transfusion transmission in Australia is considered to be 0.14 per million fresh products and 0.54 per patient episode [2].

Early concerns about a high mortality and morbidity from HCV were biased by natural histories being developed from patients referred to liver clinics; more recently published data from longitudinal studies have yielded a much less malignant picture, important at both the individual and the population levels.

In 1998, a model of the natural history of hepatitis C was used [3] to estimate cost benefit of the introduction of testing for HCV Ab and PCR. It is of interest to revisit the model in light of updated reports of longevity from Seeff [4,5] on young low risk people with HCV. Seeff had reported in 1992 [6] that there was no excess mortality from all causes 17 years after transfusion-associated non-A non-B hepatitis. He has revisited the data in 2002 [7] and confirmed his earlier observations. In other reports, of 704 young Irish women given anti D immunoprophylaxis contaminated with HCV 17 years before and found to be HCV Ab positive, only 55 % were HCV RNA positive, and cirrhosis was found in 7 (2 %), two of whom were heavy alcoholics [8]. In East Germany, of 1018 women given contaminated anti-D and recalled, 917 had developed increased ALT values at 4 weeks, but after 20 years, 53 % had normal ALT values, and although 85 % still had HCV Ab, only 55 % still had detectable HCV RNA and none had cirrhosis [9]. In an Australian study [10], of 95 patients with acute hepatitis who had HCV Ab in serum stored 25 years earlier, only 6 (2 %) had developed cirrhosis in the mean time, again suggesting that the progression of disease to cirrhosis is slower and in a smaller proportion of those infected with HCV than originally thought.

Model of HCV Infection

The Brown and Crofts model starts with intravenous drug users (IVDUs) exposed to HCV and was developed to estimate health care costs of the epidemic. In the model, of each cohort of 1000 patients exposed to HCV, 200 will not be infected or will clear the virus. Of the remaining 800, 50 % will progressively develop chronic hepatitis over 15 years, and the rest will remain well. Of those who develop chronic hepatitis, all will develop cirrhosis at a steady rate of 2 % per year. Of those who develop cirrhosis, 25 % will develop liver failure and 10 % will develop hepatocellular carcinoma at a steady rate of 3.5 % per year. All cases of liver failure and hepatocellular cancer are fatal within 2 years. All other cases of cirrhosis die at a steady rate of 10 % per year.

Rate of Seroconversion in Transfusion Recipients

In Victoria in 1997-8 [11], lookback identified 1340 patients likely to have received fresh blood components in the previous five years from 358 donors who returned to give blood after the introduction of the screening test and who were found to be infective for hepatitis C. The majority (58 %) were deceased. Of the 424 recipients of at-risk blood components traced in whom HCV results were available, 199 (47 %) were HCV Ab positive, 8 (2 %) were HCV Ab indeterminate and 218 (51 %) were HCV Ab negative. All donations traced were from donors who were PCR reactive or consistently reactive on three different antibody screening tests. All reactive recipients in Victoria were tested by PCR to confirm their status. In general, donors were regarded as infective for the lookback if they met the interpretation developed in Victoria [12] and published in 1995.

In the UK, Dike reported that 55/104 (53 %) seroconverted [13]. The entire English lookback program, including Dike's figures, reported that of 1,223 tested recipients of donations from donors subsequently found to have antibodies for HCV, 492 were found to be negative for antibodies to HCV, 677 (55.4 %) were positive and 54 were indeterminate [14]. Seroconversion rates in the English lookback study were significantly higher among sub-sets of recipients who had received a transfusion from a donor with a positive test result for HCV RNA (68 %), and who had confirmation in their hospital notes that the lookback unit number was transfused (odds ratio 1.50, 95 % CI 1.08-2.07).

Despite the above evidence, Ismay et al [15] reported a seroconversion rate of 27 % of recipients of 26 HCV Ab reactive (retrospective) samples, but the rate increased to 100 % if only RIBA positive samples had been transfused. This reflects the expected improved effectiveness of screening tests.

It is evident that the expected seroconversion rate depends on the source of experience and, for blood transfusion, lies between the Victorian experience of 53 % and the UK experience of 68 % for HCV RNA positive donors. However, both are rather lower than the 80 % proposed for an IVDU population.

Outcome of Acute Hepatitis in Seroconverters

Post transfusion hepatitis is often subclinical and difficult to detect unless specifically sought [16]. Starting with patients who developed acute post transfusion hepatitis defined as a raised ALT, Ismay et al reported an Australian cohort that was transfused before HCV Ab screening became available and had a complete sample array [17]. They reported that 7 of 8 (88 %) post transfusion hepatitis subjects later seroconverted for HCV. In the Australian cohort, 7 of 26 recipients of HCV Ab positive blood developed acute hepatitis, but all the 6 RIBA positive samples caused acute hepatitis and seroconversion. The Australian study suggests that most and possibly all recipients of transfused blood positive to second & third generation HCV Ab screening tests will develop acute hepatitis. Of the Australian patients who received 7 HCV Ab positive blood (samples tested by RIBA when it became available), 6 seroconverted.

In a Canadian cohort [18], there was a rate of 20.2 per 1000 of post transfusion hepatitis before the introduction of HCV Ab screening, similar to 2 % in an Australian study reported in 1982 [19], but the rate of hepatitis in the recipients of HCV reactive donations (pre HCV samples subsequently tested) is not available. Overall, however, 8.8 % of 799 recipients received a donation with at least one NANB marker, and 5.7 % developed hepatitis, of which 0.4 % was due to HCV.

On the other hand, in donors with chronic HCV infection, based on second generation HCV Ab results (HCV-2), about 23 % have raised ALT results on a single estimation. An Australian study of the incidence of post transfusion hepatitis in the late 1980's reported that 4 of 21 HCV reactive donations had an ALT > 45 iu/L (20 %), implying that 20 % otherwise well donors with chronic HCV infection had biochemically active hepatitis at the time of testing [20]. Of donors since 1990 both HCV-2 and Western blot positive, 31 % of 119 males had an ALT > 60 iu/L and 24 % of 83 females had ALT > 45 iu/L [21]. If HCV-2 positive and Western blot indeterminate donors are also included, similarly low proportions of males 42/152 (28 %) and females 22/123 (18 %) had raised ALT levels. In other words, 23 % of donors reactive for HCV-II antibody have evidence of active hepatitis at the time of testing.

Seeff quotes levels of clearance of the virus after acute hepatitis of 14-46 % with a long chronic phase, accelerated in the presence of concomitant infection with hepatitis B or HIV or by heavy alcohol intake [22]. The effect on quality of life was heavily influenced by whether or not a person was aware of their hepatitis status [23]. It was also apparent that only a small portion (14.6 %) of young children undergoing cardiac surgery had persistent antibody to HCV and that 45 % of those had cleared the virus 20 years later, suggesting a greater ability of children to eliminate the virus after infection [24]. One of the infected patients had cirrhosis on biopsy.

Long Term Outcomes of HCV from Transfusion

The proportion of patients developing acute hepatitis after seroconversion is uncertain, but the progression of HCV to cirrhosis seems to be lower than in the Brown & Crofts model.

Starting from acute HCV hepatitis, Freeman et al in Australia reviewed all studies of the natural history of HCV infection and concluded that selection bias was probably responsible for the high rates of progression reported from liver clinics and that 7 % was the most likely progression rate, but with a variable follow up period [25].

Bennett et al have used a Markov model based on their own liver clinic experience that assumes a rather higher 7.3 % annual conversion from chronic hepatitis to cirrhosis and a 0.1 % development of hepatocellular carcinoma, which has an 86 % progression to death per year [26]. In those developing cirrhosis, 1.5 % will develop hepatocellular cancer and 4 % per year will develop ascites, variceal bleeding or hepatic encephalopathy, suggesting a fairly slow progression. This is lower than the rate suggested in textbooks, where cirrhosis is less well defined in natural history terms [27].

A projection of the hepatitis C epidemic in 1998, *Estimates and projections of the hepatitis C epidemic in Australia* [28], uses the assumption that around 75 % of all people exposed to HCV will develop chronic HCV infection [29,30], similar to the model, but that between 3 % and 11 % will progress to cirrhosis after 10 to 24 years [31-34], whereas Brown and Crofts expected half of 2 % per year or 10 %-14 % would progress after 10-24 years. This is much less than Bennett's clinical experience.

The Brown and Crofts model also postulates that all IVDU cirrhotics will die at 10 % per year. However, there is a definitional problem in that, apart from clinic experience not reflecting a population sample: "cirrhosis" is often used as a clinical term with variable intensity on biopsy [35-40] and therefore different life expectancies.

Three reports of the progression from cirrhosis to hepatocellular cancer, together suggest that the rate of progression is about 0.1 % per year, rather less than the model (2.5 %) and Bennett (1.5 %) [41-43].

In summary, a model of post transfusion hepatitis C based on this evidence is shown below with Brown and Crofts estimates in parentheses:

- seroconversion rate of 60 % (80 %);
- 100 % seroconverters develop acute hepatitis C;
- acute hepatitis C resolves in 30 % (50 %);
- all acute hepatitis C which does not resolve progresses to chronic hepatitis;
- chronic hepatitis progresses to clinical cirrhosis at a rate of 0.3 % pa (2 %);
- Hepatocellular cancer (HCC) develops in patients with chronic hepatitis at a rate of 0.1 % pa (0.1 %);
- people who develop clinical cirrhosis will have a mortality of 10 % pa (13.5 %);
- people who develop HCC will die in 2 years (2 years)

Survival of the Transfused Population

There were two studies available in 1999 of total transfused populations for estimating the survival of fresh blood components by Whyte (1988) [44] from New Zealand and Vamvakas (1994) [45] from the Mayo Clinic in the United States. Whyte's study found a weighted average age of recipients of 60.0 years. Vamvakas reported a median age of transfused patients of 63.0 yrs.

The survival of all patients at successive anniversaries was different in each study: Whyte reported that 78.7, 75.1, 72.9, 70.7 and 69.0 % of transfused patients would be alive on successive anniversaries of their transfusion, on the assumption that the age specific rates revert to those of the general population after the second year. On the other hand, Vamvakas reported that 75.7, 70, 60 and 48.3 % of patients were alive after 1, 2, 5 and 10 years, but with 6.1 % (mostly younger and fitter patients) lost to follow-up. The lower survival may be due to an older and more referred (and therefore sicker) population at the Mayo clinic.

Using data from the two series, a model of survival of recipients of transfusion with red cells was constructed for the purpose of modelling outcomes of transfusion.

The mean age of transfusion will be taken to be 55 years. Survival at 1 and 2 years will be assumed to be 75.7 % and 70.0 %, and survival at 5 and 10 years will be assumed to be 60.0 % and 48.3 %. Survival at 3 and 4 years will assumed to be proportionate and taken as 66.7 % and 63.3 %, respectively. At 6, 7, 8 and 9 years, survival will also be assumed to be proportionate between 5 and 10 years, with an outcome of 57.7, 55.3, 53.0 and 50.6 % respectively. After 10 years, it was assumed that there would be no further effect of the condition for which they were transfused, i.e. survival will revert to age specific death rates in 94/95 as provided by the Australian Bureau of Statistics [46].

Model for HCV in Transfusion Recipients

Table 1: The effects of modelling two sets of assumptions (B & C and PTH) about the natural history of hepatitis C on 1000 young women and on 1000 transfused (Tx) patients of 55 years exposed to the virus blood products.

Years from exposure		**0**	**5**	**10**	**15**	**20**	**25**	**30**	**35**
Women of 25 years	General survival	1000	997	993	990	985	974	960	933
	HCV (B & C)	1000	987	961	929	896	858	821	775
	HCV (PTH)	1000	996	991	986	979	966	950	920
General population of 55 years	General survival	1000	961	923	826	713	495	272	25
Transfused patients of 55 years	Transfused patient survival	1000	600	480	430	371	257	142	13
	Tx & HCV (B & C)	1000	594	464	403	337	227	121	11
	TX & HCV (PTH)	1000	600	479	428	368	255	140	13

B & C refers to the model of Brown & Crofts.
PTH refers to the modified model constructed by a review of the literature in this paper.

A table can be constructed that shows the effects of applying the Brown and Crofts model (B & C) and the revised model for transfusion to the expected survival of young women of 25 years and to the transfused population. Table 1 clearly demonstrates that the B & C model is overly pessimistic about the rate of development of clinical cirrhosis when compared to the real events described by Seeff and others. On the other hand, the revised assumptions derived for post transfusion hepatitis (PTH), are rather more compatible with the observed long term natural history of post transfusion hepatitis.

Acknowledgements

I would like to thank Dr. Angela Robinson for assistance with the English figures for HCV lookback and the Australian Red Cross Blood Service for permission to use the Victorian lookback figures.

References

1 Marshall DA, Kleinman SH, Wong JB, AuBuchon JP, Grima DT, Kulin NA, Weinstein MC: Cost-effectiveness of nucleic acid screening of volunteer blood donations for hepatitis B, hepatitis C and human immunodeficiency virus in the United States. Vox Sanguinis 2004; 86: 28-40.

2 Australian Red Ross Blood Service Quick Reference Guide: Obtaining informed consent – Blood & Blood Products www.transfusion.com.au/Transfusionpocketguides/Pocket_RiskConsent.asp (accessed 30 Nov 2005).

3 Brown K, Crofts N: Health care costs of a continuing epidemic of hepatitis C virus infection among injecting drug users. Aust NZ Jnl Pub Health 1998; 22 (3 supp): 384-388.

4 Seeff LB: Natural History of Chronic Hepatitis C. Hepatology 2002; 36: S35-S46.

5 Seeff LB, Miller RN, Rabkin CS, Buskell-Bates Z, Straley Eason KD, Smoak BL, Johnson LD, Lee SR, Kaplan EL: 45 Year follow up of hepatitis C virus infection in healthy young adults. Ann Int Med 2000; 132: 105-111.

6 Seeff LB, Buskett-Bates Z, Wright E et al: Long-term mortality after transfusion associated non A, non B hepatitis. N Engl Jnl Med 1992; 327: 1906-1911.

7 Seeff LB: Natural History of Chronic Hepatitis C. Hepatology 2002; 36: S35-S46.

8 Kenny-Walsh E for the Irish Hepatology Research Group: Clinical outcomes after hepatitis C infection-from contaminated anti D immune globulin. N Engl Jnl Med 1999; 340: 1228-1233.

9 Wiese M, Berr F, Lafrenz M, Porst H, Olsen V: Low frequency of cirrhosis in a hepatitis C (genotype 1b) single source outbreak in Germany: a 20 multicenter study. Hepatology 2000; 32: 91-96.

10 Rodger AJ, Roberts S, Lanigan A, Bowden S, Brown T, Crofts N: Assessment of long term outcomes of community – acquired hepatitis C infection in a cohort with sera stored from 1971-1975. Hepatology 2000; 32: 582-587.

11 Victorian HCV: Lookback Steering Committee Transfusion-associated hepatitis C (HCV) lookback: lessons from a state-wide donor-targeted program in Victoria Draft report.

12 Strasser SI, Watson KJR, Lee CS et al: Risk factors and predictors of outcome in an Australian cohort with hepatitis C infection. Med J Aust 1995; 162: 355-358.

13 Dike AE, Christie JML, Kurtz JB, Teo C-G: Hepatitis C in blood transfusion recipients identified at the Oxford Blood Centre in the national HCV lookback programme. Trans Med 1998; 8: 87-95.

14 The English National Blood Service HCV Lookback Collation Collaborators: Transfusion transmission of HCV infection prior to anti-HCV testing of blood donations in England: results of the national HCV lookback programme. Transfusion 2002 Sep; 42 (9): 1146-1153.

15 Ismay SL, Thomas S, Fellows A et al: Post transfusion hepatitis revisited. Med Jnl Aust 1995; 163: 74-77.

16 Seeff LB: Natural History of Chronic Hepatitis C. Hepatology 2002; 36: S35-S46.

17 Ismay SL, Thomas S, Fellows A et al: Post transfusion hepatitis revisited. Med Jnl Aust 1995; 163: 74-77.

18 Blajchman MA, Bull SB, Feinman SV: Post-transfusion hepatitis: impact of non-A, non-B hepatitis surrogate tests. Lancet 1995; 345: 21-21.

19 Cossart YE, Kirsch S, Ismay SL: Post-transfusion hepatitis in Australia: report of the Australian Red Cross study. Lancet 1982; 319: 208-213.

20 Ismay SL, Thomas S, Fellows A et al: Post transfusion hepatitis revisited. Med Jnl Aust 1995; 163: 74-77.

21 Wong P-Y, Dodd R, Keily P, Carroll C, Whyte G: Characteristics of hepatitis positive blood donors in Victoria, Australia. Transfusion Medicine 1999; 9:15-19.

22 Seef LB: Natural History of Chronic Hepatitis C. Hepatology 2002; 36: S35-S46.

23 Rodger AJ, Jolley D, Thompson SC, Lanigan A, Crofts N: The impact of diagnosis of hepatitis C on quality of life. Hepatology 1999; 30: 1299-1301.

24 Vogt M, Lay T, Frosner G, Klingler C, Sendl AF, Zeller A, Wiebecke B et al. Prevalence and clinical outcomes of hepatitis C infection in children who underwent cardiac surgery before the implementation of blood donor screening. N Engl Jnl Med 1999; 341: 866-870.

25 Freeman AJ, Dore GJ, Low MG, Thorpe M, Van Overhede J, Lloyd AR, Marinos G et al: estimating progression to cirrhosis in chronic hepatitis C virus infection. Hepatology 2001; 34: 809-816.

26 Bennett WG, Inoue Y, Beck JR, Wong JB, Pauker SG, Davis GL: Estimates of the cost-effetiveness of a single course of interferon alpha 2b in patients with histologically mild chronic hepatitis C. Ann Int Med 1997; 127: 855-865.

27 LaMont JT, Koff RS, Isselbacher KJ: Cirrhosis Harrison's Principles of Internal Medicine. (10th ed) McGraw-Hill 1983:1807.

28 Australian National Council on AIDS and related diseases, Hepatitis C sub-committee Hepatitis C virus projections working group: Estimates and projections of the hepatitis C virus epidemic in Australia August 1998 National Centre in HIV Epidemiology and Clinical Research.

29 Van der Poel CL, Cuypers HT, Reesink HW: Hepatitis C virus six years on. Lancet 1994; 334: 1475-1479.

30 Dore GJ, Kalsor JM, McGaughan GW: Systematic review of role of polymerase chain reaction in defining infectiousness among people infected with hepatitis C virus. Br Med Jnl 1997; 315: 333-337.

31 Alter HJ, Conry-Cantilena C, Melpolder J et al: Hepatitis C in asymptomatic blood donors. Hepatology 1997; 26 (3S): 29S-33S.

32 Soto B, Sanchez-Quijano A, Rodrigo L et al: Human immunodeficiency virus infection modifies the natural history of chronic parenterally-acquired hepatitis C with an unusually rapid progression to cirrhosis. J Hepatology 1997; 26: 1-5.

33 Tefler P, Sabin C, Devereux H et al: The progression of HCV-associated liver disease in a cohort of haemophiliac patients. Brit J Hepatol 1994; 87: 555-561.

34 Rodger A, Crofts N: The Macfarlane Burnet Centre for Medical Research Hepatitis C retrospective cohort study, 1998 Internal Technical Report. 1998 MBCMR.

35 Mattson L, Sonnerborg A, Weiland O: Outcome of acute symptomatic non-A, non-B hepatitis: a 13 year follow up of acute hepatitis C markers. Liver 1993; 13: 274-278.

36 Di Biscegle AM, Goodman ZD, Ishak KG et al: Long-term clinical and histological follow-up of chronic post-transfusion hepatitis. Hepatology 1991; 14: 969-974.

37 Hopf U, Moller B, Kuther D, et al: Long-term follow-up of post-transfusion and sporadic chronic hepatitis non-A, non-B and frequency of circulating antibodies to hepatitis C virus (HCV). Jnl Hepatology 1990; 10: 69-76.

38 Tremolada F, Casarin C, Alberti A et al: Long-term follow-up of non-A, non-B (type C) post-transfusion hepatitis. Jnl Hepatology 1992; 16: 273-81

39 Yano M, Kumada H, Kage M et al: The long -term pathological evolution of chronic hepatitis C. Hepatology 1996; 23: 1334-1340

40 Poynard T, Bedossa P, Opolon P: Natural history of liver fibrosis progression in patients with chronic hepatitis C. Lancet 1997; 349: 825-832.

41 Di Biscegle AM, Goodman ZD, Ishak KG et al: Long-term clinical and histological follow-up of chronic post-transfusion hepatitis. Hepatology 1991; 14: 969-974.

42 Tremolada F, Casarin C, Alberti A et al: Long-term follow-up of non-A, non-B (type C) post-transfusion hepatitis. Jnl Hepatology 1992; 16: 273-281.

43 Koretz RL, Abbey H, Coleman E, Gitnick G: Non-A, non-B post transfusion hepatitis; looking back in the second decade. Ann Int Med 1993; 119: 110-115.

44 Whyte GS: The transfused population of Canterbury, New Zealand, and its mortality. Vox Sanguinis 1988; 54: 65-70.

45 Vamvakas EC, Taswell HF: Long-term survival after blood transfusion. Transfusion 1994; 34: 471-477.

46 Australian Bureau of Statistics Causes of Death, Australia 1995 AGPS Canberra 1996.

Prof. G. Whyte, International Education Development Unit, Faculty of Medicine, Nursing and Health Sciences, Monash University, Victoria 3800, Australia.
E-mail: gordon.whyte@med.monash.edu.au

Dax EM, Farrugia A, Vyas G (eds): Advances in Transfusion Safety – Volume IV.
Dev Biol (Basel). Basel, Karger, 2007, vol 127, pp 215-224.

Is Haemovigilance Improving Transfusion Practice? – The European Experience

P.F.W. Strengers

Sanquin at CLB, Amsterdam, The Netherlands

Key words: Haemovigilance, transfusion practice, adverse events, Europe, European Haemovigilance Network.

Abstract: Improving transfusion practice for a donor means a safer donation process and maximal use of the donation. From the clinical perspective, it includes the production of the right type of blood component of adequate quality, administered at the right dose at the right moment to the right patient in order to obtain the expected or anticipated effect in absence of harm. Transfusion practice involves not only the complete blood chain, i.e. from the donation to clinical usage, but also the input from the competent authority that bears responsibility for the concepts of improving health care practice. In Europe, experience has shown that haemovigilance offers an effective tool in improving transfusion practice.

INTRODUCTION

Blood components and plasma derivatives are used for the treatment of a great number of hereditary and acquired diseases and are prescribed by almost all medical specialists. For a blood system to function well with high quality supply, an organised system for donor selection, blood drawing, safety and compatibility testing with a controlled production, and optimal clinical usage of blood products, including the vigilance for adverse events, is required. Like any other medical intervention, treatment with a blood product implies potential adverse reactions. Because the products are of a biological nature, the adverse reactions should be limited mainly to immunological reactions or infections with transfusion transmittable agents.

HAEMOVIGILANCE

The aim of haemovigilance is to detect and analyse all untoward effects of blood transfusion in order to correct their cause and to prevent recurrence, thus improving the safety of blood transfusion.

Haemovigilance has been defined as "a set of surveillance procedures covering the whole transfusion chain from the collection of blood and its components to the follow-up of its recipients, intended to collect and assess information on unexpected or undesirable effects resulting from the therapeutic use of labile blood products, and to prevent their occurrence and recurrence" [1]. Haemovigilance focuses on complications related to transfusion in donors and patients and includes failures in the production line, complications in donors related to blood donation, "near-miss" events, retrospective registration of unwanted events, and prospective action with early warning in a rapid alert system of new threats. The word haemovigilance is derived from the word pharmacovigilance, which encompasses activities and systems to collect information useful in supervising medicinal products with particular reference to adverse drug reactions in human beings, and to evaluate such information scientifically. Adverse reactions are defined as reactions that are harmful and unintended and that occur at doses normally used in man for prophylaxis, diagnosis or treatment or modification of physiological function(s). Haemovigilance concerns the follow-up of blood components: whole blood, red cell concentrates, platelets and plasma for transfusion (Fresh Frozen Plasma, FFP). Pharmacovigilance in transfusion medicine concerns clinical usage of the plasma derivatives, such as clotting factor concentrates, immunoglobulins, albumin and other fractionated products. In Europe, since January 1, 1993, plasma derivatives are considered to be pharmaceuticals, and the manufactures have to comply with the European regulations on pharmacovigilance [2].

Haemovigilance in Europe

Pioneer work on haemovigilance started in France in 1991 with the set up of monitoring systems by Blood Transfusion Committees, followed by the start of the Centre National d'Hémovigilance in 1992 [3]. On the European level, haemovigilance began three years later. The European Council published its Resolution of June 2, 1995, and a Communication on "Blood Safety and Self-Sufficiency in the Community," with the objective of improving public confidence in the safety of the blood supply. The word "haemovigilance" appeared in documents of the European Commission, and an invitation to tender was published to carry a feasibility project on the establishment of a haemovigilance network in the European Community. Three goals were identified for the project: identification of objectives, methods and means related to the establishment of a Community-wide haemovigilance network that would also serve to improve exchange of information between the Member States; promotion of co-operation between the Member States on the systematic monitoring of risks and hazards associated with blood collection and transfusion and provide guidance for this; and determination of measures that added value to the actions and measures of Members States and that needed to be proposed to the European Commission in order to enhance the safety of the blood chain. Four years later, the European Commission published the resulting report (the Haeman Report). Also in 1995, at the ISBT 5th Regional (4th European) Congress in Venice, Italy, the symposium "Haemovigilance procedures in Transfusion Medicine" was organised. The conclusion of this symposium was that haemovigilance should be considered as part of the quality assurance process in transfusion medicine. Collection of data, the key to quality assurance in medicine, was recognised as essential, but it was also recognized that not all data are equally important and that those which are really important should be given prominence [4]. In 1996, the European Commission organised at an informal meeting of Ministers of the European Commission in Adare, Ireland, a Colloquium on Blood, which resulted in the document "Blood Safety and Self-Sufficiency: an Agenda for the European Community." It covered six areas of action, including haemovigilance. Haemovigilance systems were then launched in a number of countries.

In 1997, the first European Seminar on Haemovigilance (EHS) was organised by the Agence Française du Sang in Bordeaux, France. In February 1998, this meeting resulted in the initiative to set up a European Haemovigilance Network (EHN), which subsequently gave rise to the organisation of EHN Seminars.

After 2000, the number of countries where haemovigilance systems were developed increased (Table 1), and the annual European Seminar on Haemovigilance served in some cases as a starting point for the haemovigilance organisation in a specific country. At the Seminars, results were presented on the organisation of haemovigilance systems (voluntary or compulsory), definitions, the required (type of) data, the data on adverse events related to blood donations, the data on the actual usage of blood components or on specific plasma derivatives like Anti (D) Immunoglobulin, material-vigilance, and the security of systems.

In the European Blood Directive (EU Blood Directive), adverse event reporting in transfusion medicine is mandatory, and the need for a common procedure for notifying serious adverse reactions and events and notification format is mentioned in three of the articles [5].

Article 14:

Traceability requires a unique identification system, and archiving of data in relation to full traceability must be guaranteed for at least 30 years.

Article 15:

1. Members States shall ensure that:

- any serious adverse events (accidents and errors) related to the collecting, testing, processing, storage and distribution of blood and blood components which may have an influence on their quality and safety, as well as any serious adverse reactions observed during or after transfusion which may be attributed to the quality and the safety of blood and blood components are notified to the competent authority,
- Blood establishments have in place a procedure accurately, efficiently and verifiably to withdraw from distribution blood or blood components associated with the notification referred to above.

2. These serious adverse events and reactions shall be notified in accordance with the procedure and notification format referred to in Article 29 (i).

Article 29:

The following technical requirements and their adaptation to technical and scientific progress shall be decided in accordance with the procedure referred to in Article 28 (2):

- (i) Community procedure for notifying serious adverse reactions and events and notifying format.

Table 1 : The haemovigilance systems in Europe [11].

2003	Germany	Austria	Belgium	France	Finland	Greece	Ireland	Luxem-burg	Norway	Nether-lands	Portugal	U.K.
Start of system	June 1994	January 2003	Under develop-ment	January 1994	Under develop-ment	November 1995	October 1999	January 1996	January 2004	January 2003		October 1996
Guidelines	yes	yes	EU Direct.	yes	yes	no	yes	yes		no	no	yes
Units distributed	5 million			2,587,581	400,000	951,611	169,688	31,928	192,470	709,947		3,399,988
Number of SAR	450			265	31	20				50		457
SAR / 1000 Units	0.09			0.10	0.07	0.02				0.7		0.13
Number of AR				7,619		319	155	9		1,092		
AR / 1000 Units				2.94		0.34	0.91	0.28		1.53		

SAR = Serious Adverse Reactions + Adverse Reactions.

After the issuing of the EU Directive in 2002, in 2005 two other directives have been published where the implementation of the EU Directive as regards to a quality system for blood establishments and the traceability requirements and notification of serious adverse reactions and events have been specifically addressed [6,7].

The focus within haemovigilance in the EU Blood Directives is product-related adverse events reporting. Reporting on complications in donors related to blood donations is included, as well as 'near-miss' events. Based on retrospective registration of unwanted events and prospective action with early warning in a rapid alert system of new threats, actions in order to improve transfusion practice should be taken. Most blood banks are producing blood components to be delivered to hospitals. They provide therapeutic advice but have no real insight in the actual use in clinical care. The usage of blood components is wide-spread in many different departments, administered for the treatment of the elderly, adults and children, and in a great number of clinical indications. Haemovigilance reports have clarified that most blood banks and blood transfusion centres are not taking part in regular transfusion medicine because of insufficient access to hospitals. Lack of feed-back can create dangerous situations for the production of safe blood components. By implementing the EU Blood Directive in national legislation, the national competent authorities have been forced to build structures in order to be able to inspect haemoviglance systems, and this has thus contributed to improvement of transfusion practice.

European Haemovigilance Network

The EHN has been set up in order to increase blood safety at a European level and to develop and maintain in Europe a common structure with regards to safety of blood and blood products [8]. Information on adverse events is being pooled, as well as epidemiological data collected systematically to evaluate differences between countries and to investigate the reasons for the differences. Material-vigilance of blood transfusion devices has been developed because it was recognised that specific devices were marketed in several EU countries at the same time, and reports were received that locally recalled devices were re-marketed elsewhere in Europe. An inventory in all countries showed that legislation and regulation in the field of haemovigilance was either non-existent or not equal. In Austria, France, Germany, Netherlands, Sweden and Switzerland, notification of adverse events to the authorities is mandatory. In Denmark, only notification of viral transmission by blood is required. Further, it was recognised that in a mandatory system, adverse events are not always reported and that underreporting exists.

In order to improve communication, EHN exchanges valid information between members, increases rapid alert and/or early warning between the members, encourages joint activities between the members, and undertakes educational activities. EHN assists in standardisation of processes and forms by developing common "mother" matrixes, assists in the compilation and analysis of European data generated by national systems, and assists in the implementation of the European Blood Directive.

The EHN has developed forms for a Rapid Alert/Early Warning System (RAS) and for Adverse Reactions to blood component transfusion reporting in order to standardise the information process needed to take appropriate action, and aiming to implement a single format for documents to report adverse events in all European haemovigilance systems. The objective of RAS is to enable corrective actions to be taken in the shortest periods of time. RAS is being used for signalling the appearance of clusters of clinical signals after transfusion, hidden or apparent defects of disposable materials such as leakage of filter housings, holes in blood bags, defects in aphaeresis material and problems with equipment. RAS has allowed quick and safe transmission of correct and precise data to the persons responsible for quality assurance in blood transfusion centres and to competent authorities.

The report Form for Adverse Reaction to Blood Component Transfusion was developed by EHN to assist in the investigation of the clinical adverse event in order to define the course of action and to try to define the adverse event in the treatment (in most cases complex) of the patient involved.

As a tool for optimal connection and information exchange, the Internet website www.ehn-org.net has been developed with two zones of information, a public domain with general information on blood transfusion organisations, data on donors, data on donations, data on blood components, and a protected domain with the Rapid Alert System. The Rapid Alert System, where only one person per country has access, is used for rapid dissemination of (emerging) threats, detecting clusters of adverse events, and for material-vigilance.

Adverse Events after Transfusion

For some years, a number of reports have been published on the occurrence of adverse events after transfusion, including transfusion-associated deaths. The risk of the occurrence of an adverse event, absolutely or relatively based on the number of actual cases divided by the number of units of blood products issued or transfused, is low compared to other medical interventions. However, from the public and the medical-scientific point of view, the perception of risk related to blood is quite different and not correlated with the actual magnitude of the risk. This difference might be explained by the history of transmissions of blood-borne viruses by blood transfusions and, in particular, by the social and legal consequences of these transmissions for patients and their relatives, and in some cases also for professionals in the field of blood transfusion and transfusion medicine and even politicians. Inadequate responses from blood transfusion establishments and lack of communication have contributed to this unfortunate situation. Already in 1990, it was advised that "management systems for transfusion facilities should be created (see Chapter xxx) or revised to include the specific identification of personnel eligible to administer transfusions, to provide written guidance and appropriate training, including recognition and management of errors, and to implement measures that target safe transfusion practice" [9].

If errors in the handling process with blood products in a hospital are occurring, the effect on the clinical outcome might be dramatic. Reports of transfusion incidents in the State of New York in 1990-2000 and in Annual Reports on Haemovigilance from a number of European countries like the United Kingdom, Ireland, France, and The Netherlands have shown that more than 40 % of the reported incidents were caused by administrative failures [10-14]. Of these administrative failures, 10-50 % was the result of a wrong blood drawing or of wrong identification of the blood sample. Errors in prescription, sampling and request were found in more than 25 % of the reported cases. In the blood centres themselves, the occurrence of distribution errors was rather small (2 %), in contrast to the hospital blood banks (31 %). These reports showed that wrongly identified blood samples are the most important source of blood transfusion incidents, and incorrect blood component transfusion is the main cause of morbidity and mortality.

Participation of hospitals in haemovigilance systems is relatively important, as shown by an analysis in the UK, where 53 % of the hospitals that reported an IBCT incident received 74 % of the blood supply [15]. Notification of side effects and/or incidents related to the clinical use of blood components has given information on the actual usage and on unwanted effects. Acute transfusion reactions (ATR), delayed transfusion reactions, transfusion associated Graft versus Host Disease, transfusion related acute lung injury (TRALI), post transfusion purpura, bacterial contamination, post transfusion viral infection, incorrect blood component transfusion (IBCT), autologous incidents and other events may occur after transfusion, but were not the main reason for mortality or morbidity. Analysed results from SHOT showed that almost 70 % of the reports concerned incorrect blood component transfusions (IBCT) as the main cause of adverse transfusion events (Fig. 1). ICBT is defined as the transfusion of a blood component that does not meet appropriate specifications or was intended for another patient.

In the period 1996-2004 there were 1,832 reports, including 20 deaths and 92 major morbidity events, which were all preventable. These results were not different from those in other countries like those collected in the DART system in Denmark. They showed that the problems are not isolated to one country alone and do not depend on the size of the blood programme [16] (Tables 2 and 3).

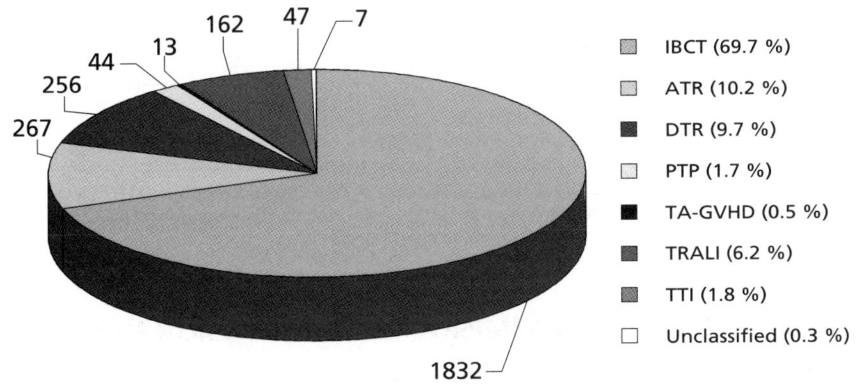

Fig 1: SHOT total analysed reports 1996-2004 (n = 2628) [13].

Table 2: Comparison of haemovigilance reported events (%) of two EU countries [14].

Reports (%)	**SHOT – U.K. (1996-2003)**	**DART – Denmark (1999-2003)**
IBCT	67	53
ATR	11	16
DTR	10	16
PTP	2	1
GVH	1	1
TRALI	7	9
TTI	2	4
Total numbers (%)	2080 (100)	105 (100)

IBCT: Incorrect Blood Component Transfusion; ATR: Acute Transfusion Reaction; DTR: Delayed Transfusion Reaction; PTP: Post Transfusion Purpura; GVH: Graft Versus Host reaction; TRALI: Transfusion Related Acute Lung Injury; TTI: Transfusion Transmitted Infections.

Table 3: Haemovigilance and clinical outcome (data from SHOT – U.K. 1996-2003 and DART – Denmark 1999-2003) [14].

	Death (percentage)		**Major morbidity (percentage)**	
	SHOT	DART	SHOT	DART
IBCT	18	50	34	33
ATR	11	0	2	37
DTR	9	25	9	0
PTP	2	0	5	3
GVH	14	25	0	0
TRALI	37	0	36	19
TTI	9	0	14	7
Total numbers (%)	90 (100)	4 (100)	249 (100)	27 (99)

IBCT: Incorrect Blood Component Transfusion; ATR: Acute Transfusion Reaction; DTR: Delayed Transfusion Reaction; PTP: Post Transfusion Purpura; GVH: Graft Versus Host reaction; TRALI: Transfusion Related Acute Lung Injury; TTI: Transfusion Transmitted Infections.

Haemovigilance and Improving Transfusion Practice

Haemovigilance has improved transfusion practice. The reports on the circumstances surrounding adverse events have increased understanding of the root causes. Failures occur mainly at the interface between the blood transfusion centre and the ward and are related to wrong patient data on samples, resulting in incorrect blood component transfusion. Educational programmes have started because of differences in cultures on wards and lack of education and knowledge of those giving the transfusion. Following cases of bacterial contamination, measures such as improved donor arm cleaning and not using the first 5 ml of the blood drawn from the donor have been more vigilantly practised. For prevention of further cases of TRALI, exclusion of implicated donors or the usage of FFP from only male donors has been introduced. In order to prevent cases of incorrect blood component transfusion, better identification of patients with improved control of the wrist band identifiers has been instituted. The role of hospital transfusion committees has been better defined, including the objectives to define transfusion policies according to hospital activities and proceeding to regular evaluations of the transfusion practices by analysing side effects of blood transfusion and by being more active in taking necessary measures in order to prevent them. In addition, technical aspects in the transfusion process have been improved, including improved quality follow-up of devices and reagents and organising meetings with the producers of these devices.

In particular, information concerning close incidents or near misses has been shown to be important. Owing to the morbidity following incorrect blood transfusion, general aspects of incidents, including the time of the incident, the usage of protocols, information on the circumstances under which blood was drawn, the procedures of proper identification checks, the number of persons in the room where the near incident happened and so on, were studied and subsequently improved.

In most blood transfusion centres, a single donation will be processed into different components, i.e. a unit of red cells, a unit of platelets, and a unit of Fresh Frozen Plasma, and these units might be divided or processed into more products with different specifications. The shelf life of these products is not the same, and therefore the time of actual use of the different products from the same donor may differ. In case the unit of platelets harms the recipient, due to a bacterial contamination for example, the introduction of a Rapid Alert/Early Warning system (RAS) that warns the blood transfusion centre or the ward of the hospital not to transfuse the unit of red cells or the unit of FFP prepared from the same donation because of the potential adverse reaction, which was detected during or after the transfusion of the first unit used, has been shown to be effective.

Safe incident reporting must be blame-free [17]. By creating a failures management culture where physicians and nurses are not afraid to report incidents and where reporting is not anonymous but is done in an atmosphere of confidence, transfusion practice is improved. In an open and transparent culture with the objective of reporting incidents in order to improve quality and safety, a change in culture can be made. It is important that the person who encountered the incident and who is often very disappointed because he/she has made a failure which could seriously harm the patient is consulted. Patient safety is partly a function of employer safety and partly of the improving processes.

Conclusion

Haemovigilance has an important function in safeguarding transfusion medicine. Errors have to be prevented, and improvement in the use of blood products might be achieved through an audit process based on simple indicators, providing the responsible clinicians with continuous feedback of results obtained. Twelve years ago, the Sanguis Study showed that in a three-year period such an audit programme reduced both excessive preoperative requesting and actual transfusion of red cell units and plasma in elective surgical patients by 22 %, 20 %, and 70 %, respectively [18].

Continuous feedback of data in laboratory medicine reduces excessive ordering of laboratory tests and other resources. More importantly, intensive "marketing" of accepted practice guidelines is required to produce changes in clinical transfusion practice.

Uniform Rapid Alert Forms and Adverse Reaction Forms are important means of communication for rapid dissemination of information on adverse events in blood transfusion. Fax, e-mail and the Internet are tools to be used to inform all parties involved and all parties that may benefit from this information. It has to be realised, however, that dissemination of this information may have legal consequences regarding privacy and liability if not handled with care. All players involved in a rapid alert are potentially prone to be held liable for any damage to one of or many of the parties involved. These legal aspects should be taken into account, but in no way should it hold back persons from taking the necessary measures to prevent the occurrence or recurrence of an adverse event.

References

1 Faber J-C: Haemovigilance around the world. Vox Sang 2002; 83 (suppl 1): 71-76.

2 Committee for Proprietary Medicinal Products: Guideline for competent authorities on the undertaking of pharmacovigilance procedures. (III/3963/92), EN, 1994.

3 Salmi R: Les supports épidémiologiques de l'hemovigilance. Transf Clin Biol 1994; 6: 421-424.

4 Strengers PFW, Heier H-E: Haemovigilance procedures in Transfusion Medicine, in Rossi U, Massaro AL, Sciorelli G (eds): Proceedings of the ISBT 5th Regional (4th European) Congress, 1997, p 953.

5 Directive 2002/98/EC of the European Parliament and of the Council of January 2003 setting standards of quality and safety for the collection, testing, processing, storage and distribution of human blood and blood components and amending Directive 2001/83/EC. Off Journal EU, L 33/30, 8.2.2003.

6 Directive 2005/61/EC of 30 September 2005 implementing Directive 2002/98/EC of the European Parliament and of the Council as regards traceability requirements and notification of serious adverse reactions and events. Off Journal EU, L 256/32, 1.10.2005.

7 Directive 2005/62/EC of 30 September 2005 implementing Directive 2002/98/EC of the European Parliament and of the Council as regards Community standards and specifications relating to a quality system for blood establishments. Off Journal EU, L 256/41, 1.10.2005.

8 Faber J-C: Haemovigilance in Europe: the European haemovigilance network. Transf Clin Biol 2001; 8: 285-290.

9 Sazama K: Reports of 355 transfusion-associated deaths: 1976 through 1985. Transfusion 1990; 30: 583-590.

10 Linden JV et al: A report of 104 transfusion errors in New York State. Transfusion 1992; 32: 601-606.

11 Serious hazards of transfusion (SHOT) Annual report 2003.

12 National Haemovigilance Office. Annual report 2003.

13 AFSSAPS. Rapport annuel Hémovigilance 2003.

14 TRIP rapport 2003.

15 Stainsby D, Jones H, Cohen H, Chapman J: 8 years of SHOT data 1996-2004: a view of transfusion safety in the UK. Vox Sanguinis 2005; 89 (1): 18-19.

16 Jorgensen J: The use of haemovigilance data to increase safety in transfusion. Vox Sanguinis 2005; 89 (1): 3.

17 Strengers PFW: Reporting of transfusion errors: ethics and risks. Vox Sanguinis 2005; 89 (1): 18.

18 Sirchia G, Giovanetti AM, McClelland B, Fracchia GN: Safe and Good Use of Blood in Surgery (Sanguis). European Commission, 1994.

Dr. P.F.W. Strengers, Sanquin at CLB, Plesmanlaan 125, NL-1006 AD Amsterdam, The Netherlands.
E-mail: p.strengers@sanquin.nl

Dax EM, Farrugia A, Vyas G (eds): Advances in Transfusion Safety – Volume IV.
Dev Biol (Basel). Basel, Karger, 2007, vol 127, pp 225-233.

Product Traceability and Lookback: Assuring the Integrity of the Transfusion Process

P. Flanagan

New Zealand Blood Service, Auckland, New Zealand

Key words: Traceability, lookback, materiovigilance, blood components, leucodepletion.

Introduction

The principle that each individual blood donation represents a unique batch in manufacturing terms has underpinned many of the systems developed to assure quality in blood product manufacture. The biological nature of the raw material, human blood or plasma, used to manufacture blood products and recognition of the propensity for transmission of infection reinforces the importance of being able to trace the fate of blood donations and the components or products derived from them. The concepts of traceability and lookback are natural consequences of these principles.

Whole blood is now used only rarely. The nature of blood component manufacture has changed significantly over the last decade. Increasingly, additional manufacturing steps are involved in the production of components. This may involve additive solutions or blood filters. The changing nature of production and improved understanding of the range of adverse effects associated with transfusion of blood products inevitably have an impact on the requirements of traceability. The existence of effective systems for traceability thus becomes a significant underpinning requirement for effective Materiovigilance and Haemovigilance.

Traceability

Blood Services are highly regulated organisations. Understanding of the requirements of traceability can be derived from standards developed by various regulatory authorities.

The Council of Europe Guide for the preparation, use and quality assurance of blood components (the Guide) includes lookback and traceability as part of Haemovigilance. A descriptive approach is used. The 11th Edition of the Guide [1] states that "Haemovigilance consists of the detection, gathering and analysis of information regarding untoward and unexpected effects of transfusion". It goes on to state that one of the key roles of haemovigilance involves "Warning hospitals and blood transfusion services about adverse events that could involve more individuals than a single recipient, including those related to the transmission of infectious diseases and those related to blood bags, solutions or blood processing". The Guide indicates that "traceability is the ability to identify the actual recipients of every component released and conversely the ability to identify all blood donors involved in the transfusion of a given patient".

The AABB Standards take a more prescriptive approach to defining the elements of information that must be included in traceability. The 22nd edition of the standards [2] defines requirements for identification and traceability of process or procedural steps, traceability of blood, components and tissues and general labelling requirements. Detail is provided in Table 1.

Table 1: AABB standards relating to identification and traceability.

Standard	Description
5.1.6.1 Process and procedure steps	For each critical step in collection, processing, compatibility testing and distribution of blood and blood components there shall be a mechanism to identify the individual performing the step and when it was performed
5.1.6.2 Traceability of blood, components and tissue	The blood bank or transfusion service shall ensure that all blood, components, tissue, derivatives and critical materials used in their processing, as well as laboratory samples and donor and patient records, are identified and traceable
5.1.6.3 General labelling requirements	The blood bank or transfusion service shall have a labelling process. This process shall include all steps taken to: 1) identify the original unit, any components, and any component modifications; 2) complete the required reviews; and 3) attach the appropriate labels

The Australian Therapeutics Goods Administration includes specific requirements in its Code of GMP for Blood and Tissues [3]. These are shown below.

Clause 600 The system should provide an unambiguous means of collating and providing confirmation of performance and traceability.

Clause 602 The record system must demonstrate that there is a complete history of the donation from the donor selection/registration to the release for use as a final product and should include:

- identification and traceability to all critical manufacturing steps;
- traceability to a location, including transportation between sites;
- accountability for records which have been withdrawn and archived.

Taken together, these three sources enable the definition of a framework for traceability. This extends beyond the classical approach of donor to donation to component and recipient to include the capture of critical materials and personnel involved in the manufacturing process. This is shown in Figure 1.

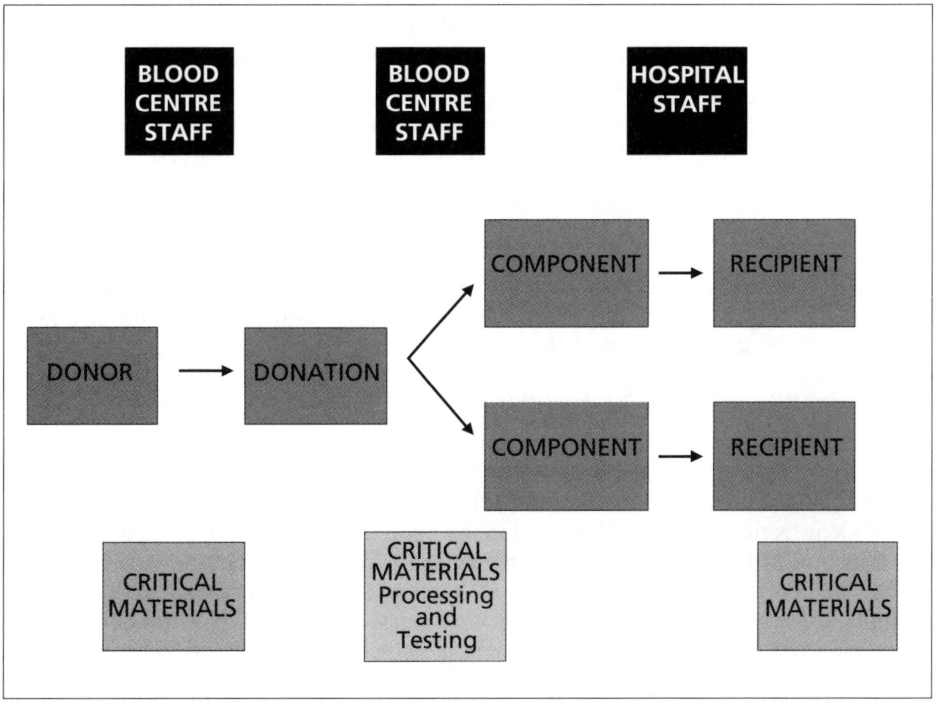

Fig. 1: A schematic approach to the definition of traceability.

Lookback and Notification

Effective traceability systems act as enablers for Lookback and Notification of recipients. Lookback is the process whereby information identified in one part of the traceability chain is used to investigate the possibility that patients might have been harmed by the transfusion process. Classically, this applied primarily to investigations of possible transfusion transmitted infection. More recently it has also been applied to improve overall understanding of non-infectious complications of transfusion of blood components.

Different types of lookback can be defined. One way to achieve this is by definition of the trigger for lookback (Table 2).

Table 2: Lookback definitions.

Lookback type	Description
Recipient triggered	Occurs in response to information provided by clinicians relating to the outcome of a transfusion e.g. Transfusion transmitted infection TRALI
Donor triggered	Occurs in response to information provided by or about a donor that might have influenced the decision to allow the individual to donate had it been known at the time e.g. Post donation information Results of donor assessment or test results found at subsequent donation
Institutionally triggered	Decision to notify or lookback triggered by a wider concern in relation to safety e.g. recent decision by UK authorities to notify donors whose donations were transfused to individuals who subsequently developed vCJD

The principles of lookback and traceability are well embedded in modern blood systems. Indeed, many of the recent successes in transfusion medicine are good examples of the effectiveness of these approaches.

Traceability and lookback and infectious hazards of transfusion

Traceability and lookback have contributed to our understanding of the threat posed to the blood supply by emerging infections. West Nile Virus (WNV) and Variant Creutzfeldt-Jakob disease (vCJD) are excellent examples of this.

WNV infection was first identified in the United States in 1999 [4]. The ability of the infection to be transmitted by transfusion of fresh blood components was confirmed in 2002 [5]. Recipient triggered lookback was used to establish the link. Patients, especially those with laboratory evidence of recent WNV infection within four weeks of receipt of a blood component transfusion, were identified by physicians and reported initially to blood collection agencies or state and local health departments. The blood collection agencies identified the donors of blood components transfused to the infected recipients. Other blood components derived from the same donations along with any remaining samples from the donation were retrieved and tested for evidence of WNV infection (WNV RNA and IgM). In the event that a donor was subsequently found to have been infected at the time of donation, recipients of other components derived from the donation were also followed up. The results of the study clearly confirmed that WNV was a transfusion transmissible infection. Rapid introduction of Nucleic Acid Testing (NAT) for WNV followed. Similar approaches were used to demonstrate that pooled NAT was only partially effective at reducing transmission of the agent. This led to the definition of protocols for implementation of single donation NAT during periods of high levels of infection.

Prevention of vCJD is another good example of the value of effective lookback systems. Variant CJD was first described in the United Kingdom in 1996. The UK authorities had a high index of suspicion that this infection might be transfusion transmissible. In 1977 an active surveillance system was established jointly by the United Kingdom CJD Surveillance Unit (UKCJDSU) and the UK National Blood Services [6]. The Transfusion Medicine Epidemiology Review (TMER) was set up as a two-way surveillance system. The aim of the system was to identify possible transfusion-associated vCJD infection. Donor and recipient triggered lookback approaches were put in place. In the forward study (donor triggered) the CJDSU notified Blood Services of individuals who had developed vCJD. Blood Service computer systems were scrutinized to identify if these individuals had donated blood. In the event that they had, the details of recipients of components derived from their donations were checked against the CJDSU database. In the reverse study (recipient triggered), the transfusion history of patients who developed vCJD was investigated. The Blood Service computer systems were interrogated to identify donors who had contributed to the transfusion. Details of the implicated donors were then checked against the CJDSU database.

To date, the TMER has identified two possible cases of transfusion-associated transmission of the disease. The first case reported in early 2004 [6] involved a recipient who developed symptoms of vCJD 6.5 years after receiving a transfusion of non-leucodepleted red cells donated by an individual 3.5 years before the donor developed symptoms of vCJD. The second case [7] raised a number of questions in relation to our understanding of the disease. The case involved a patient dying of a ruptured aortic aneurysm in 2004. The patient had no signs of neurological disease. The patient had received a transfusion of non-leucodepleted red cells in 1999. One of the donors subsequently developed vCJD some 18 months following the implicated donation. A post mortem examination was carried out on the recipient, identifying the presence of PrP^{Sc} in the spleen but not in the central nervous system. The case raises the possibility of either pre-clinical disease or an asymptomatic carrier state. This is of particular interest since the patient was found to be heterozygous at codon 129 whereas all symptomatic cases of vCJD to date have been methionine homozygotes.

During 2005 the UK authorities introduced a series of measures to inform recipients who are considered at risk of vCJD based on receipt of blood components derived from donors who subsequently developed vCJD. More recently, a similar approach has been taken with donors who have contributed to transfusion of patients who have subsequently developed the disease. Effective traceability systems underpin these initiatives, which are examples of institutional triggered lookback.

The recent availability of HBV DNA assays suitable for screening of blood donations has increased awareness of occult Hepatitis B infection. This involves individuals whose blood contains HBV DNA in the absence of hepatitis B surface antigen. Such assays have the potential to further reduce the risk of transfusion-associated hepatitis B infection. Interestingly, some donors with HBV DNA do not appear to transmit the infection to recipients of blood components [8]. Donor and recipient triggered lookback systems have the ability to improve our overall understanding of occult HBV DNA and the factors that determine transmissibility.

Traceability and lookback and non infectious hazards of transfusion

Transfusion Related Acute Lung Injury

Haemovigilance studies have identified that Transfusion Related Acute Lung Injury (TRALI) is one of the most significant complications of transfusion. Recipient triggered lookback systems are commonly used in investigation cases of TRALI, enabling identification of donors who are considered to be the likely source of the complication. Donor triggered lookback has also been used to increase our understanding of TRALI. This involves follow up of the recipients of components derived from donors who have been implicated in cases of TRALI. In one such study 103 patients who had received components from a donor implicated in a case of TRALI were followed [9]. The donor had multiple HLA antibodies. Review of case records of the recipients showed only one case of TRALI. Lookback investigations of this type will assist in gaining an improved understanding of the pathophysiology of this serious complication of transfusion.

Traceability and blood component manufacture

During the last five years a number of blood services have implemented universal leucodepletion of blood components. Pre-storage leucodepletion is a significant development in component manufacture. Systems have been developed to monitor the effectiveness of leucodepletion against defined specifications. The introduction of pre storage leucodepletion has not been without problems. In New Zealand, for example, problems have been identified with both filtration associated haemolysis and failure of leucodepletion i.e. a failure to meet the defined specification for residual leucocytes. Effective traceability systems will be essential in determining whether identified problems are manufacturer specific, batch specific or more unpredictable in nature.

Filtration induced haemolysis

Prompted by reports of haemolysis following the introduction of universal leucodepletion, Gyongyossi-Issa and co-workers undertook a study to investigate the level of haemolysis in leucodepleted versus non-leucodepleted red cell units [10]. The study indicated that the level of haemolysis seen in leucodepleted red cell units was less than that seen in non-leucodepleted units. They concluded that leucodepletion is beneficial for red cells and that it does not cause haemolysis or enhance fragility.

The New Zealand Blood Service (NZBS) introduced universal prestorage leucodepletion in 2000. In early 2003 problems were identified in pre-acceptance testing of a batch of Pall Whole Blood Packs. Sixteen of 52 units processed showed "visible haemolysis". Closer inspection also provided evidence of haemolysis in two further units from other batches. Initial investigation excluded centrifuges as the source of the problem. Validation of the implicated batch was stopped. The manufacturer was informed and an alternative batch provided. Further investigation by the manufacturer identified a mechanical, rather than biological, problem as the source of the haemolysis. This related to "intermittent flow restriction, possibly in association with an air-lock within the filter media" as the likely problem. The manufacturer introduced a "surrogate test" as an interim measure aimed at analysing a statistically selected proportion of bulk non-sterile filters to identify "any trending towards a longer filtration time or flow restriction".

In 2004 the Pall Corporation issued a voluntary recall of 24 batch numbers of the BPF4 Leukotrap filtration system. This is a stand-alone filter that is connected to blood packs during processing using a sterile docking procedure. The recall followed reports to the FDA of haemolysis of red cells and whole blood products following leucodepletion using the BPF4 High Efficiency Filter [11]. Investigation by

Pall identified an incidence of 0.27 %, a portion of which was related to older blood (> 15 days). Pall reported that several causal items were revealed during the investigation and process modifications were made. However, no single root cause was identified [12].

This is a good example of the difference between scientific studies where variables can be well controlled and traceability linked to routine blood component production that allows investigation to focus on system variables. Systems that work well in defined settings can perform poorly when external variables change.

Failure of leucodepletion

NZBS utilises the buffy coat method to manufacture platelet pools. Platelet pools are leucodepleted using the Pall Leucotrap filter on the Compomat processing system. The system has been in place since 2000 and had proved to be very reliable. In early 2005 a number of reports were received involving platelet pools failing routine quality control testing for residual white cell counts. NZBS has four processing sites. The problem was initially seen in one processing site, and later in a second site. At any one time at least two batches of any filter system will be in place. The two sites reporting the problem were using the same batch of filters. The other two sites had not identified problems.

Initial investigation identified no obvious cause for the problem. NZBS utilises the NWA Quality Analyst system for statistical process control (SPC) of residual white cell counts. Review of results of SPC for platelet pools demonstrated a gradual increase in recorded values for residual white cells over the previous two years (2003-2005) with an increasing number of "rule violations" recorded. Confidence reports provided by the NWA Quality Analyst software indicated that the process was moving out of control. In contrast, the data for 2000-2002 appeared to be stable and in control. Review of data identified similar results at all four processing sites indicating that it was not a batch-associated problem. Further investigation did not identify any change in the system that might explain the change in capability of the system. The manufacturer was informed. It was initially thought that the problem coincided with a change in filter assembly between Pall manufacturing sites. Interestingly, the National Blood Service in England was using the same filter batches. They had not noticed any problems. Pall reviewed the NZBS manufacturing system and recommended that the final filtration step in manufacture of the platelet pools be changed to stop the use of the Compomat and introduce manual filtration. This resulted in a significant improvement in system performance. Further investigation then identified that the settings on the Compomat processors were suboptimal. The platelet pool was being filtered too quickly, resulting in the lack of system capability. The Compomat settings were modified to reflect those used in the English National Blood Service. Automated processing was re-introduced with excellent results. Further review identified that the manufacturer had set the Compomat settings in 2000 when prestorage leucodepletion was initially introduced. These had been modified overseas as the filter systems developed. However, no changes had been made in New Zealand.

Filtration failure

New Zealand is a long, thin country. Weather patterns are markedly different in the upper North Island (sub-tropical) from those in the lower South Island where more extreme conditions arise. Whole blood destined for processing is normally transported by road in temperature monitored storage containers. Recurrent reports of filtration failure have been identified in the lower South Island. The problem relates specifically to NPBI whole blood filtration systems in the colder winter months. The problem is seen with all batches of the product. In extreme situations up to 10 % of units fail to pass through the filter. This appears to relate to prolonged, slow cooling of the units during transportation. Nevertheless, the temperature specification for transportation is met. Pall filtration systems appear to work satisfactorily in this environment. The problem is sufficiently problematic to avoid use of the NPBI system during the colder winter months. Considerable effort has been devoted to working with the manufacturer to address the problem. The filter could be modified to improve flow. However, this is likely to lead to increased levels of leucodepletion failure.

Lessons learned from prestorage leucodepletion

The introduction of prestorage leucodepletion marked a significant change to routine component production. Previously, routine component manufacture utilised simple centrifugation and application of controlled pressure to achieve separation of components. Prestorage leucodepletion introduces a more complex variable into the system. Experience has shown that the filtration systems currently available are heavily influenced by environmental factors and processing variables. The above examples amply demonstrate this. Manufacturers strive to improve their systems. Changes to individual filtration systems are validated prior to routine introduction. Validation studies often rely on relatively small numbers of units in well-controlled conditions. The challenges posed by routine component production are, however, very different. Changes in environmental conditions and processing methods can have a significant impact on filtration system performance. Close scrutiny of system performance is necessary to ensure that it remains capable and in control. Traceability is essential to support thorough investigation of incidents as they occur. In order to be maximally effective, traceability needs to extend beyond the traditional donor to donation to recipient approach. It needs to encompass environmental monitoring and materiovigilance. Collaborative efforts between manufacturers and blood services will be needed to ensure thorough and effective investigation of incidents as they occur.

Future developments in component production are likely to lead to increasingly complex manufacturing processes. The availability of new technologies such as pathogen reduction systems and prion filters provide opportunities to manufacture potentially better and safer components. Effective systems for Lookback and traceability will be increasingly necessary to ensure that incidents can be fully evaluated and potential adverse effects of the technologies quickly identified. In this context the introduction of prestorage leucodepletion might be seen as the "coming of age" of component production. Lessons learned from this provide an opportunity to improve systems to support introduction of future technologies.

Concluding Comments

Lookback and traceability systems have played important roles in improving our understanding of both manufacturing and clinical issues in transfusion medicine. Further development of these systems will assist in ensuring the overall safety of blood components and of clinical transfusion systems.

References

1 Guide to the preparation, use and quality assurance of blood components. Strasbourg. Council of Europe Publishing, 11th Edition, 2005.

2 AABB Standards for Blood banks and Transfusion Services 22nd edition, 2003.

3 Australian Code of Good Manufacturing Practice – Human Blood and Tissues, 2000. http://www.tga.gov.au/docs/html/gmpbltic.htm

4 Dodd RY: Emerging Infections, Transfusion Safety and Epidemiology. New England Journal of Medicine 2003; 349: 1205-1206.

5 Pealer LN, Marfin AA, Petersen LR, Lanciotti RS, Page PL, Stramer SL, Stobierski DVM, Kimberley Signs DVM, Newman B, Kapoor H, Goodman JL, Chamberland ME: Transmission of West Nile Virus through Blood Transfusion in the United States in 2002. New England Journal of Medicine 2003; 349: 1236-1245.

6 Llewelyn CA, Hewitt PE, Knight RSG, Amar K, Cousens S, Mackenzie J, Will RG: Possible transmission of variant Creutzfeldt-Jakob disease by blood transfusion. The Lancet 2004; 363: 417-421.

7 Peden AH, Head MW, Ritchie DL, Bell JE, Ironside JW: Preclinical vCJD after blood transfusion in a PRNP codon 129 heterozygous patient. The Lancet 2004; 264: 527-529.

8 Flanagan P, Charlewood R, Horder R, Dravitsky M, Hollis H: Reducing the risk of transfusion transmitted hepatitis B in New Zealand. Vox Sanguinis 2005; 89 (Supp 2): 23.

9 Toy P, Hollis-Perry KM, Jun J, Nakagawa M: Recipients of blood from a donor with multiple HLA antibodies: a lookback study of transfusion related acute lung injury. Transfusion 2004; 44: 1683-1688.

10 Gyongyossy-Issa MIC, Weiss SL, Sowemino-Coker SO, Garcez RB, Devine DV: Prestorage leucoreduction and low-temperature filtration reduce hemolysis of stored red cell concentrates. Transfusion 2005; 45: 90-96.

11 FDA Announcement www.fda/cber/safety/pallhem121004.htm Potential Haemolysis in Red Blod Cells and Whole Blood Leukocyte Reduced Products Manufactured with the Pall BPF4 Filter.

12 AABB Regulatory Update June 2005. Pall Reports Decline in Hemolysis Associated with Filtration System.

Dr. Peter Flanagan, New Zealand Blood Service, Auckland, New Zealand.
E-mail: peter.flanagan@nzblood.co.nz

Dax EM, Farrugia A, Vyas G (eds): Advances in Transfusion Safety – Volume IV.
Dev Biol (Basel). Basel, Karger, 2007, vol 127, p 235.

SESSION VII

Emerging Risks and their Communication

Chair: *A. Farrugia*

Dax EM, Farrugia A, Vyas G (eds): Advances in Transfusion Safety – Volume IV.
Dev Biol (Basel). Basel, Karger, 2007, vol 127, pp 237-248.

Emerging Infections and Global Blood Safety

R.Y. Dodd

Research and Development, American Red Cross, Holland Laboratory, Rockville, MD, USA

Key words: Emerging infections, blood transfusion, safety, human behavior, international.

" We have met the enemy, and he is us " – Pogo (Walt Kelly)

INTRODUCTION

The broad concept of emerging infections developed when it became apparent that victory against infectious diseases had not been achieved. In the context of blood safety, it is also true that, at least in the developed world, the major transfusion-transmissible diseases are almost completely under control, but that emerging infections offer an increasing threat. The most dramatic of the emerging infections to affect blood safety in the past 25 years was undoubtedly HIV/AIDS. This outbreak resulted in profound changes in the way that blood safety was regarded and managed – perhaps the silver lining in this terrible cloud. More subtly, however, it generated an assumption that future transfusion-transmissible infections would have similar properties: a prolonged blood borne stage and a predominantly parenteral and/or sexual transmission route. To date, this prediction has proven largely unfounded. Indeed, the biggest unexpected outbreak of transfusion transmitted infection in the past few years has involved an acute, mosquito-borne infection that primarily affects birds: namely, West Nile virus.

EMERGING INFECTIONS

There are a number of factors that underlie the emergence of any given infectious disease, although a broad common theme is that emergence ultimately results from some perturbation of an ecological balance, brought about by human behaviors (Table 1). In the context of transfusion-transmissible infections, emergence has

Table 1 : Human behaviors potentially involved with emergence of selected infectious agents.

Agent	Behavior
HIV	Bush meat, sexual behavior, travel
Malaria	Global climate change, travel
Chagas' disease	Population migration
West Nile virus	Unknown (travel ?), irrigation practice
SARS	Exotic diet ? Air travel
Monkeypox	Exotic pets
vCJD	Intensive agricultural practice and export of feed, cattle
LCMV	Non-exotic pets
Leishmania	Military adventures

been a consequence of factors that include: the appearance of an infection new to humans, infections imported from other locations, infections that are expanding in their range, and infections that are reappearing in areas from which they had previously been eliminated. Outside the field of transfusion, a number of infections are emerging as a result of the appearance of drug-resistant strains, and it could perhaps be argued that the development of mutants that evade screening tests might be a comparable phenomenon in the field of blood safety. Fortunately, although such mutants or variants do exist, they have had only a minor impact on blood safety to date. Two other circumstances deserve comment, although they do not truly reflect emergence. The first is the recognition of existing but previously unknown or uncharacterized infectious agents as a result of new technology. Recent examples include the human herpes viruses 6, 7 and 8 and the GBV-C and SEN-V/TTV agents. Although only recently recognized, it seems likely that all of these viruses have been endemic in human populations for hundreds or perhaps even thousands of years. The other circumstance is the extent to which aggressive (and particularly immunosuppressive) therapies may exacerbate the effects of infection with normally benign agents, such as CMV.

Elements of a Program

There should be effective programs to manage the threat of emerging infections to blood safety. Such programs should include mechanisms to identify agents that may impact the blood supply and to assess their overall relevance. Such evaluations have two major dimensions. The first is the actual risk to patients, involving the likely frequency of transmission of the agent and severity and treatability of the resultant disease. The second dimension is that of public concern, which is not necessarily congruent with risk itself. It might be argued, for example, that the response to vCJD has been disproportionate to the overall public health risk to blood recipients, although it must be acknowledged that it is really not possible to define the actual risk at this time. In any event, this raises the next point, which is that, if possible, there should be some attempt to measure the actual risk of transmission of the agent in question. This could be done by performing prevalence studies on the donor population, for example. Ideally, this may also provide an opportunity to evaluate an appropriate intervention. The intervention could then be implemented, but there should be provision for evaluation of its efficacy and its subsequent modification or elimination.

HIV

It is generally accepted that HIV originated as a simian virus that entered human populations in Africa. It is not known exactly how this happened, but a plausible hypothesis is that it could have been a result of the preparation of so-called bushmeat from wild primates. Thereafter, the virus was likely transmitted person-to person by sexual routes. In the US and some other developed nations, there was rapid spread through networks of highly mobile and sexually active homosexual men, whereas in many less-developed countries, the predominant transmission route appears to be heterosexual. Although the infection likely moved from continent to continent as a result of travel by infected individuals, it seems possible that in some cases, it was actually introduced through clotting factor concentrates. In the US, about 2 % of all AIDS cases in the early years of the epidemic were attributable to transmission by blood transfusion, but this source was rapidly minimized by the use of serologic tests for HIV antibodies to screen blood donations. In fact, from the perspective of transfusion safety, HIV can no longer be considered to be an emerging infection in the developed world. However, the epidemic continues to expand in many parts of the world, notably sub-Saharan Africa, Southeast Asia, India and some of the former Soviet Republics. At least at the end of 2002, not all countries were testing all their blood for HIV, and one reportedly did not test any [1]. Unfortunately, the areas with the highest prevalence of HIV infection are frequently also those with the lowest available resources.

HBV

HBV is not regarded as an emerging infection. In fact, in many locations, its incidence is declining, in large part due to successful vaccination programs. In addition, serologic tests for HBsAg have achieved a very high level of sensitivity and, in parts of the developed world, nucleic acid testing (NAT) for HBV DNA is in place or is under consideration. In the developed world, in some areas of low HBV prevalence, testing for anti-HBc is used, further reducing transfusion associated transmission risk. However, in many other parts of the world, there is a very high prevalence of HBV infection, which is maintained in the population by both vertical and horizontal transmission. This is exacerbated by the high likelihood of persistent infection among those with neonatal infections. An issue of potential concern is the apparently increasing frequency of vaccine escape mutants of HBV. Some of these mutants generate HBsAg that cannot be detected by all currently available serologic tests. However, tests that are appropriately configured with multiple capture and detection antibodies are less affected by the mutants.

HCV

It is also clear that HCV is really not an emerging infection at this time. However, as with HIV and HBV, its prevalence and incidence rates do vary by region. In some cases, the reasons are known – for example, the very high prevalence in Egypt has been attributed to a schistosomiasis control program that was based upon inappropriate injection procedures [2]. It is unfortunate that the high cost of HCV tests have limited their availability and use in areas of highest need. The current risk for these agents in the US is presented in Table 2.

Table 2: Prevalence, incidence and risk of transfusion-transmissible infections among American Red Cross blood donors over the two-year period 2000-2001*.

	Prevalence among first-time donors (n = 3.055 million)		Incidence among repeat donors (4.182 million person-years)		
	Number confirmed positive	**Rate per hundred thousand**	**Number confirmed positive**	**Rate per hundred thousand person-years**	**Risk of infectivity per donation**
HBsAg	2229	72.9	53	1.27	1: 144,000
HCV	9420	308.3	79	1.90	1: 1,390,000
HIV	313	10.2	65	1.55	1: 1,525,000
HTLV	299	9.8	10	0.24	1: 2,230,000

* Adapted from [3,4].

Malaria

Malaria is a parasitic disease, caused by an intraerythrocytic protozoan parasite of the genus *Plasmodium*. Four species affect humans. The disease is transmitted by mosquitoes and is prevalent throughout the tropics. Each year, there are 300 to 500 million cases, although some authorities suggest that the number may actually be almost twice as great. Most cases occur in Africa. There are some 1.5 to 2.7 million deaths each year. The parasite is readily transmitted from affected individuals by transfusion of blood. In non-endemic areas, the transmission of malaria is controlled mainly by deferring donors who have traveled to endemic areas, a policy that is quite effective. For example, in the United States, there are about 1000 cases of imported malaria each year, but usually there are 2 or fewer transfusion-transmitted cases [5]. However, the deferral policy results in the unnecessary rejection of large numbers of donors – perhaps as many as 100,000 each year in the US. The problem is greater in some other countries, and a policy of testing deferred donors for malaria antibodies has been implemented in some countries such as England and Australia. Those donors with a positive travel history but a negative serological test may be permitted to donate.

Although malaria is not strictly an emerging infectious disease, it has the potential to reemerge in locations that had previously eliminated it. It is already apparent that malaria is occurring at greater elevations, probably due to global warming. In order to transmit the parasite, mosquitoes need to survive for a defined amount of time, which requires a particular temperature. There is also concern that the parasite could be reintroduced into countries such as the US. Indeed, there have been quite a number of cases of mosquito-borne malaria in the US that are not readily explained. If such cases were to increase in number, or were to form a nexus for epidemic spread, then current methods for protecting the US blood supply would be ineffective.

Babesia

Babesia is another intraerythrocytic protozoan parasite. Although various species of babesia are globally distributed, reported cases of transmission by transfusion are confined almost exclusively to the US, where well over 50 such cases have been recorded. A single case of transfusion transmission has been reported from Japan [6]. In the US, *B. microti* infects mice and deer and is transmitted by Ixodes ticks. Humans are an accidental host. The agent is defined as emerging because its geographic range is increasing. In addition, humans are being exposed more frequently as a result of their choices for housing locations. Many individuals are choosing to live in outer suburbs in areas that are encroaching on the habitat of wild deer. Additionally, in many areas, the deer themselves are multiplying with little to restrict them. Currently, *B. microti* is endemic in coastal districts of the Northeastern United States and in the upper Midwest, specifically Wisconsin and Minnesota. However, other piroplasms have been isolated in Missouri (MO1) and in California and Washington (WA1). The latter has also been shown to be transmissible by transfusion. In Connecticut, the seroprevalence rate for *B. microti* among blood donors is about 1.5 % [7]. It has been shown that individuals can be parasitemic and thus infectious for relatively long periods – six months in some cases. In some areas of Connecticut, the demonstrable risk of transfusion transmission is approximately one case per 1800 units [8]. Although the disease is usually relatively mild and treatable, it is more severe in the aged, those who are immunocompromised, and particularly, those who are asplenic. There have been a number of deaths attributable to transfusion transmitted babesiosis. Currently, there is little available in the way of an intervention. There is no readily accessible serologic test, and there is no effective strategy for questioning donors to identify risk of exposure. In fact, although it might be anticipated that a history of tick bites would correlate with babesia infection, this is not the case [9]. This is probably because Ixodes ticks are very small, and because those who recognize that they have been bitten probably remove the tick during the grace period prior to transmission of the parasite.

Chagas' Disease

Chagas' disease is caused by the protozoan parasite *Trypanosoma cruzi*. The parasite occurs in the continental Americas between latitudes 40°S and 40°N. However, the conditions that are conducive to transmission to humans are generally found only in Latin America. The parasite normally infects a wide range of mammals and is transmitted to humans by the bite of infected reduvid bugs. The parasite is present in high titer in the bug's feces, which are shed as the bug takes a blood meal. The affected individual is infected as he or she accidentally rubs the feces into the bite site or the mucous membranes. The bug lives in cracks, crevices and roofing of substandard housing and usually bites at night. Many infections occur in childhood, either through being bitten or by maternal-child transmission. Most infected individuals develop a lifelong chronic infection, which may result in serious or fatal cardiac or digestive tract disease, as the parasite has an affinity for smooth muscle. While acute disease may be treatable with investigational drugs, chronic infections are not responsive to treatment. Chronically infected individuals have antibodies to the parasite, but studies using PCR and parasite culture indicate that about 60 % of seropositive individuals are parasitemic and therefore potentially infectious [10]. Data from South America suggest that 12 % to 49 % of recipients of blood from an infected donor will themselves become infected.

Chagas' disease is regarded as an emerging infection in non-endemic countries, despite successful efforts to control it in Latin America. It is recognized that such efforts (based largely on the use of insecticidal sprays in affected housing) cannot be completely effective because of the natural sylvatic cycle of the vector insect. The basis for the emergence of Chagas' disease in countries like the USA is population movement. Because infection is lifelong and often occurs in childhood, members of immigrant populations may be silently infected. Such individuals may transmit their infection via blood transfusion or vertically from mother to child. In the US, the prevalence rates of *T. cruzi* antibodies among blood donors are relatively high in cities with Hispanic populations, and prevalence rates in Los Angeles have progressively increased among donors as a result of increased Hispanic representation in the donating population [11]. There have been relatively few (7) reported cases of transfusion-transmitted Chagas disease in the US and Canada, although such cases are poorly recognized. Indeed, in one case, the transmission was only recognized because an exposed patient was carefully followed up [12].

The most effective intervention to prevent the transmission of *T. cruzi* by transfusions is by the use of serologic testing. Such testing is routinely performed in many countries in Latin America, although it is generally accepted that most tests are insensitive and, therefore, two tests are often used additively. At the time of writing (end of 2005), no test is licensed by the FDA for donor screening in the US, although major manufacturers are developing and clinically evaluating such tests. It seems likely that only a single test will be used in the US. Another strategy that has been used in countries at risk of infection through transfusion is to rely on a travel history, followed by testing only those donors who have had exposure risk. However, it is clear that risk questions for exposure to *T. cruzi* are neither sensitive nor specific [11,13].

Leishmania

Again, Leishmania is not generally regarded as an emerging infectious agent, but there are circumstances that have brought it to the attention of the transfusion medicine community. A variety of Leishmania species are found throughout tropical areas of the world. In general, there is little evidence for transmissibility by conventional blood transfusion, although there have been a small number of reports. Concern about the potential for transfusion-transmission originally arose in the US as a result of an unusual visceral presentation of *L. tropica* among troops deployed in conflict areas in Persian Gulf countries in 1990-91 [14]. The reaction was to defer individuals who had been in the conflict area until a specific future date. Once this date passed, no further action was taken. During the second Gulf conflict, there was a high incidence of Leishmania among troops and others deployed to Iraq and Afghanistan. A limited deferral for all returnees from Iraq was implemented. No specific action was taken with respect to Afghanistan, since the affected areas are also malarious and returnees would be deferred according to routine practices.

West Nile Virus

Perhaps one of the most dramatic examples of an emerging infection has been the outbreak of West Nile virus (WNV) in the US. It is a mosquito-born flavivirus that is endemic in parts of Africa, Southern Europe and the Middle East. Prior to 1999, this virus had been absent from the Western Hemisphere. However, during that year, there was a relatively small outbreak in Queens, New York. In the following two years, the virus spread up and down the entire East Coast of the US, although there were relatively few human cases. In 2002, there was an explosive outbreak, with over 4000 human cases occurring across the US as far West as the Rocky Mountains [15]. During that year, 23 well-documented cases of transfusion-transmission of the virus occurred, although there were undoubtedly many more infections by this route [16]. This led directly to the rapid development and implementation of NAT for WNV RNA, which was in place by the beginning of the WNV season in 2003, a year with a record number of cases [17]. By 2005, the virus had been found in humans, birds, mammals or mosquitoes in every one of the continental states and in much of southern Canada. It was also present in Mexico and some of the Caribbean islands.

The actual source of this extraordinary outbreak is unknown. The strain of virus occurring in the US was very closely related to one that was isolated in Israel in 1998. There has been speculation that the virus entered the US via import of an infected exotic bird. It is unlikely that the virus was introduced by an infected human, as the levels of viremia are not adequate to sustain mosquito transmission from mammals. In any event, it seems likely that the infection was brought as a result of rapid air transportation. In the US, the outbreak has been remarkable for its size and rapid spread and for the number of humans that have been infected (estimated to be many hundreds of thousands). In part, this may be due to the absence of any inherent immunity among human or avian populations. It has also been suggested that mosquito behavior in the US may differ from that elsewhere with respect to the number and density of species that habitually bite both birds and humans. It also appears that, in some parts of the US, irrigation practices may have favored extensive mosquito breeding, and apparently numerous untended swimming pools had the same effect in parts of Arizona.

With respect to transfusion transmission, WNV challenged the concept that such transmission was largely confined to agents with a prolonged asymptomatic carrier state. WNV causes an acute disease and there is only a short period (around one to two weeks) when virus circulates in the blood at a relatively high titer. Some other acute infections are known to be transmitted by transfusion (for example, hepatitis A and E viruses), but this is uncommon. What differed for WNV was the overall size of the epidemic – in fact, although there were 23 well-authenticated cases of transfusion-transmitted WNV in 2002, there were also thought to have been over 400,000 human infections. The intervention, which has proven to be highly successful, was the implementation of NAT for WNV RNA. This was only possible because the blood providers in the US had already implemented NAT for HIV and HCV. The transfusion community's response to WNV is described in much greater detail elsewhere in this volume (Stramer SL, pp. 43-58).

HHV-8

Human herpesvirus-8 (HHV-8), also called Kaposi's sarcoma-associated herpesvirus (KSHV), is perceived as an emerging virus largely because of its association with HIV. As indicated above, it is a virus that, although only recently characterized, has probably affected humans for hundreds of years. It is a herpesvirus that is known to be the causative agent of Kaposi's sarcoma (a condition first described in 1872). The classical and endemic forms of Kaposi's sarcoma occur around the Mediterranean in Jewish individuals (mostly men) of Eastern European origin, and in Africa. Epidemic Kaposi's sarcoma is found among individuals with AIDS: within that population, it appears to be transmitted mainly by male to male sex. The virus has been shown to be transmitted by organ transplantation [18], and elevated prevalence rates for antibodies to the virus have been found among some intravenous drug users [19] and populations of blood recipients [20,21]. At the time of writing, there has been no direct evidence of transfusion transmission, although unpublished studies in Africa may demonstrate such transmission. There continues to be a concern about this possibility. Currently, there is no satisfactory serologic test for HHV-8 infection, but it seems likely that the risk of transfusion transmission might be reduced by leukoreduction.

SARS

Severe acute respiratory syndrome (SARS) was an entirely new human disease that emerged in Southern China in late 2002. It spread extremely rapidly to other countries as a result of intercontinental air travel. By July 2003, the epidemic was over, but more than 8500 cases had been recorded. The causative agent, a coronavirus novel to humans, was rapidly isolated and characterized [22,23]. It is thought that the infection passed to humans as a result of preparation of exotic mammals as a food source. The virus was extraordinarily infectious, and SARS had a high mortality rate. Although there were no recorded cases of transfusion transmission, there was considerable concern about the possible impact of SARS on blood safety. These concerns were aggravated by findings that showed that the virus was present in the blood, at least during symptomatic disease. Temporary deferral measures were implemented for individuals who had suffered from SARS, contacted cases, or who had traveled in areas where SARS was known to have occurred. These deferrals extended even to very remote levels of risk, such as having traveled through the Toronto airport. It is possible that some aspects of the response to SARS will be a model for managing an influenza pandemic.

vCJD

Variant Creutzfeldt-Jakob disease (vCJD) is another new disease that has emerged recently in human populations. In common with other transmissible spongiform encephalopathies, it is a prion disease that is uniformaly fatal and untreatable. It resulted from the consumption of tissues from animals infected with bovine spongiform encephalopathy (BSE) primarily in the United Kingdom where BSE originated. In turn, BSE arose from intensive agricultural practices involving the use of meat and bone meal to feed cattle. It is not known how the infection actually originated, but it is clear that it was extensively amplified by further rendering of carcasses from infected cattle. Although the practice of feeding cattle with meat and bone meal had been in place for many years, changes in the rendering process were thought to have resulted in survival of the infectious agent. It is unfortunate that cattle feed, beef and live cattle were extensively exported from the UK during the peak periods of infection, probably introducing the bovine, and perhaps the human disease, to many other countries.

To date, there have been about 200 cases of vCJD worldwide, with the vast majority occurring in the UK or as a probable result of exposure in the UK. Although classical CJD does not appear to be transmissible by blood transfusion, little was known about vCJD, which clearly differed from the classical form in a number of ways, including its transmission route and association with lymphoid tissue. In addition, animal model studies demonstrated transmission of the agent by blood. Early measures were taken to try to reduce the risk of transmission, including the implementation of leukoreduction and, outside the UK, deferral of donors who had spent significant amounts of time in selected areas affected by BSE. Subsequently, surveillance studies in the UK have identified one case in which blood from a donor who subsequently died of vCJD had been given to a patient who subsequently developed the disease [24]. It was thought that there was only a 1 in 30,000 likelihood of this occurring by chance. Subsequently, the vCJD prion was detected at post-mortem in another patient who had received blood from a donor who later developed vCJD [25]. More recently, a third case of transfusion-associated transmission has been reported. Thus, it is almost certain that the agent can be transmitted via blood transfusion. Unfortunately, it is not possible to define the actual risk of transfusion transmission, as the size and nature of the human epidemic of vCJD is currently unknown, although the frequency of new cases is currently decreasing.

Existing interventions are briefly described above. Many presume that there will be a test to detect infectious prions in the blood, but this is a formidable technical challenge. In addition, the ethical problems associated with the implementation of such a test are profound. Some progress has been made in an alternate approach, which is to develop affinity filters designed to remove prions from blood components.

Other Agents and Bioterrorism

A number of other infectious agents offer actual or potential risk to blood safety and should be subject to some degree of surveillance and perhaps preparedness. *Anaplasma phagocytophilum* is a small, intracellular bacterium, previously classified as an Ehrlichia species. In the US, it is transmitted by Ixodes ticks and is epidemiologically associated with Lyme disease and babesiosis. One potential transfusion-transmission has been reported [26]. Of greater potential concern is dengue, a mosquito-born virus common to the tropics. In many ways, it behaves very much like WNV, with very large outbreaks (hundreds of thousands of cases) and with a presymptomatic or asymptomatic viremic period. At least in theory, it could readily spread to non-endemic countries where its vector mosquitoes (*Aedes* spp.) exist. Relatively recently, dengue was introduced into parts of Queensland, Australia, as a result of tourist travel. However, only one well authenticated case of transfusion-transmission of dengue has occurred (in Hong Kong).

Another interesting case is that of simian foamy virus. This is a retrovirus that appears to be non-pathogenic. However, it has been transmitted to a number of animal handlers. Some lookback studies have been performed that suggest the virus was not transmitted by transfusion [27]. However, there is concern that transmission of this virus to animal handlers could be a sentinel event potentially heralding the emergence of a mutant or strain that would be pathogenic to humans. Consideration has been given to deferring certain animal handlers from donating blood in some countries.

An area of increasing concern is the impact that pandemic influenza will have on the blood supply. Although influenza infection is not normally thought to result in presymptomatic viremia, there are some data suggesting that this could occur on occasion. It is not generally anticipated that donor deferral will be necessary in the event of a pandemic, but nevertheless, some regulatory authorities may choose to implement a brief deferral. However, the greatest problem is likely to be a shortage of blood components as a result of the reduced availability of donors and of blood center staff. It is possible that this may be somewhat offset by reduced blood needs.

A final area for consideration is the impact of bioterrorism on the blood supply. The organisms considered most likely to be used in an organized attack are anthrax, plague, smallpox, tularemia and viral hemorrhagic fevers. In addition, botulinum toxin has also been identified. With the exception of botulinum toxin, each of these agents has some potential to compromise the safety of blood products as a result of donor infection. In the event of a major attack on a city, it seems likely that the best solution would be to shut down the blood supply and provide support from unaffected areas. However, in the event of a limited attack, it may be necessary to implement appropriate quarantine and deferral policies.

Commentary

There is a very high standard of blood safety in countries with a high human development index (HDI), at least with respect to the major transfusion-transmitted infections, HBV, HCV, HIV and syphilis. In contrast, in many countries with a low HDI it has not been possible to assure the same degree of safety for these agents, although the situation is certainly improving. However, the combination of high frequencies of infection and minimal available resources is very hard to overcome. The situation with respect to emerging infections is much less clear, particularly for developing countries. The example of WNV has shown that surveillance systems already in place in countries such as the USA, along with a network of alert clinicians, can identify a major outbreak rapidly and effectively. In addition, the transmission of disease by transfusion was identified quite early and a preventive measure was developed and implemented in short order. In the context of surveillance, it is of interest that some potentially transfusion-transmissible infectious diseases are also recognized among organ transplant recipients; recent examples are Chagas' disease [28], rabies [29], LCMV [30] and HHV-8 [18]. In marked contrast to WNV, some other emerging infections have not received as much attention, although they have been known for many years; a prime example is babesiosis. Others, like vCJD, have been recognized and have generated much concern but have proven to be somewhat intractable.

There is little doubt that infectious diseases will continue to emerge and reemerge. In many cases, this can be traced to human impacts or behaviors. An increasingly mobile society generates numerous opportunities to move diseases across national borders, emphasizing the need for both global and local surveillance. Where necessary, appropriate interventions to prevent transfusion transmission should be developed and implemented. Ideally, such interventions should not focus exclusively upon travel-based deferrals.

References

1 WHO: Global database on blood safety. Report 2002-2002. http://www.who.int/bloodsafety/GDBS_Report_2001-2002.pdf.

2 Frank C, Mohamed MK, Strickland GT, et al: The role of parenteral antischistosomal therapy in the spread of hepatitis C virus in Egypt. Lancet 2000; 355: 887-891.

3 Dodd RY, Notari EP, Stramer SL: Current prevalence and incidence of infectious disease markers and estimated window-period risk in the American Red Cross blood donor population. Transfusion 2002; 42: 975-979.

4 Dodd RY: Current safety of the blood supply in the United States *Int J Hematol* 2004; 80: 301-305.

5 Mungai M, Tegtmeier G, Chamberland M, Parise M: Transfusion-transmitted malaria in the United States from 1963 through 1999. N Engl J Med 2001; 344: 1973-1978.

6 Matsui T, Inoue R, Kajimoto K, et al: First documentation of transfusion-associated babesiosis in Japan [article in Japanese with English summary]. Rinsho Ketsueki 2000; 41: 628-634.

7 Leiby DA, Chung APS, Gill JE, Houghton R L, Persing DH, Badon S, Cable RG: Demonstrable parasitemia among Connecticut blood donors with antibodies to Babesia microti. Transfusion 2005; 45: 1804-1810.

8 Cable RG, Badon S, Trouern-Trend, et al: Evidence for transmission of Babesia microti from Connecticut blood donors to recipients. Transfusion 2001; 41 (Suppl): 12S-13S (Abstr.)

9 Leiby DA, Chung APS, Cable RG, et al: Relationship between tick bites and the seroprevalence of Babesia microti and Anaplasma phagocytophila (previously Ehrlichia sp.) in blood donors. Transfusion 2002; 42: 1585-1591.

10 Dodd RY, Leiby DA: Emerging infectious threats to the blood supply. Annual Review of Medicine 2004; 55: 191-207.

11 Leiby DA, Herron RM, Read EJ, Lenes BA, Stumpf RJ: Trypanosoma cruzi in Los Angeles and Miami blood donors: Impact of evolving donor demographics on seroprevalence and implications for transfusion transmission. Transfusion 2002; 42: 549-555.

12 Leiby DA, Lenes BA, Tibbals MA, et al: Prospective evaluation of a patient with Trypanosoma cruzi infection transmitted by transfusion. N Engl J Med 1999; 341: 1237-1239.

13 Leiby DA, Fucci MH, Stumpf RJ: Trypanosoma cruzi in a low- to moderate-risk blood donor population: seroprevalence and possible congenital transmission. Transfusion 1999; 39: 310-315.

14 CDC: Viscerotropic Leishmaniasis in persons returning from operation Desert Storm – 1990-1991. MMWR 1992; 41: 131-134.

15 Petersen LR, Hayes EB: Westward ho? – the spread of West Nile virus. N Engl J Med 2004; 351: 2257-2259.

16 Pealer LN, Marfin AA, Petersen LR, et al: Transmission of West Nile virus through blood transfusion in the United States in 2002. N Engl J Med 2003; 349: 1236-1245.

17 Stramer SL, Fang CT, Foster GA, Wagner AG, Brodsky JP Dodd RY: West Nile virus among blood donors in the United States, 2003 and 2004. New Engl J Med 2005; 353: 451-459.

18 Regamey N, Tamm M, Wernli M et al: Transmission of human herpesvirus 8 infection from renal-transplant donors to recipients. N Engl J Med 1998; 339: 1358-1363.

19 Cannon MJ, Dollard SC, Smith DK et al: Blood-borne and sexual transmission of human herpesvirus 8 in women with or at risk for human immunodeficiency virus infection. N Engl J Med 2001; 344: 637-643.

20 Mbulaiteye SM, Biggar RJ, Bakaki PM et al: Human herpesvirus 8 infection and transfusion history in children with sickle-cell disease in Uganda. J Natl Cancer Inst 2003; 95: 1330-1335.

21 Dollard SC, Nelson KE, Ness PM, et al: Possible transmission of Human herpesvirus 8 by blood transfusion in a historical United States cohort. Transfusion 2005; 45: 500-503.

22 Marra MM, Jones SJM, Astell CR et al: The genome sequence of the SARS-associated coronavirus. Science 2003; 300: 1399-1404.

23 Rota PA, Oberste MA, Monroe SS et al: Characterization of a novel coronavirus associated with severe acute respiratory syndrome. Science 2003; 300: 1394-1399.

24 Llewelyn CA, Hewitt PE, Knight RS et al: Possible transmission of variant Creutzfeldt-Jakob disease by blood transfusion. Lancet 2004; 363: 417-421.

25 Peden AH, Head MW, Ritchie DL et al: Preclinical vCJD after blood transfusion in a PRNP codon 129 heterozygous patient. Lancet 2004; 364: 527-529.

26 Eastlund T, Persing D, Mathiesen D et al: Human granulocytic ehrlichiosis after red cell transfusion (abstract). Transfusion 1999; 39 (Suppl): 117S (Abstr).

27 Boneva RS, Grindon AJ, Orton SL, et al: Simian foamy virus infection in a blood donor. Transfusion 2002; 42: 886-891.

28 CDC: Chagas disease after organ transplantation – United States, 2001. MMWR 2002; 52: 210-212.

29 CDC: Investigation of rabies infections in organ donor and transplant recipients – Alabama, Arkansas, Oklahoma, and Texas, 2004. MMWR 2004; 53: 586-589.

30 CDC: Lymphocytic choriomeningitis virus infection in organ transplant recipients – Massachusetts, Rhode Island, 2005. MMWR 2005; 54: 537-539.

R.Y. Dodd, Research and Development, American Red Cross, Holland Laboratory, 15601, Crabbs Branch Way, Rockville, MD 20855, USA.
E-mail: dodd@usa.redcross.org

Dax EM, Farrugia A, Vyas G (eds): Advances in Transfusion Safety – Volume IV.
Dev Biol (Basel). Basel, Karger, 2007, vol 127, pp 249-258.

Management of Transfusion Related Risks: Is Risk Communication to Non-Experts at all Possible?

C. Hossenlopp

Etablissement Français du Sang, EFS – Direction of International Affairs, Paris, France

Key words: Hazard, risk communication, risk perception, behaviours, beliefs, patient information.

Abstract: Blood transfusion medicine has to confront the challenge of ensuring maximal safety in spite of minimal but real risks, emerging risks, or potential risks, all of which must be prevented and avoided. Continuous searching for maximum safety of blood products should remain a constant goal for all professionals involved in blood transfusion medicine. Over the last decade, those involved have considered in depth the questions of risk assessment and then risk management, concentrating first and foremost on technical (biological) approaches, a little less on economy and least of all on the social aspects of risk. Transfusion therapy is probably safer than it has ever been. However, public perception and the increase in litigations may suggest the opposite. Transfusion professionals must re-inspire confidence in the field through the management of the perception of risk, real or otherwise. However, risk management requires instigation of changes both in terms of the organisations and professional behaviour. Changes can generate fear unless their advantages are immediately apparent. Thus, the acceptance of a proposed change can only be achieved when the issue and its risks are fully understood.

Introduction

In transfusion medicine, appropriately informing both the donor and the recipient patient is part of the fundamental relationship that associates the duties of the physician with the patient's rights. It has been shown that the basic principles of the communication process constitute a transfer of information. In order to be effective, the communication process should include a feedback loop, i.e. the communication is verified. In so doing, true dialogue between the sender and the receiver of the information is shown to have occurred.

The present paper first introduces the notion of risk and the theories around its perception. It then attempts to explain the effectiveness of the communication process between the "public" (donor/patient) and a physician in charge, emphasizing the basic principles of the communication process. Risk communication is then approached more specifically. In the discussion the author considers how an efficient communication can shape the perception of risks and make blood transfusion risks "socially acceptable".

The Concept of Risk

Uncertainety related to permanent changes

According to the Committee on Risk Perception and Communication of the National Research Council (NRC), hazard is "an act or phenomenon posing potential harm to some person(s) or thing(s)"; the extent of harm is called magnitude. Risk is defined as the quantification of a hazard in terms of the probability that harm or undesirable results will be realized. This does not incorporate the magnitude of the hazard, just the probability of its occurrence. For example, people building their home on a field that experiences a flood once every 20 years face the same hazard as those building in a similar area that experiences a flood once in 100 years, but the former face five times the risk. However, the damage of the hazard (the flood) may vary, causing greater or lesser harm depending on its magnitude. The harm relates both to the magnitude of the hazard and the risk.

Over the centuries, the word "risk" has changed its meaning and use. It is assumed here that the concept of risk appeared in the Middle Ages. At that time risk was perceived to be a natural event (storms, floods, epidemics etc). It excluded the idea of human responsibility.

With modernity, i.e. beginning of the 17th and 18th centuries when the industrial revolution occurred, the key to human progress became bound with scientific knowledge and rational thinking. Through these, social and natural laws could be measured. Probabilities and statistics were developed during the 19th century and the introduction of the concept of human responsibility was incorporated into the concept of risk.

In contemporary western societies, an enormous body of research has been developed in the last decade that includes risk analysis, risk assessment, risk communication and risk management. All this research is used to measure and control risks in public health, finance, law, business as well as in medicine and blood transfusion. This era of post-modernity is characterized by uncertainty related to permanent changes and the breakdown of rules, norms and traditions. This uncertainty has implications on how we think about ourselves, others, organisations, institutions and governments. Risk is everywhere. Risk strategies are attempts to tame uncertainty but often have the paradoxical effect of increasing anxiety about risk because of the intensity of their focus and concerns.

Cognitive sciences versus social sciences

In the literature on risk perception there are a number of ways in which risk is addressed. Two main approaches are (a) that of cognitive sciences and (b) that of social sciences.

- *Cognitive sciences* present a realist approach, which represents the most common perspective and is mainly expressed in technical and scientific views. The question is, "How do people respond cognitively to risk?" Strategies are developed with a or some measurement(s) as a basis.

- *Social sciences* offer an alternative approach called social constructionism. This approach concerns the social and cultural aspects of risk, rather than their measure. The key question here is, "How is risk understood in different socio-cultural contexts?"

Between these two main approaches there may obviously be a range of combinations corresponding to whether it relates to self or to a collective approach of risk [1].

Risk perception is a subjective process with what is identified and responded to as risk. It is often said that we live in a "risk society" [2]. The topic of risk itself is very broad and beyond the scope of the present paper. We therefore refer the reader to further information for broader scope on this topic per se [3,4].

Community perception of risk is influenced by a number of that which are not based on scientific evidence (Table 1).

Table 1 : Risk perception*.

Risk is accepted	Risk is not accepted
An everyday accident (household)	Unusual risk (unknown chemical pollution)
Natural risks	Artificial risks
Ethical risks	Risks which are considered unethical
Voluntary risks (such as smoking)	Involuntary risks
Random (a car accident)	Catastrophic events (an airplane crash)
Information coming from a trustworthy source	Information coming from unreliable source
Fair risks	Unfair risks
Risks under personal control (driving a car)	Not under control (travelling as a passenger in a plane)
Detectable risks	Undetectable risks
Risks that scientists can explain	Risks for which scientists recognize uncertainty

* Adapted from Baker F, J Public Health Policy, 1990.

Risk Communication

The context of blood transfusion

Few disciplines of medicine have attracted as much media attention as transfusion in recent decades. The attention has been evident everywhere in the world. As a result of the media campaigns, the lay public has developed a high concern about transfusion-related risks. Although it can be readily assessed that tremendous efforts have been made to ensure safe blood supplies, little has been done or at least accomplished by blood transfusion professionals to communicate the actual residual risks to patients and lay public. The public do not perceive that they have any control over the risk.

At a time when generalised informed consent is required in blood transfusion, it is of the utmost importance that the "patient" is truly and properly informed. Physicians who prescribe blood products should be able to understand the probabilities of occurrence of risks, but should also be in a position to explain them to their patients in a clear manner which is understandable to them.

Blood transfusion services everywhere encounter difficulties because on one hand blood donations have decreased, and individuals are hesitant about receiving blood transfusions even when recommended to do so by their physicians on the other. It remains essential that potential recipients of blood and blood products be informed correctly and accurately about risks that are quantitative despite their being determined by risk perception that is highly dependent on factors that cannot be qualified such as fear, emotion and degree of trust. Broadly speaking, the public, with each of its members being a potential transfusion recipient, has two main sources of information about health and, more specifically, about blood transfusion. First there is the media, and second the medical establishment and healthcare workers in general.

Information " which will not be understood "

Most public knowledge about residual risks in health care comes from the media. The results of a study on the written press and concerning the transmission of biomedical information [5] have shown that researchers and physicians are reluctant to provide journalists with clear, accessible and regular information. It is shown that it is extremely important to avoid an emotional approach and consequently sensationalist headlines. For risks associated with blood transfusion this can only be achieved by anticipating needs for communication and regularly communicating on the daily issues of transfusion medicine. It is the only way for experts to be understood and to educate effectively both the press and the lay public. Too often experts limit their actions concerning the media to answering questions asked by journalists and mostly under urgency.

As to the second main source of information, i.e. the medical professionals, the results of very few studies lead us to think that there is a reluctant attitude of physicians toward informing their patients. Using frank language to focus on the risks, a patient may be frightened and less likely to accept a perceived risk. Thus, there has been a tendency to speak to the patient in emotional language, which tends to hide its message and the patient may perceive the risks as unimportant.

On one hand the potential patient would like to know the risks (but what would he like to know ?), and on the other the medical professional who would like to inform but may not know what to say or how to say it or does not want to give information which a priori "will not be understood". However, when no information is given, assumptions are made and these, over time, become certainties and myths.

The basic principles

A major means by which a physician can understand and appreciate the level, type and nature of information expected by the patient is to listen carefully to him or her. Effective communication between doctor and patient is a major principle that cannot be delegated to somebody else.

Informing people about advances in biological and medical research involves particular difficulties in comparison to other areas of health. Human beings are affected by such information in a number of ways ; their worries, fears, suffering or hopes all come into play.

Once the listening time has been completed, the communication process begins. The communication process has three basic elements : the sender, the message and the recipient.

Additionally, there are filters which will alter the message at either end of the channel through which it passes.

The basic scheme of sending, message transfer and receiving represents a simple transfer of information (Fig. 1). The quality of the reception is not checked. The comprehension of the receiver is not evaluated. Some would say that the message has been transmitted, just as some others would consider they have obtained consent from a patient in merely distributing an information sheet.

A more advanced approach is the follow-up of this scheme of "listening first". It is the notion of obtaining "feedback" which enables the sender to check whether his message has been received, and how it has been received. It is the necessary step to achieve the the full two-way communication process.

Each communication process will take place in a environment at a given time and with given constraints. This is why, in addition to the application of the communication process, it is very useful to think about the tools relevant to specific situations. For instance, a person to person communication process will not necessitate the same channel (tool) as communicating information to staff of an organization, although the issue to be communicated could be the same. In other words, a written leaflet for helping a patient to make his decision is one tool, a verbal discussion is another. Ideally, whether the audience is big or small, the sender of the information has to elaborate a communication plan and to choose the most relevant message(s) and tool(s).

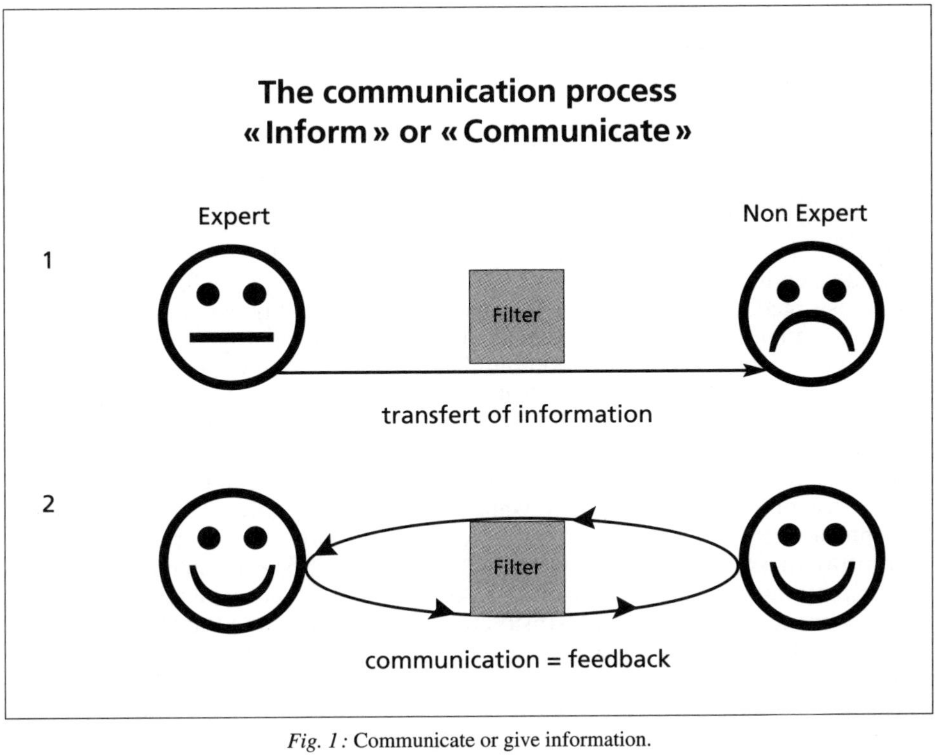

Fig. 1 : Communicate or give information.

Risk communication

Risk communication is defined by Plough and Krimsky [6] as follows: risk communication consists of experts intentionally conveying information about health or environment risks, obtained from scientists and technical experts, to a targeted audience of non-experts through designated channels. To simplify things and to come back to the broader process of communication, a narrower definition of "information channelled intentionally from experts to a general audience" will be used here.

Who are these experts? Are we talking about communicators or about physicians? Their competence in channelling information is different. Furthermore, it has been shown that 54 % of patients' complaints and 45 % of patients' concerns are not answered by medical doctors. Fear and stress in the patient is generated by uncertainty, particularly by lack of feedback from the physician [7,8]

Intentionally refers to the communication strategy: in order to set up an intentional communication strategy to induce health promoting behaviour, the following steps should be followed [as in any communication plan]:

- assess the risks;
- set goals;
- assess the target audience;
- assess the socio-cultural context;
- choose the approach;
- build the communication plan;
- implement the plan and evaluate the effects.

The strategy should have one objective of including people in the decision-making process. However, in some instances such a plan has proved that the aim was to persuade the public to adhere to the experts' views, which should not be the case.

Information about health: Efficient communication about risks is far more complex and difficult than is generally appreciated. Some topics may be so technical as to be confusing to laypersons. These persons include journalists who pick out only those pieces of information that they understand. Misunderstandings often come from attempts to communicate scientific and technical topics. This is particularly acute with an objective like communicating about blood with all the associated symbolism and myths of life and death. Tools to make the communication more efficient have been created, for example the Paling scale [9], and there seem to be no good reasons not to use it. This will only be effective when the intention of communicating is made an objective and not a compulsory constraint.

Because one cannot manipulate when communicating effectively, communicators (physicians) have an important ethical responsibility to determine what the appropriate message(s) to give are. The message(s) should be arranged in a way that will help promote health, e.g. the risks associated with transfusion medicine.

In the present example of transfusion medicine, information transfer (communication) and the patient's consent to receive blood products are part of the fundamental relationship that associate the duties of the physician with the patient's rights. It is often feared by the medical world that rights newly obtained by patients could lead to a consumer-patient demanding more and more. Mutual confidence must be preserved between physician and patient. A buyer-vendor relationship cannot be envisaged by most physicians, and as a consequence a certain number of them seem to choose not to inform patients, or avoid facing delicate situations of a consumerist nature [10]. In addition, medicine based on curing and treating diseases rather than prevention, as is the case in France, can also explain the silence of physicians, especially when facing uncertainties such as emerging risks.

Communication: A science that can be taught

Several studies now show that problems in physician-patient communication are very common and affect management of the situation for a patient [11]. To reiterate the important example, 54 % of patients' complaints and 45 % of patients' concerns are not settled by physicians. In addition, it is also noted that most complaints about physicians do not deal with clinical issues but with communication problems [12]. Is this a consequence of not educating the patient? Possibly, because it has also been shown that a very high proportion of patients do not understand or remember what the physician tells them about diagnosis and treatment.

Other studies have shown that fear and stress in the patient is related to their uncertainty and the lack of feedback from the physician. Physicians often do not fully appreciate the quantity and type of information or extent of explanation a patient is expecting. The level of distress to receiving adverse information in patients with severe diseases is less when they feel they receive adequate and appropriate information [13].

Despite the importance of effective medical interviewing, few physicians have had either formal training in communication skills or have been formally observed when communicating with patients [14]. Some believe that communication skills are dependent on personality and/or natural talent and therefore cannot be improved; others believe that any physician will improve his communication ability with time and experience. Nevertheless, studies have demonstrated that the deficiencies in communication skills are similar for experienced physicians, recent graduates and medical students [15]. There is therefore an urgent need to teach communication skills to all physicians from those who are experienced to those in medical-school training. Communication skill training should be incorporated into medical school curricula as well as into continuing education programs. When effective communication skills are well taught, changes are maintained and skills enhanced.

There are many articles about communication skills training for health care professionals [16]. However, very often isolated techniques that have not been properly evaluated are used in evaluations. Furthermore, most of this literature is published in non-medical journals and tends not to be read by medical professionals. One by Fallowfield et al [17] describes the difficulties reported by senior oncologists who attended a short intensive training course. It shows that the substantial improvements in communication reported immediately after the course were maintained after three months. It concludes that resources for educational initiatives are needed to help both patients and their physicians improve their communication skills.

To communicate efficiently about risks of a procedure is far more complex and difficult than is generally appreciated [18]. If very clear language is used to focus on the risk, a patient may be frightened and less likely to accept a risk that he/she perceives as a consequence; the communicator tends to speak to the patient in emotional language in which the message is "hidden" and then the patient may not perceive the "communicated" risks as important.

Successful communication to patients and their relatives depends on five factors:

- estimate of the patient's current knowledge;
- estimate of the patient's ability to receive and understand the information;
- ability to give appropriate and correct information;
- will to verify that the patient understands the information and therefore make an informed consent;
- recognition of the need to follow up and to keep the patient informed of any progress or change.

The point of this paper is to relate these findings about communications to blood safety. Blood safety has reached such a high level today that it is difficult to envisage further technical progress making highly significant increases. On the other hand, it seems timely to consider improvements that may be realized through the social sciences in the areas of communication and training methods in communication as a potential resource for restoring confidence in the whole system.

How can perception, beliefs and behaviours be shaped or changed?

Any communication process entails an "influence" dimension. There are three major ways in which our attitudes and reactions can be "manipulated" by verbal or non-verbal messages.

- *Presentation:* The order in which information is given to patients may influence perceptions and behaviours. Research has shown [18] that when the topic is important or relevant to the person, he/she will remember the information given at the beginning and forget what is presented at the end of a conversation. There is a sort of "shut down" once the major information has been given. For instance, cancer patients often tell the story that when their doctor first told them about their diagnosis, they did not remember anything beyond the information of "you have cancer". Research has shown [19] that when someone is overwhelmed with frightening information, he stops listening or processing subsequent messages.
- *Amount of information:* The quantity of information given on a topic influences perceptions. As research is progressing, it is obvious that it is not possible to "fully" inform individuals about health risks. Moreover, time and space for adequate presentation are generally scarce and consequently the amount of information given to patients or others is necessarily limited. It has been reported that practitioners interrupt patients after an average of 18 seconds in a medical interview. Alternatively, [20] public health practitioners have from 30 to 60 seconds to inform and make a recommendation on health risk during an interview with a patient. Therefore, communicators should give some thought as to what information should or should not be presented. The central question in terms of ethics is what "information" should be chosen to influence health positively.
- *Framing the message(s):* Because of the limited quantity of information that can be given it is essential that the physician chose the wording of his message consciously and strategically. This will enhance the chance of achieving the intended outcome. Physicians (or communicators) who do not make the effort to

consciously consider word choices could produce harmful outcomes. Indeed, when using one word over another, one aspect of a message is emphasised over another, intentionally or unintentionally. Researchers strongly support the position that framing messages has profound influence on perceptions and, hence, on decisions [21]. They found that patients would choose proposed treatments very differently according to how the associated risks were presented, e.g. presented as chances of survival or chances of dying. Slovic et al [22] also demonstrate that subtle changes in the ways that risks are presented can have a major consequence on decisions. It is also clear that the way communicators frame their health risk messages may manipulate individuals' perception and ultimately their behaviours [23].

Today's communicators have theories and tools (technology) to build up messages that produce positive outcomes, and they should use them [24]. If messages are presented in an arbitrary manner, the chances of attributing negative outcomes to message presentation are greatly increased.

There are now many opportunities for health care professionals to train in communication skills that may be utilized (Fallowfield, op. cit, Kraan, op. cit).

Conclusion

Reluctance to appropriately inform the lay public or patients has been shown among medical professionals. Health care workers or physicians have the primary objective of transfusing the right product at the right moment to achieve adequate treatment. Traditionally, they have been less concerned that patients understand risks and consequences of procedures. However, patients today claim their right to know about these things. They claim their right to choose whether the procedure should be carried out and why. To be effective, evidence shows that communication must involve an interactive exchange. There are proven techniques and methods to establish efficient communication programs. It is time for blood transfusion professionals to promote them. Whether the consequences of an individual's choices are favourable or unfavourable to their clinical outcomes may depend on the quality of information available to them. It is precisely behaviour at this level which will alter trends in public health. Like the costs of poor quality in products and services, the costs of ignorance are enormous.

However, risk perception is a subjective process that one identifies and responds to. Blood transfusion" experts'" responses to risks have so far been purely biological. Although social responses to blood transfusion risks (i.e. communication, marketing) would be more difficult to implement, they do not appear to represent an additional key to restoration of confidence in blood transfusion organisations and toward achieving and maintaining an adequate blood supply.

References

1 Lupton D: Risk, in Hamilton P (ed): London, Routledge, 1999, pp 181.

2 Beck U: From industrial society to the risk society: questions of survival, social structure and ecological environment. Theory, Culture and Society 1992; 9: 97-123.

3 Giddens A: Risk society, the context of British politics, in Franklin J (ed): The politics of risk society. Cambridge, Polity Press, 1998, pp 23-24.

4 Beck U: Risk society and the provident state, in Lash S, Szerszinski B, Wynne B (eds): Risk, Environment and Modernity: Towards a New Ecology. London, Sage, 1996, pp 27-43.

5 Hossenlopp C: Communication scientifique et médicale, difficultés de la médiatisation. Humanisme et Entreprise 1997; 56: 45-59.

6 Plough A, Krimsky S: Emergency of Risk Communication Studies: Social and Political Context. Scientific and Technical Human Values 1987; 2:4-10.

7 Stewart MA, McWhinney IR, Buck CW: The Doctor-Patient Relationship and its Effect Upon Outcome. Journal of the Royal College of General Practitionners 1979; 29: 77-82.

8 Ley P: Communication with Patients: Improving Satisfaction and Compliance. London, Croom-Helm, 1988.

9 Lee DH, Paling JE, Blajchman MA: A new tnool for communicating transfusion risk information transfusion 1998; 38: 184-188.

10 Hossenlopp C: Communication about blood transfusion risks ESTM residential course on risk perception and risk assessment in transfusion practice; how to achieve a sound transfusion practice based on scientific truth? Brussels, 26-29 February 2000.

11 Fallowfield L, Lipkin M, Hall A: Teaching senior oncologists communication skills: Results from phase I of a comprehensive longitudinal program in the United Kingdom. Journal of Clinical Oncology 1998; 16 (5): 1961-1968.

12 Richards T: Chasms in communication. B.M.J. 1990; 301: 1407-1408.

13 Fallowfield LJ, Hall A, Maguire GP, Baum M: Psychological outcomes of different treatment policies in women with early cancer outside a clinical trial. B.M.J. 1990; 301: 575-580.

14 Fallowfield LJ: Giving sad and bad news. The Lancet 1993; 341: 476-478.

15 Gordon GH, Rost K: Evaluating a faculty development course on medical interviewing, in Lipkin M, Putnam NM, Lazare A (eds): The Medical Interview: Clinical Care, Education and Research. Frontiers of Primary Care. New York, NY, Springer-Verlag, 1995, pp 436-447.

16 Kraan HF, Crunen AAM, van der Vleuten CPM, et al: Evaluation instruments for medical interviewing skills, in Lipkin M, Putnam NM, Lazare A. (eds): The Medical Interview: Clinical Care, Education and Research. Frontiers of Primary Care. New York, NY, Springer-Verlag, 1995, pp 460-472.

17 Fallowfield L, Lipkin M, Hall A: Teaching senior oncologists communication skills: results from phase I of a comprehensive longitudinal program in the United Kingdom. J Clin Oncol 1998; 16: 1961-1968.

18 Lundgren RE: Risk communication: A handbook for communicating environmental, safety and health risks. Columbus, OH, Battelle Press, 1994.

19 Bostrom RN: Persuasion. Englewood Cliffs, NJ, Prentice-Hall, 1983.

20 Witte K: Putting the fear back into fear appeals: the extended parallel process model. Communication monographs 1992; 59: 329-349.

21 Rice RE, Atkin CK: Public communication campaigns. Newbury Park, CA, Sage, 1989, (2nd edition).

22 McNeil BJ, Pauker SG, Sox HC, Tversky A: On the elicitation of preferences for alternative therapies. The New England Journal of Medicine 1982; 306: 1259-1262.

23 Slovic P, Fishoff B, Lichtenstein S: Behavioral decision theory perspectives on risk and safety. Acta Psychologica 1984; 56: 183-203.

24 Pratkanis A, Aronson E: Age of propaganda: the everyday use and abuse of persuasion. 1991, New York, Freeman.

25 Roper WL: Health communication takes on new dimensions at CDC. Public Health Reports 1993; 108: 179-183.

Dr. C. Hossenlopp, Etablissement Français du Sang, EFS – Direction of International Affairs, 100 avenue de Suffren, FR-75015 Paris, France.
E-mail: claudine.hossenlopp@efs.sante.fr

Dax EM, Farrugia A, Vyas G (eds): Advances in Transfusion Safety – Volume IV.
Dev Biol (Basel). Basel, Karger, 2007, vol 127, pp 259-265.

Blood Safety in the New Millenium – Scientific Purity and Political Reality – Can They be Synthesised for the Public Good?

D. Starr

Boston University Department of Journalism, College of Communication Boston University, Boston, MA, USA

INTRODUCTION

These are times of emerging dangers, both man-made and natural, from microscopic pathogens to political violence to natural disasters that sweep entire regions. In response to these terrors, the public can become, paradoxically, both alarmed and unmotivated: alarmed by the stream of frightening messages put out by government and the media, unmotivated by a sense of helplessness or even disconnection.

Clearly, there is a need for more education about blood – or rather, an updated education about blood that takes into account the confusing times in which we live. In order to accomplish that task, it is essential to understand today's evolving media landscape and how it affects the messages the public receives.

This chapter follows my book, BLOOD: An Epic History of Medicine and Commerce. The book portrays the history of biologics as a long narrative arc, beginning with the earliest transfusions and ending with the storm of litigation that arose from the AIDS epidemic. It describes that history as a series of transformations – from a magical humor to a biological substance, with the development of the first reliable transfusions; from a biological substance to a wartime materiel, with the development of blood banks just prior to World War II and the mass usage of blood and component therapy; and from a wartime materiel to a global commodity, with the growth of the international biologics industry (Fig. 1). Then, of course, came the AIDS epidemic, which traumatized the field as nothing before. Indeed, so frightening were the AIDS years that a kind of backward transformation took place in the public mind, with the re-introduction of medieval thinking about the dark and dangerous properties of blood.

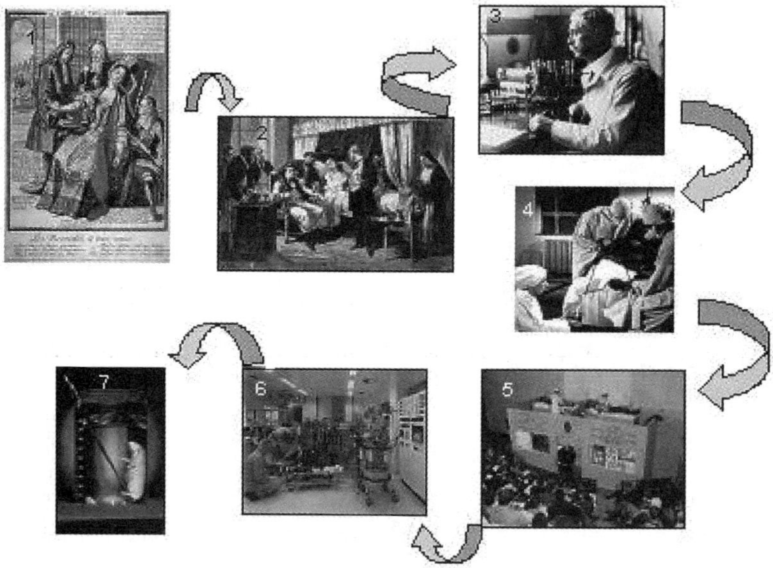

Fig. 1: From alchemical concept – 1. to therapeutic intervention – 2. made possible by the discovery of blood groups – 3. blood has become an increasingly complex therapy, now increasingly subject to pharmaceutical operations after blood harvesting and storage – 4. enabled innovators such as Edwin Cohn – 5. to fractionate blood plasma to its individual fractions – 6. We now hope for substitutes to blood – 7. to minimize the very small residual risks and assist in coping with the problem of supply. So – the process is complex, demanding a nuanced message to communicate its importance.

Happily, the response to AIDS and other health challenges has reassured people to a large extent. Today blood, at least in the advanced nations, is remarkably safe. Since 1980, nine new tests have been added to ensure the safety of blood collection, and rigorous screening measures have been put in place. People with hemophilia, once the unintentional canaries in the cave, are safer today because of the development of recombinant clotting products. The risk of contracting AIDS, hepatitis or other diseases is infinitesimal.

In today's post-AIDS era of biologics, blood bankers and regulators have shown progress not only in the tools they use, but in the way they go about their business. Countries have formed hemovigilance committees, not only to respond to problems, but also to monitor their systems and anticipate problems in the earliest possible stages. When new problems have arisen, such as CJD, the industry tackled them quickly and pro-actively, even at great sacrifice to supply. The response to emerging pathogens such as SARS and West Nile virus was quick, smart and effective. The embrace of the precautionary principle, while sometimes controversial, has made blood and blood products safer than almost any other medical procedure.

Yet if public behavior is any indication, people still don't understand what blood centers do and how they should participate. Donor rates seem frozen at five percent or less – in many places those figures are declining. Return rates are not what they should be. People donate blood paradoxically: they line up to give during the kind of emergencies when blood is not needed, but stay away during the precise times when it is.

THE NEW MEDIA LANDSCAPE

Experts in blood products understand the biological challenges facing them today. You understand the problems of emerging pathogens that can travel across the world in 24 hours, the difficulty in harmonizing safety standards across many diverse nations, and the eternal balancing act between maximum safety and sustainable supply. What you may not be aware of is the new communication challenges you face – how changes in the landscape of public communication affect your role in the public mind.

Today's media outlets are undergoing radical and painful business transformations. Not long ago, media companies were often family-owned. However, a succession of developments, including aging owners and the promise of the financial benefits of taking companies public, have created an avalanche of corporate buyouts (Fig. 2). Newspapers have been consolidated into ever-larger chains and the electronic media into global networks. Meanwhile, at the same time that profitability in media has become increasingly important, the key source of revenue – advertising – has declined.

These business pressures have affected journalism largely in a negative way. The consolidation of major news media has resulted in fewer independent voices covering and interpreting major news developments. In order to meet profit goals,

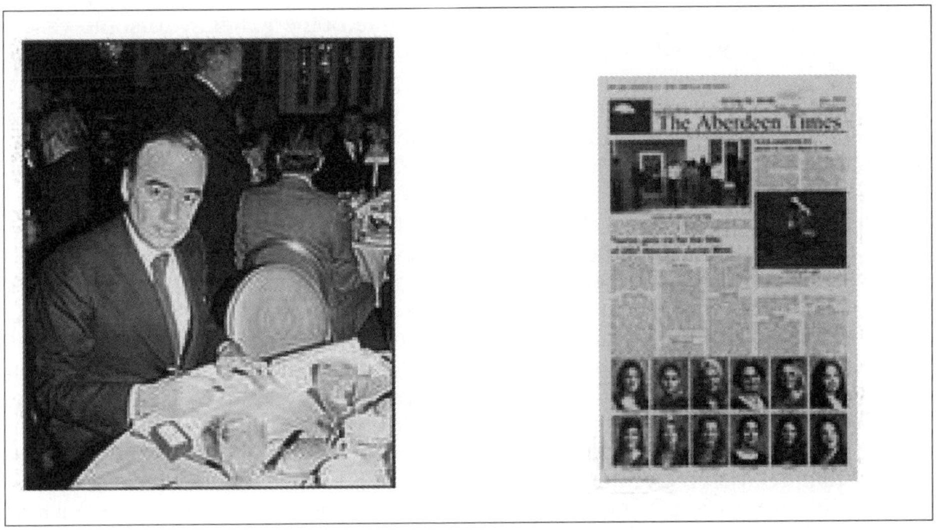

Fig. 2: The new media landscape is more related to the increasing consolidation represented by the Murdoch news empire than the small-town family owned newspaper of the past.

news operations save money by laying off staff, leaving fewer reporters to cover more stories. The companies also expect reporters to write for a variety of media, from newspapers to television to on-line editions. As a result, what little time reporters have to spend on a story is increasingly spent on formatting the story for various media rather than reporting the substance of the story. Not only are reporters increasingly harried, but many are younger and more poorly paid as well. As part of some companies' cost-cutting measures, middle-aged reporters – those who'd developed considerable expertise in their fields – have been replaced at lower salaries by younger, less experienced journalists. Although it may not be the case at the large national news outlets, it is likely that on the regional and local levels some of the reporters one deals with may be inexperienced, naïve, and have less time to report on a story than before.

Meanwhile, other changes have altered the media landscape in which blood banks now operate. In the USA for example, a cynical administration portrays scientists not as the seekers of observable evidence, but as just another interest group. The news media have been unwitting accomplices in this practice with their traditional portrayal of "both sides" of a given issue. That custom might work when two politicians argue against each other, but it does not accurately portray the multi-faceted issues of science, medicine, and public health. In such cases, the appropriate practice would be to portray not only the spectrum of opinions on an issue, but also the evidence and the weight of scientific consensus. By clinging to their traditional practices, news media have portrayed national controversies such as global climate change or the teaching of evolution as debates between equal and opposite sides, even though one side may represent only a small number of outliers. As a result, the scientist's presentation of observable data has been misrepresented as just one voice of many in a "marketplace of ideas" in which anyone's word is as good as anyone else's.

The final complication in today's media landscape involves the sense of a continuing crisis. Ever since 9/11, the public (especially the American public) has been bombarded with messages about real and imagined emergencies. In some cases, officials have announced various states of color-coded states of emergency without explaining what they mean or what actions people could take in response. In other cases, officials suggested incorrect protective measures, such as sealing windows with duct tape in the event of a biological attack. In still other cases, officials and news media have naively encouraged the public to take useless measures to help the larger community. The result is a public that doesn't know which warnings to listen to or what actions to take and retreats into apathy or even cynicism.

Such was the case following the 9/11 attack, when public figures encouraged people to donate blood despite the fact that no blood was needed. Days after blood bankers tried to stop the donations, news anchors and politicians (including members of Congress and the President) urged Americans to continue giving blood. Not only was an enormous amount of donated blood wasted, but the over-reaction caused a prolonged slump in donations as people rebounded into a sustained apathy. Supplies throughout the nation declined. By December, many blood centers were issuing emergency appeals. Indeed, even in New York – Ground Zero for the attack – fewer than ten percent of the people who lined up to give blood returned, plunging the city into a sustained period of critical shortages. As one blood banker told me: "People came out of the woodwork to donate… and then they went back into the woodwork."

Communicating Effectively in the New Media Landscape

Given today's complicated and flawed media landscape, how can you successfully engage the public? How can you communicate issues involving safety and risk to a public battered by confusing messages? How can you communicate effectively and clearly when it most matters – during a public health emergency?

The answer lies in a pro-active engagement with the media. Public health emergencies, from blood shortages to emerging diseases, frequently occur. But if you wait until the emergency to exchange business cards with your local reporters, you've waited to long.

The best way to pro-actively educate reporters in your area is to hold educational seminars to brief them on issues they need to understand. (It's amazing how rarely this simple undertaking is performed). In this effort, you'll find natural allies in your area's health department, hospitals, medical schools and universities. Presenting yourselves as part of a collaborative group will help journalists see the work you do and the decisions you make, not in the isolated context of a blood bank but in the larger context of public health and emergency response.

The seminars should feature a collection of experts, such as epidemiologists from the local medical school, infectious disease specialists from the local or regional health department, and representatives from your blood bank, all explaining their roles in a given issue or area of public policy. It's useful to have a notable journalist discuss how he or she reports effectively in this area to serve as a role model for the less experienced reporters. You'll distribute fact sheets, lists of websites for quick reference, phone lists of people reporters should contact, and phone numbers for the public to call. The ideal is not to have a one-way discussion in which you and your colleagues download information, but to stimulate a lively give and take, in which you and the local journalist explore areas of mutual concern. By the end of the event, reporters will have a better grasp of the complexities of the issues and the basic science underlying your decisions. Most importantly, they would have developed the beginnings of a working relationship with you and your institution.

Although time consuming to plan, such pro-active seminars will help avoid sensationalized, inaccurate reporting or one-side-versus-the-other scenarios. Should a controversy or emergency later occur, you and the journalists will share a common body of knowledge and a contextual understanding. You'll be able to focus on updating reporters on changing developments rather than providing elementary background.

Contrary to what advertising executives and politicians might tell us, communicating with the media does not mean trying to shape or "spin" the truth, especially during a controversy or emergency. The best communicators are those who speak forthrightly and honestly. (Dr. C. Everret Koop, a famously blunt and straight-talking surgeon general during the Reagan administration, is one of the publicly admired people to hold that office – precisely because of his refusal to "spin"). Yet, in an evolving situation with reporters on deadline, it's difficult to convey the most complete information at any given moment. The following suggestions may help you in that effort during emergency situations:

- Use press conferences wisely. Holding a press conference is an excellent way to update the media about an evolving situation in a public and forthright way. Because of press deadlines, you can't wait until you have all the information before you hold a press conference; if you do wait, people will make assumptions (often incorrect ones) to fill the void. Consider press conferences as updates in which you honestly tell the public what you know at a given point. The ideal press conference pairs a policy spokesperson with a medical specialist to give both broad context and the details of whatever problem you and your community face, such as the outbreak of a disease. You should tell reporters what you know and how you know it (such as the number of cases, where and when those cases were reported, the condition of the patients, and how communicable the disease is known to be based on other outbreaks in the past). You should also tell them what you don't know (such as how communicable this particular strain might be), what you're doing to find out (what kind of lab tests you're conducting), and when you'll know more (how long you expect the lab tests to take). Tell the reporters when to expect the next update. Try to make sure that each successive press conference is more substantive than the previous one. Don't use press conferences to fend off, but to inform.

- Understand the language of risk. How many times have we picked up the paper or looked at the TV and heard or seen the phrase: "Worst case scenario?" By definition, worst case scenarios are rare; life consists more of likely scenarios, or possible scenarios. It's important to clearly communicate risk. By all means, answer clearly when a reporter asks about a worst case scenario, but be sure to describe that which is most likely to occur. When the most likely scenario eventually happens, it will preserve your credibility and help reduce cynicism about public health announcements.
- Pair a warning with an action whenever possible. One of the problems with America's color-coded homeland security advisory system is that the colors do not clearly correspond to specific actions. The government maintains a website explaining the significance of each color, but the actions are vague ("be alert for suspicious activity...") and often not communicated during public announcements. This, like vague or overstated communication about risk, leads to public inattention, apathy or cynicism.

An effective communication strategy is to pair each announcement about risk with specific actions people can take. Should people stay home, or evacuate certain neighborhoods? If so, what modes of transportation and routes should they take? What phone numbers should they call for more information? Should people give blood, and if so, where? (After 9/11 many donors showed up at non-collecting hospitals). Should the recipients of certain blood products suspend their treatments for non-life threatening conditions? The more specifically you can designate actions, the more people will listen.

Of course, those of you in the blood business face many enduring, non-emergency challenges. You struggle continually to widen your donor base. Many of you are discussing previously taboo subjects such as reconsidering the lifetime ban on gay donors. Some blood banks are also making it easier to collect from people with hemachromatosis, which is another possible source of donations.

You're working creatively to strengthen your return rate. Some notable efforts include Zimbabwe's Club 25, now being adopted by several nations, which incorporates blood donation into young people's lives, inculcating them with enduring habits of good health and altruism. Some places, like the Oklahoma Blood Institute, are re-casting themselves not only as blood centers, but as components of an individual's healthy, upscale lifestyle, with free cholesterol testing and on-line results.

You also struggle with an enduring public habit that, while well-intentioned, needs to be reversed. Ever since the first mass blood drives in the Second World War, the public has associated blood-giving with emergencies (Fig. 3). However, as we know from 9/11 and similar disasters, giving blood at such times can be useless and even harmful. Meanwhile, people neglect to give blood during holiday and vacation times, when supplies become dangerously low.

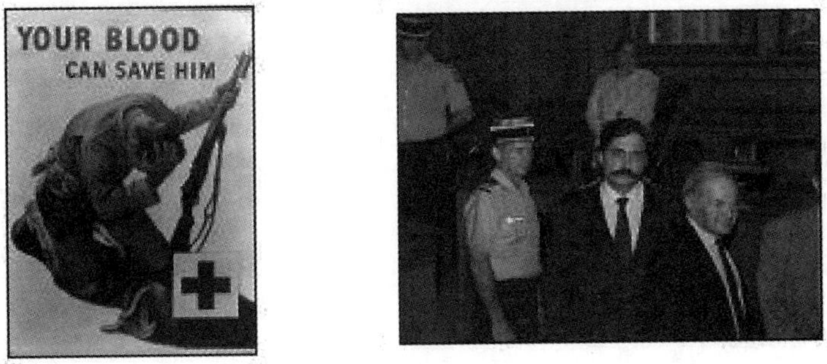

Fig. 3: Between a donor paradigm shaped by war (left – WWII recruitment poster) and recipient paradigm dominated by the AIDS crisis (right – French blood service head Michel Garetta is tried for negligence by the French courts), the blood system needs to initiate a new and more meaningful engagement with the media if it is to communicate its mission and purpose.

One step in reversing this pattern would be to change the enduring metaphor of your enterprise. People have always known your centers as blood banks – a useful metaphor invented by the Chicago physician Bernard Fantus, who coined the phrase to describe a center for deposits and withdrawals. But the enterprise of blood is so dynamic today that the metaphor has outlived its usefulness. After all, people think of a bank as a relatively static place that holds a valuable substance (money or blood). They don't think they can cause harm by overflowing a blood bank and tend not to hear your warnings in times of crisis.

A number of experts have suggested changing your central metaphor from "bank" to a pipeline – in image if not in name. It's a more accurate and dynamic description of your function: the blood comes into your center continually; you process it and send it out. When the flow is low, during holidays and vacations for example, you need to replenish it. Yet, as the public needs to learn, if too many people come in at once, it overflows the figurative pipeline, overtaxing the system and causing problems along the way.

The field of biologics will never be an easy one. You deal with a critical biological substance, laden with imagery as well as medical importance. Because of the voluntary nature of donation, you're utterly dependent on the public's good will. The future will hold endless and difficult decisions. But if you could actively engage the public, both directly and through the media, they'll become your allies in weighing decisions, as opposed to your adversaries. And they may even share responsibility for some of the outcomes.

Mr. D. Starr, Boston University Department of Journalism, College of Communication Boston University, 640 Commonwealth Avenue, Boston, MA 02215, USA.
E-mail: dstarr@bu.edu

List of Participants

ALLAIN Jean-Pierre, Cambridge Blood Centre, National Blood Service, Long Road, Cambridge CB 2PT, U.K.

AENO Umuli, PO Box 1174, Boroko, New Guinea.

ARMSTRONG Vee, Australian Red Cross Blood Service, 290 Wellington Street, Perth, WA 6000, Australia.

ARTHUR Margaret, Abbott Diagnostics, Unit D, 31 – 33 Sirius Road, Lane Cove NSW 2066, Australia.

AYOB Yasmin, National Blood Centre, Jalan Tun Razak, Kuala Lumpar 50400, Malaysia.

BARDZAMIAN Sylvia, Roche Diagnostics, 31 Victoria Avenue, Castle Hill, NSW 2154, Australia.

BARTLETT Jane, Baxter Healthcare, PO Box 71, Brunswick, VIC 3056, Australia.

BLACK Diane, CSL Bioplasma, 189-209 Camp Road, Broadmeadows, VIC 3047, Australia.

BOND Andrew, CSL Bioplasma, 189-209 Camp Road, Broadmeadows, VIC 3047, Australia.

BONDAR Noemi, Red Cross Blood Service Australia, 153 Clarence Street, Sydney, NSW 2000, Australia.

BOYCE Robin, Department of Health & Ageing, GPO Box 9848, Canberra, ACT 2601, Australia.

BROUMIS Connie, CSL Bioplasma, 189-209 Camp Road, Broadmeadows, VIC 3047, Australia.

BULT Jan Menso, PPTA, 147 Old Solomons Island Rd, Suite 100, Annapolis, MD 21401, USA.

BUSCH Michael P, Blood Systems Research Institute, 270 Masonic Avenue, San Francisco, CA 94118, USA.

CARIS Sharon, Haemophillia Foundation Australia, 1624 High Street, Glen Iris, VIC 3146, Australia.

CARTY Ray, National Blood Authority, Level 1, 19-23 Moore Street, Turner ACT 2601, Australia.

CASS Yael, Dept of Health & Ageing, GPO Box 9848, Canberra, ACT 2601, Australia.

CHOQUET Christian, 1800 Acta Vista Drive, Ottawa, ONT K1G 4J5, Canada.

COGHLAN Patrick, ARCBS National, PO Box 5103, Melbourne, VIC 3001, Australia.

COSTE Joliette, EFS Pyrenees-Mediterranee, FR-34397 Montpellier, France.

COWLEY Nathalie, ARCBS, PO Box 10325, Brisbane, QLD 4000, Australia.

CUMMINS Barbara, GPO Box 48, Brisbane, QLD 4000, Australia.

DALY Rodney, CSL Bioplasma, 189-209 Camp Road, Broadmeadows, VIC 3047, Australia.

DAX Elizabeth, National Serology Reference Laboratory, 4TH Floor Healy Building, 41 Victoria Parade, Fitzroy, VIC 3065, Australia.

DELETOILLE Patrice, Bio-Rad Laboratories, PO Box 210, Regents Park, Sydney, NSW 2143, Australia.

DE NATRIS Theo, BioMerieux, Boseind 15, NL-5281 RM Boxtel, The Netherlands.

DE SAINT MARTIN Guillaume, MacoPharma, PO Box 5335, West, NSW 1515, Australia.

DHINGRA Neelam, World Health Organisation, 20 Ave Appia, CH-1211 Geneva, Switzerland.

DODD Roger, American Red Cross Holland Lab, 15601 Crabbs Branch Way, Rockville, MD 20855, USA.

EARNGEY James, 22 Cadow Street, Frenchs Forest, NSW 2086, Australia.

EPSTEIN Jay, US Food and Drug Administration, HFM-300, 1401 RockvillePike, Rockville, MD 20852, USA.

EVANS Roger, Bio-Rad Laboratories, PO Box 210, Regents Park, NSW 2143, Australia.

EVERS Theo, IPFA, Plesmanlaan 125, NL-1066 CX Amsterdam, The Netherlands.

FARRUGIA Albert, Office of Devices, Blood and Tissues, PO Box 100, Woden ACT 2606, Australia.

FLANAGAN Peter, New Zealand Blood Service, PO Box 26611, Epsom, Auckland, New Zealand.

FERREIRA Mada, South African National Blood Service, 442D Mimosa Ave., Lynnwood 0081, South Africa.

FLETCHER Anne, Growing Your Knowledge, PO Box 716, Spit Junction, NSW 2088, Australia.

FLOWER Robert, ANZ SBT, Level 4 Bld 1 RNSH, Pacific Highway, St Leondards, NSW 2065, Australia.

GLEN Tony, National Blood Authority, Level 1 19-23 Moore Street, Turner, ACT 2601, Australia.

HARBOUR Colin, University of Sydney, Dept Infectious Diseases, Camperdown, NSW 2006, Australia.

HARTMAN Mariah, Chiron Blood Testing, 456 Horton Street, Emeryville, CA 94608, USA.

HIROSE Toru, 2-8-16-503, Ashi-Gaoka, Hino-City, Tokyo 191-0655, Japan.

HOSSENLOPP Claudine, Etablissement Français du Sang, Direction of International Affairs, 100 avenue de Suffren, FR-75015 Paris, France.

HUME Sandy, Bio Merieux Australia, PO Box 897, Baulkham Hills, NSW 2153, Australia.

HYLAND Catherine, Australian Red Cross Blood Service, 480 Queen Street, Brisbane, QLD 4000, Australia.

ISBISTER James, Royal North Shore Hospital of Sydney, University of Sydney, Sydney, NSW 2000, Australia.

ISMAY Sue, Australian Red Cross Blood Service, 153 Clarence Street, Sydney, NSW 2000, Australia.

JANKELOWITZ Gary, Novo Nordisk, L3, 21 Solent Ct, Baulkham Hills, NSW 2153, Australia.

JARDINE Darren, National Serology Reference Laboratory, 4th Floor Healy Bldg, 41 Victoria Parade, Fitzroy, VIC 3065, Australia.

JENNINGS Helen, ARCBS, PO Box 10325, Brisbane, QLD 4000, Australia.

JOYCE Kathryn, 26 Surrey Street, Pascoe Vale, VIC 3044, Australia.

KEE Glenda, ARCBS, 153 Clarence Street, Sydney, NSW 2000, Australia.

KEILY Phil, Australian Red Cross Blood Service, PO Box 354, South Melbourne, VIC 3205, Australia.

KELLER Anthony, Australian Red Cross Blood Service, GPO Box 880, Perth, WA 6000, Australia.

LAMBERT Nadine, Bio-Rad, 3 Bd Raymond Poincaré, FR-92430 Marnes-La-Coquette, France.

LENNOX Elizabeth, Sullivan Nicolaides Pathology, PO Box 344, Indooroopilly, QLD 4068, Australia.

LIM Che-Kit, Health Sciences Authority, 11 Outram Rd, Singapore 169078, Singapore.

LYNCH Garry, Australian Red Cross Blood Service, 153 Clarence Street, Sydney, NSW 2000, Australia.

MAHER Darryl, CSL Bioplasma, 189-209 Camp Road, Broadmeadows, VIC 3047, Australia.

MASTERS Colin, Department of Pathology, University of Melbourne, Australia.

MAY Philip, Abbott Diagnostics Division, Unit D, 31-33 Sirius Rd, Lane Cove, NSW 2066, Australia.

MAZURE Huber, Cellabs Pty Ltd, 7/27 Dale Street, Brookvale, NSW 2100, Australia.

MC CLELLAND Brian, SNBTS, Ellen's Glen Road, Edinburgh EH17 7QT, Scotland, Great Britain.

MEALEY Lilly, Baxter Healthcare, PO Box 88, Toongabbie, NSW 2146, Australia.

MOORE Graeme, 9 Sirius Road, Lane Cove, NSW 2066, Australia.

MUELLER Norbert, Institut für Transfusionmedzin, Univ-Klinik Essen, Hufelandstr, DE-45122 Essen, Germany.

NICK Sigrid, Paul-Ehrlich-Institut, Paul-Ehrlich-Str. 51-59, DE-63225 Langen, Germany.
NORRIS Sarah, Therapeutic Goods Administration, PO Box 100, Woden, Symonston, ACT 2606, Australia.
NUITTA Silvana, Therapeutic Goods Administration, PO Box 100, Woden, Symonston, ACT 2606, Australia.

PADILLA Ana, World Health Organisation, 20 Avenue Appia, CH-1211 Geneva, Switzerland.
PEMBREY Richard, Therapeutic Goods Administration, 136 Narrabuudala Ave, Woden ACT 2606, Australia.
PETRUS Maturbongs, JL Bungur Besar Raya # 49, Jakarta 10610, Indonesia.
PILLAI Patricia, Seals Haemotology, St George Hospital, Gray Street, Kograh, NSW 2217, Australia.
PRY Christine, Abbott New Zealand, Ground Floor, Building D, 4 Pacific, Mr Wellington, Auckland, New Zealand.

RAJASEKARIAH Raj, Cellabs Pty Ltd, 7/27 Dale Street, Brookvale, NSW 2100, Australia.
RATNA Hendardji, JL Bungur Besar Raya # 49, Jakarta 10610, Indonesia.
RIBEIRO Gus, MacoPharma, PO Box 5335, West, NSW 1515, Australia.
ROHWER Robert, Molecular Neuroviral, 10N. Greene Street, Mailstop 151, Baltimore, MD 21201, USA.

SAEED Awad, Riyadh Armed Forces Hospital, C/- Cellabs Pty Ltd, 7/27 Dale Street, Brookvale, NSW 2100, Australia.
SCHOCHETMAN Gerald, Abbott Laboratories, 100 Abbott Park Rd, Abbott Park, IL 60064, USA.
SCHRAMM Wolfgang, University Hospital of Munich, Ziemssenstr. 1, DE-80336 Munich, Germany.
SCHULLER Margaret, Bio-Rad Laboratories, PO Box 210, Regents Park, Sydney, NSW 2143, Australia.
SCOTT Ray, New Zealand Blood Service, PO Box 26611, Epsom, Auckland, New Zealand.
SEED Clive, Australian Red Cross Blood Service, PO Box 880, Perth, WA 6000, Australia.
SEITZ Rainer, Paul-Ehrlich-Institut, Paul-Ehrlich-Str. 51-59, DE-63225 Langen, Germany.
SHANG Guifang, Therapeutic Goods Administration, PO Box 100, Woden, ACT 2606, Australia.
SIVAPALAN Nivethan, National Blood Authority, 19-23 Moore Street, Turner, ACT 2601, Australia.
SMITH Meredith, New Zealand Blood Service, PO Box 26611, Epsom, Auckland, New Zealand.
SMITH Glenn, Therapeutic Goods Administration, PO Box 100 Woden, Symonston, ACT 2606, Australia.
SOBOLL Heidi, Paul-Ehrlich-Institut, Paul-Ehrlich-Str. 51-59, DE-63225 Langen, Germany.
STARR Douglas, The Center For Science, Boston University, 640 Commonwealth Ave, Boston, MA 02215, USA.
STAUBER Edward,
STRAMER Susan, American Red Cross Blood Services, , 9315 Gaither Rd, Gaithersburg, MD 20877, USA.
STRENGERS Paul F.W., ISBT, J.Van Goyenkade 11, NL-1141 AR Amsterdam, The Netherlands.

TADOKORO Kenji, Japanese Red Cross Society, 1-1-1-3 Shiba-Daimon, Minato-Ku, Tokyo, Japan.
TEO Diana, Centre For Transfusion Medicine, Health Services Authority, Health Sciences Authority 11, Singapore 169078, Singapore.
TURNER Alison, National Blood Authority, Locked Bag 8430, Turner, ACT 2601, Australia.

UDECHUKU Nnambi, Novo Nor Disk, Level 3, 21 Solent Circuit, Balkham Hills, NSW 2153, Australia.
UNAL Aytac, CSL Bioplasma, 189-209 Camp Road, Broadmeadows, VIC 3047, Australia.

VYAS Girish, University of California School of Medicine, 513 Pamassus Ave, Rm S-561, San Francisco, CA 94143-0100, USA.

WAI-POI Irene, New Zealand Blood Service, Private Bag 92071, Auckland, New Zealand.

WALKER Sandy, National Serology Reference Laboratory, Australia, 4th Floor Healy Building, 41 Victoria Parade, Fitzroy, VIC 3065, Australia.

WENDEL Silvano, Hospital Sirio Libanes-Blood Bank Rua Dona Adma Jafet, 91-3, Bella Vista, Sao Paulo, 01308-05, Brazil.

WHITBREAD Lel, Therapeutic Goods Administration, PO Box 100, Woden, Symonston, ACT 2606, Australia.

WHITE Catherine, Roche Diagnostics, 31 Victoria Avenue, Castle Hill, NSW 2154, Australia.

WHYTE Gordon, International Education Development Unit, Faculty of Medicine, Nursing and Health Sciences, Monash University, VIC 3800, Australia.

WILLIAMS Joanne, Medtel Pty Ltd, 5 Orion Road, Lane Cove NSW 2066, Australia.

WYLIE Brenton, Transfusion Services, PO Box 1701, Double Bay, NSW 2028, Australia.

YOUNG Suzanne, Medtel Pty Ltd, 5 Orion Road, Lane Cove NSW 2066, Australia.

ZHU Yong Ming, Shanghai Blood Center, #1191 Hongqiao, Shanghai 200051, Rep. of China.

Index of Authors

Developments in Biological Standardization

Vol. 67: Melbourne 1986	Standardization in blood fractionation including coagulation factors
Vol. 68: Geneva, 1986	Cells – Products – Safety
Vol. 69: London, 1987	Cytokines Laboratory and Clinical Evaluation
Vol. 70: Arlington, VA, 1988	Continuous Cell Lines as Substrates for Biologicals
Vol. 71: Utrecht, 1989	Monoclonal Antibodies for Therapy, Prevention and In vivo Diagnosis of Human Disease
Vol. 72: Annecy, 1989	Progress in Animal Retroviruses
Vol. 73: Shizuoka, 1990	Pertussis: Evaluation and Research on Acellular Pertussis Vaccines
Vol. 74: Bethesda, MD, 1990	Biological Product Freeze-Drying and Formulation
Vol. 75: London, 1990	Virological Aspects of the Safety of Biological Products
Vol. 76: Bethesda, MD, 1991	Continuous Cell Lines - An International Workshop on Current Issues
Vol. 77: Annecy, 1991	Standardization of the Immunopharmacology of Natural and Synthetic Immunomodulators
Vol. 78: Bethesda, MD, 1991	Poliovirus Attenuation: Molecular Mechanisms and Practical Aspects
Vol. 79: Ploufragan, 1992	The First Steps Towards an International Harmonization of Veterinary Biologicals: 1993 and Free Circulation of Vaccines within the EEC
Vol. 80: Heidelberg, 1992	Transmissible Spongiform Encephalopathies - Impact on Animal and Human Health
Vol. 81: Cannes, 1992	Virological Safety Aspects of Plasma Derivatives
Vol. 82: Albany NY, 1993	Recombinant Vectors in Vaccine Development
Vol. 83: Annecy, 1993	Genetic Stability and Recombinant Product Consistency
Vol. 84: Langen, 1993	Non-Target Effects of Live Vaccines
Vol. 85: Santa Fé, NM, 1994	Genetics of Streptococci, Enterococci and Lactococci
Vol. 86: Langen, 1994	Replacement, Reduction and Refinement of Animal Experiments in the Development and Control of Biological Products
Vol. 87: Geneva, 1995	New Approaches to Stabilisation of Vaccines Potency
Vol. 88: Bethesda, MD, 1995	Viral Safety and Evaluation of Viral Clearance from Biopharmaceutical Products
Vol. 89: Rome, 1995	Pertussis Vaccine Trials
Vol. 90: Oslo, 1996	Fish Vaccinology
Vol. 91: San Francisco, CA, 1996	Development of Specifications for Biotechnology Pharmaceuticals Products
Vol. 92: Bergen, 1996	Modulation of the Immune Response to Vaccine Antigens
Vol. 93: Annecy, 1996	Safety of Biological Products Prepared from Mammalian Cell Culture
Vol. 94: Bethesda, MD, 1997	Simian Virus 40 (SV40): A Possible Human Polyomavirus
Vol. 95: Paris, 1997	Preclinical and Clinical Development of New Vaccines
Vol. 96: Washington, DC, 1995	Characterization of Biotechnology Pharmaceutical Products
Vol. 97: London, 1997	Biological Characterization and Assay of Cytokines and Growth Factors
Vol. 98: London, 1997	Inactivated Influenza Vaccines Prepared in Cell Culture
Vol. 99: Strasbourg, 1998	Animal Sera, Animal Sera Derivatives and Substitutes Used in the Manufacture of Pharmaceuticals: Viral Safety and Regulatory Aspects
Vol. 100: Geneva, 1998	A Celebration of 50 Years of Progress in Biological Standardization and Control at WHO
Vol. 101: London, 1998	Alternatives to Animals in the Development and Control of Biological Products for Human and Veterinary Use

Developments in Biologicals

Vol. 102: San Francisco, CA, 1999	Advances in Transfusion Safety
Vol. 103: Annecy, 1999	Physico-Chemical Procedures for the Characterization of Vaccines
Vol. 104: Langen, 1999	Development and Clinical Progress of DNA Vaccines
Vol. 105: Paris, 2000	Progress in Polio Eradication: Vaccine Strategies for the End Game
Vol. 106: Rockville, MD, 2000	Evolving Scientific and Regulatory Perspectives on Cell Substrates for Vaccine Development
Vol. 107: London, 2000	The Design and Analysis of Potency Assays for Biotechnology Products
Vol. 108: Langen, 2001	Advances in Transfusion Safety
Vol. 109: Washington, DC, 2000	Biologics 2000 – Comparability of Biotechnology Products
Vol. 110: Palm Cove, 2001	Orphan Vaccines – Bridging the Gap
Vol. 111: Utrecht, 2001	Advancing Science and Elimination of the Use of Laboratory Animals for Development and Control of Vaccines and Hormones
Vol. 112: Bethesda, MD, 2001	Immunogenicity of Therapeutic Biological Products
Vol. 113: Berlin, 2001	Process Validation for Manufacturing of Biologics and Biotechnology Products
Vol. 114: Ames, IA, 2002	Vaccines for OIE List A and Emerging Animal Diseases
Vol. 115: Bergen, 2002	Laboratory Correlates of Immunity to Influenza – A Reassessment
Vol. 116: Los Angeles, CA, 2003	Development of Therapeutic Cancer Vaccines
Vol. 117: Langen, 2003	Consideration of Alternative Licensing Procedures for Vaccines for Minor Species, Minor Indications and Autogenous/Autologous Products
Vol. 118: Langen, 2003	PDA/EMEA European Virus Safety Forum
Vol. 119: Buenos Aires, 2004	Control of Infectious Animal Diseases by Vaccination
Vol. 120: Bethesda, MD, 2003	Advances in Transfusion Safety
Vol. 121: Bergen, 2003	Progress in Fish Vaccinology
Vol. 122: Bethesda, MD, 2003	State of the Art Analytical Methods for Characterization of Biological Products and Assessment of Comparability
Vol. 123: Rockville, MD, 2004	Vaccine Cell Substrates 2004
Vol. 124: Paris, 2005	OIE/FAO International Scientific Conference on Avian Influenza
Vol. 125: Kiev, Ukraine, 2005	First International Conference on Rabies in Europe
Vol. 126: Saint-Malo, France, 2005	New Diagnostic Technology: Applications in Animal Health and Biologics Controls

IMPRIMERIE MEDECINE HYGIENE
GENEVE
SUISSE

mars–2007